Neurological Disorders

Clinical Methods

Neurological Disorders – Clinical Methods

Publisher: iConcept Press Ltd.
Cover design: Pineapple Design Ltd.
Interior design: iConcept Press Ltd.
Typesetting and copy editing: iConcept Press Ltd. and Pineapple Design Ltd.

ISBN: 978-1-922227-73-7

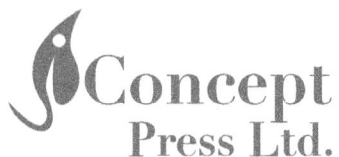

ƒConcept
Press Ltd.

www.iconceptpress.com

Contents

Preface

A neurological disorder is any disorder of the body's nervous system. Symptoms include, but do not limited to, paralysis, muscle weakness, poor coordination, loss of sensation, seizures, confusion, and altered levels of consciousness. *Neurological Disorders - Clinical Methods* brings scholars and experts who are working in the areas directly related to neurological disorder in front of you, and presents the latest research findings to you.

There are totally 9 chapters in this book. Chapter 1 reviews Temporal Lobe Epilepsy (TLE). TLE is a well-described type of epilepsy but little is known about the epidemiology. The approach to patients with temporal lobe epilepsy is complex and requires a multidisciplinary team of trained specialists. Large-scale epidemiological studies are needed for improve the understanding of TLE is a therefore necessary. Chapter 2 presents the latest knowledge on the understand of the current sources in epileptic activity in mesial areas. Current sources is a very promising tool to refine radiosurgical and improve classical surgical methods for temporal lobe epilepsy. Chapter 3 highlights the atypical co-occurrence of two genetic disorders, Cornelia de Lange syndrome and Turner syndrome, in the same individual. It focuses on the clinical methods used to explain each clinical feature, with special emphasis on neurological findings. Chapter 4 concerns the use of of probiotics to prevent fungal infection against the decrease of morbidity and mortality in ELBW, especially about long lasting neurological sequelae.

Chapter 5 describes an algorithm called Dynamic Autoregressive Neuromagnetic Causal Imaging (DANCI) which uses Granger causality to calculate effective connectivity from magnetoencephalography recordings. It also describes how this technique can be used to understand the fundamental reorganization of neural networks in neurodevelopmental disorders. Chapter 6 provides important and necessary information regarding brain herniation. Brain herniation represents a shift of brain parenchyma across the various anatomical boundaries formed by intracranial bony ridges and dural folds. This chapter emphasises on the need of emergency resuscitation and step-wise management of the patients. Chapter 7 describes spinal shortening as a new option for anterior reconstruction of the thoracic and lumbar spine after posterolateral debridment for spinal infections. Although technically demanding, this technique has a lot of advantages including short operative time, avoid morbidity of bone graft donor site, gives high biomechanical stability and high fusion rate. Chapter 8 highlights the following two aspects: (1) The increase of high alpha relative to low alpha power is a reliable EEG marker of hippocampal atrophy and it is predictive of conversion of patients with Mild Cognitive Impairment (MCI) in Alzherimer's disease (AD); (2) The MCI subjects with higher a3/a2 ratios showed minor atrophy in the impulsive disorders network bilaterally when compared to subjects with lower and middle a3/a2 ratios. It could suggest a functional hyperactivity of the cortico-accumbens-ventral striatum loop in prodromal AD explaining some early cognitive-behavioral symptoms.

Chapter 9 provides an overview of the main schools of psychotherapy, the prevalence of psychological disorders, and main cultural issues in psychotherapy. It also describes an Omani study that explored the utilization of psychotherapy within an Arabic/Islamic society, with unique value/and belief systems.

Editing and publishing a book is never an easy task. Each chapter in this book has gone through a peer review, a selection and an editing process so as to guarantee its quality. Without the supports and contributions of the authors and reviewers, this book can never be able to complete. We would like to thank all of the authors in this book and all of the reviewers who participated in the reviewing process: Catherine Abbo, Niyazi Acer, Faisal Al-Otaibi, Réza Behrouz, Atanu Biswas, Petr Bob, Alice Y. W. Chang, Sri Hari Charan, Christa Einspieler, Hedley CA Emsley, Laura Fanea, L. Fernandes, Mario Ganau, Deepak Goyal, Boret Henry, Chao-Hsien Hsieh, Laura E. Hughes, Barbara Jasiewicz, Yoshiki Kaneoke, Hee-Soo Kim, Hyeongsu Kim, Fatimah Lateef, Misha DP Luyer, Ann Manzardo, Pedro J Modrego, Giuseppe Orsitto, Jesús Pastor, Kurupath Radhakrishnan, Karthikeyan Ramalingam, Sridharan Ramaratnam, Paul E Rapp, Cornelius A Ryan, Najam-us Sahar, Muhammad Shahzad Shamim, Ghaydaa A Shehata, Dina Silva, Xenophon Sinopidis, Kathleen A Smith, Tetsuya Suzuki, Ikuo Tooyama, Olivier M. Vanakker, Wiwat Wajanavisit, Yi-Hao Weng, San-Nan Yang, G. Bryan Young and Qingbao Yu. We hope that you, the reader, will find this book interesting and useful. Any advices please feel free and are always welcome to tell us.

iConcept Press Ltd

June 2014

A Comprehensive Review of Temporal Lobe Epilepsy

Lady D. Ladino
Department of Neurology, College of Medicine
University of Antioquia, Hospital Pablo Tobón Uribe, Colombia

Farzad Moien-Afshari
Neurology Division, College of Medicine
University of Saskatchewan, Canada

José F. Téllez-Zenteno
Neurology Division, College of Medicine
University of Saskatchewan, Canada

1   Introduction

Epilepsy consists of more than 40 clinical syndromes affecting 50 million people worldwide. Approximately 30% of patients receiving medications have inadequate seizure control (Jacobs *et al.*, 2001). The International League Against Epilepsy (ILAE) defines epilepsy as "a condition characterized by two or more recurrent epileptic seizures over a period longer than 24 hours, unprovoked by any immediate identified cause". The term Temporal lobe epilepsy (TLE) was included in the classification of the ILAE in 1989 under the group of "localization-related symptomatic epilepsies characterized by seizures with specific modes of precipitation" (Commission on classification and terminology of the ILAE, 1989).

The temporal lobe is the most epileptogenic region of the human brain. Hippocampal sclerosis (HS) is the commonest cause of TLE. Therefore, mesial TLE (mTLE) is perhaps the best-characterized electro-clinical syndrome of all the epilepsies (Tatum, 2012). It is estimated that it represents about 40% of all epilepsies in adult people. It can be sporadic, commonly with a positive family history, or it can present with clear familial recurrence (Cendes, 2005). The common clinical pattern during the seizure episode includes staring and lack of responsiveness, frequently accompanied by mouth or hand automatisms. They represent approximately two thirds of the intractable seizure population requiring surgical management (Blair, 2012).

1.1   Epidemiology

There are few epidemiological studies in TLE. The majority of the studies have been generated in referral centers providing different estimates. Hauser and Kurland (Hauser & Kurland, 1975) provided the best available epidemiological data on TLE, the incidence rate was 10.4 per 100.000 and the prevalence was 1.7 per 1000 people. Few population-based studies have been published; in 1992 a study based on community physician's records reported that the frequency of TLE is only 21% within the focal epilepsy cases (Manford *et al.*, 1992). Other estimates regarding the prevalence of epilepsy have been obtained from tertiary referral centers; approximately 60-80% of patients with partial epilepsy have TLE (Oun *et al.*, 2003). In epilepsy centers the TLE prevalence usually is 60-70% (Spencer & Spencer, 1985; Semah *et al.*, 1998). The higher rates of TLE observed in epilepsy centers are probably related with its intractability. In general, patients with TLE have a better surgical outcome and a have a lower risk of neurological deficits related to excision of functional cortex compared to extratemporal lobe epilepsy (ETLE) cases. Because of this reason, neurologists and family practitioners more frequently refer patients with TLE for surgical assessment (Téllez-Zenteno & Hernandez-Ronquillo, 2012).

2   Etiology and Physiopathology

TLE could be sporadic or familial. TLE can be associated with a magnetic resonance imaging (MRI) lesion or be non-lesional (Téllez-Zenteno *et al.*, 2010). The main causes of lesional TLE are HS, benign tumors, vascular malformations, cortical development malformations, and post-traumatic or post-infectious gliosis (Cendes, 2005). The most common low-grade tumors are gangliogliomas, low-grade gliomas, and dysembryoplastic neuroepithelial tumors (Woermann & Vollmar, 2009).

2.1   Neuropathology

HS is the most common cause of TLE, representing greater than 80% of cases (Tatum, 2012). It is a combination of atrophy and astrogliosis of the amygdala, hippocampus, uncus, parahipocampal gyrus, and the entorhinal cortex (Tatum, 2012). It implies selective neuronal loss that affects various sectors to a different degree. The most vulnerable to damage are the sector CA1 (Sommer's sector) and CA3-CA4 (endfolium), whereas CA2 pyramidal and dentate gyrus granule cells are most seizure resistant (Cendes, 2005; Cendes, 2004). The majority of hipocampal specimens also reveal alterations within the dentate gyrus, i.e., granule cell dispersion. Granule cell dispersion may be associated with early seizure onset or status epilepticus at an initial stage of the disease (Blümcke, 2008). In addition, from neuroimaging and neuropathological studies it is well established that MTS can occur in combination with a second temporal lobe epileptogenic pathology such as cortical dyslamination (i.e., Focal Cortical Dysplasia type I), ectopic white matter neurons or low-grade glioneuronal tumors (Blümcke, 2008). The most common types of extra-hippocampal lesions found in dual pathology are developmental abnormalities, such as cortical dysgenesis, followed by gliotic lesions acquired in early childhood (Cendes *et al.*, 1995). Additionally, anatomic data confirm the importance of the medial thalamus in mesial TLE. Volume loss is present in ipsilateral thalamus, caudate, and amygdala in mesial TLE, and thalamic cell loss is present in epilepsy patients. Furthermore, hippocampal cell density is significantly correlated with the amount of reduction in metabolism in bilateral thalamus and basal ganglia (Spencer, 2002b).

Relation between febrile seizures (FS) and mesial temporal sclerosis (MTS) remains controversial. One theory is that the early FS damages the hippocampus and is therefore a cause of HS; another possibility is that the child has a prolonged FS because the hippocampus was previously damaged as a result of prenatal or perinatal insult or by genetic predisposition (Cendes, 2004).

2.2   Single Focus Vs. Network Model

There are many questions about the etiology of TLE. Partial epileptic seizures were traditionally thought to originate in specific areas of the cortex known as seizure onset zones (SOZ), before spreading to other areas, known as epileptogenic zones (EZ). Surgical approaches to this condition include resection or disconnection of these areas, principally the SOZ (usually identified as the epileptic focus), from the rest of the brain. This ''single focus'' model has been challenged in favor of a "network model" in which the focus would be distributed along the limbic structures (Palmigiano *et al.*, 2012).

A network is a set of cortical and subcortical brain structures and regions functionally and anatomically connected, in which activity in any one-part affects activity in all the others. Therefore, vulnerability to seizure activity in any one part of the network is influenced by activity everywhere else in the network, and that the network as a whole is responsible for the clinical and electrographic phenomena associated with seizures (Spencer, 2002b). Interruption of the network, in a structural sense, or modification of network activity by electrical, biochemical or metabolic influences will modify the seizure expression. The most common human intractable epilepsy is TLE; this entity is the result of an abnormal circuitry in the medial temporal/limbic network. It is bilateral, cortical and subcortical, and includes the hippocampi, the amygdala, the entorhinal cortices, lateral temporal neocortices, and extratemporal components of the medial thalamus and the inferior frontal lobes (Spencer, 2002b). Surgery for TLE targets a wide area in which multiple rather than single structures are resected. It is difficult to determine whether the absence of postoperative seizures is a consequence of the resection of the focus or the destruction of the network topology (Palmigiano *et al.*, 2012).

3   Semiology

Clinical semiology is the starting point to understand a seizure disorder and making the diagnosis of epilepsy. An accurate semiologic history is not only important in the diagnosis, but also relevant in localizing seizures particularly in patients with drug-resistant epilepsy (DRE) for potential surgical management (Jan & Girvin, 2008). Many times symptoms are not useful for localizing or lateralizing the seizure onset, but may give useful information about the activated network (Loddenkemper & Kotagal, 2005). Due to recall problems in many patients additional information has to be gathered from witnesses and family members. Sometimes requesting the interviewees to mimic the patient's seizures provides the most important information leading to the diagnosis (Jan & Girvin, 2008).

The temporal lobe was divided by Wieser (Wieser, 1983) into five regions: temporobasal, temporopolar, neocortical, opercular and frontobasal cingular. Nowadays the ILAE (Commission on classification and terminology of the ILAE, 1989) recognizes two syndromes, mesial and lateral or neocortical temporal epilepsy (NTE). Mesial temporal epilepsy is the best known and the most frequent (Bercovici *et al.*, 2012; Tatum, 2012).

3.1   Mesial Temporal Epilepsy

Mesial TLE is the most common form of partial epilepsy in adolescents and adults, and some studies have estimated that it represents about 40% of all epilepsies in this age range (Cendes, 2005). These patients usually have known risk factors such as perinatal injury, central nervous system (CNS) infection, FS, head trauma, and family history of epilepsy (Cendes, 2004). Up to 60% of patients with MTS may have a previous history of FS before developing seizures (French *et al.*, 1993). Typically, by the end of the first or second decade, patients present with their first FS. It is usually a complex partial seizure, although it may be a simple partial or a generalized seizure. Afterwards, some patients remain seizure-free for variable periods that range from one to two decades, or even longer (honeymoon-period). Seizures restart as adults (Tatum, 2012).

More than 80% of patients report an aura (Acharya *et al.*, 1998) with experiential and viscerosensory symptoms. Psychic phenomenon includes anxiety, *déjà vu, jamais vu* and fear. The typical aura is an indescribable rising epigastric sensation, often described as butterflies (Thompson *et al.*, 2000), and followed by staring, behavioral arrest and oroalimentary or hand automatisms, accompanied by autonomic phenomena as pupillary dilatation, hyperventilation, piloerection, and tachycardia. Contralateral dystonic posturing with ipsilateral automatisms during the seizure are reliable lateralizing signs (Tatum, 2012). Prolonged seizures, secondary generalization and status epilepticus are relatively infrequent (French *et al.*, 1993).

3.2   Neocortical Temporal Epilepsy

NTE has a different clinical profile than mesial epilepsy. A history of FS, CNS infection, perinatal complications or head injury is less common than in patients with MTS (Gil-Nagel & Risinger, 1997). Seizures in patients with NTE appear five or ten years later than in MTS (Bercovici *et al.*, 2012). Around 60% of seizures are preceded by an aura, such as auditory phenomena, psychic experiences or *déjà vu* and *jamais vu*, visual distortions, and vertiginous symptoms (Maillard *et al.*, 2004; Kennedy & Schuele, 2012). Motionless staring and unresponsiveness are the first objective clinical signs, often followed by early contralateral clonic movements and secondary generalization (O'Brien *et al.*, 1996) (see Table 1).

Mesial and Neocortical Temporal Epilepsy Clinical Features		
Clinical features	Mesial	Neocortical
Frequency	90%	10%
Risk factors	FS, CNS infections, head trauma, perinatal injuries (common)	Less frequent
Age at onset	Adolescence or young adults	Five to ten years later than MTS
Type of aura	Abdominal, olfactory, gustatory, "dreamy state" and fear feelings	Psychic, auditory hallucination, vertigo, visual symptoms, cephalic sensation, nonspecific auras
Staring and unresponsiveness	Late	Early
Ambiguous onset/offset	No	Yes
Automatisms	Early, in the first 20 seconds, oral and manual automatism, frequent searching	Late or absent. Searching less frequent
Motor	Ipsilateral automatisms followed by contralateral dystonic posturing. Leg movements and body shifting more likely	Early contralateral dystonic posturing. Clonic movements more likely, leg movements less likely
Secondary generalization	Rare	More common
Postictal cough/sigh	More likely	Less likely
Seizure duration	> 1 minute	< 1 minute
Ictal EEG	A lateralized ictal change of rhythmic 5-10 Hz sharp activity, maximally at F7/F8 or sphenoidal electrode	A lateralized ictal change of irregular polymorphic 2-5 Hz temporal rhythm
MRI	Mostly lesional epilepsy. Hippocampal sclerosis.	Mostly non-lesional epilepsy*. Tumor, AVM or CDM

Table 1: Abbreviations. FS: febrile seizures, CNS: Central Nervous System, EEG: electroencephalogram, Hz: Hertz, MRI: Magnetic resonance imaging, AVM: Arterio-venous malformation, CDM: Cortical development malformation. *Lesional neocortical temporal cases are often not reported in the literature as compared to the nonlesional cases because they may be less likely to be admitted to an epilepsy-monitoring unit (EMU) for video-electroencephalography (EEG) telemetry unless the lesion is closely associated with eloquent cortex (Bercovici *et al.*, 2012).

3.3   Auras

Auras are usually subjective symptoms without objective signs that can be documented by an observer. These usually occur at the beginning of a seizure ("warning symptoms") for seconds up to minutes, although they can be seen in isolation as well (Noachtar & Peters, 2009). Some authors have reported that auras have a good localizing value, similar to the electroencephalogram (EEG) and imaging (Palmini & Gloor, 1992). However, attempting to localize seizures based on their semiology is controversial. By definition, ictal discharges are generated in the epileptogenic zone. Theoretically, this can be any cortical region, but seizures often originate in so-called silent areas of the cortex and only become clinically manifest when they spread into areas that are able to produce symptoms (Rona, 2008). Another potential source of inaccuracy is the patient. Since auras are subjective by definition, the localizing value of the reported symptoms critically relies on the ability of the patient to describe them, which depends on the age, intellectual level and mental state of the patient (Rona, 2008). Additionally, false localization should be suspected if the onset of clinical seizures occurs earlier than the onset of ictal EEG discharge (So, 2006; Jan & Girvin, 2008). With due consideration of the above-mentioned limitations, aura semiology can still be considered to provide essential clues for the localization, lateralization and prediction of surgical success (Palmini & Gloor, 1992).

Olfactory auras classically described, as "uncinate fits" are typically unpleasant smells, often associated with gustatory phenomena (Jan & Girvin, 2008). The brain areas associated with this type of auras include the amygdala, olfactory bulb, insular cortex, and orbitofrontal cortex (Noachtar & Peters, 2009; Foldvary-Schaefer & Unnwongse, 2011). Although historically these are typical auras, they are rare phenomena occurring in only 5% of TLE patients (Chen *et al.*, 2003). Gustatory auras are hard to differentiate from olfactory sensations. Gustatory auras are even less common than olfactory auras, and are highly suggestive of a temporal onset (Noachtar & Peters, 2009; Foldvary-Schaefer & Unnwongse, 2011).

Psychic auras consist of a "strange feeling" that arises when the internal or external world is perceived in a distorted manner. These include emotional symptoms (fear, anxiety), distortions of familiarity (*déjà vu, jamais vu*) (Ebner, 1994) and multisensory hallucinations including revocation of complex memories. Patients consistently sense that the feelings are unreal and strange (Noachtar & Peters, 2009). Fear is a limbic aura, considered to be amygdaloid in origin. For this localization it must be "primary fear", and not simply the often-secondary fear that is experienced by the epileptic patient in response to the realization that "another" seizure is about to occur (Jan & Girvin, 2008).

In epileptology, a clear separation of hallucinatory, illusional, and delusional phenomena is not easily achieved. Psychiatric symptoms mimicking seizure semiology are a great diagnostic challenge. If hallucinations are a manifestation of seizures, they should occur because of activation of a localized group of neurons, which can be investigated by cerebral recording and cerebral stimulation. The 'Gold Standard' investigation in such cases has been intracranial stereoelectroencephalography (SEEG) (Elliott *et al.*, 2009a). It has also been shown that some complex psychotic states can occur because of continuous epileptic discharges. The best evidence for this can be found also in SEEG recordings showing episodes of complex partial status epilepticus with complex psychotic spells or with certain cases of apparent 'postictal' and possibly 'interictal' psychosis (Elliott *et al.*, 2009b).

Autonomic auras include cardiorespiratory (palpitations, shortness of breath), gastrointestinal, and genitourinary symptoms (urinary urgency, genital sensations) (Loddenkemper & Kotagal, 2005). The symptomatogenic zone for these symptoms is the insular cortex, anterior cingulum, supplementary motor area (SMA), amygdala and hypothalamus (Foldvary-Schaefer & Unnwongse, 2011). Abdominal aura constitutes the most common type of autonomic aura. This consists of an indescribable unpleasant feeling in the peri-umbilical area that can be static, or ascend to the chest and throat, and can also descend into the lower abdominal region (Thompson *et al.*, 2000; Foldvary-Schaefer & Unnwongse, 2011). They are often accompanied by autonomic symptoms such as nausea. The symptomatogenic zone for abdominal auras is the anterior insular cortex, frontal operculum, mesial temporal structures, and SMA (Noachtar & Peters, 2009).

Auditory auras usually manifest as auditory hallucination such as sounds, which are generated by activation of the Heschl's gyrus. Complex auditory hallucinations, such as hearing voices or tunes, can also occur. They are attributed to activation of the temporal association cortex (Loddenkemper & Kotagal, 2005). Vertiginous aura consists of sensation of rotation or movement in all planes that are usually associated with visual or auditory symptoms. These come from temporo-parietal junction (Foldvary-Schaefer & Unnwongse, 2011). The lateralizing value of these auras is poor (Jan & Girvin, 2008). Auras of right temporal origin are more commonly remembered than those from the left (Janszky *et al.*, 2004).

3.4   Automatisms

Automatisms are repetitive, involuntary, purposeless movements that are usually inappropriate, but occasionally may simulate relatively normal events. Oro-alimentary automatisms, consisting of lip smacking, sucking, swallowing or chewing movements, along with gestural automatisms such as picking or fumbling movements are suggestive of TLE (Jan & Girvin, 2008).

Automatisms occur in 70% of patients with limbic seizures compared to 10% of patients with extra-limbic seizures (Manford *et al.*, 1996). If the patient has preserved consciousness during automatisms, a non-dominant temporal focus is more likely (Ebner *et al.*, 1995). When seizure spreads to the frontal lobes, they may produce proximal automatisms such as bicycling or thrashing.

A contralateral dystonic posturing of an arm is characterized by forced unnatural limb posturing, both in flexion or extension, proximal or distal, and with a rotatory component (Foldvary-Schaefer & Unnwongse, 2011). It can follow the ipsilateral automatism (Loddenkemper & Kotagal, 2005). It is more common in TLE than in ETLE. The unilateral dystonic posturing has been attributed to spread to the ipsilateral basal ganglia (Kotagal, 1991). Unilateral automatisms without contralateral dystonia have a lower lateralizing value (Dupont *et al.*, 1999). The isolated dystonic posturing helps lateralize; however, it has no clear localizing value because it can originate from either temporal or frontal lobe (Jan & Girvin, 2008).

3.5   Motor Manifestations

In many patients, temporal seizures present only with staring, behavioral arrest, oro-alimentary and bimanual automatisms, the motor signs when present are usually related with spreading to the frontal lobe. Therefore, it is important to compare the motor and other features of seizures originating in frontal lobe versus temporal lobe (see table 2).

To be clinically significant a seizure-induced head version has to be forced, prolonged, assuming an unnatural position with the chin elevated and with the head hyperextended (Wyllie *et al.*, 1986). The head movement may be tonic or clonic, and it is associated with ipsilateral conjugate gaze deviation. The direction of head version is contralateral to the epileptogenic zone in more than 90% of cases (Foldvary-Schaefer & Unnwongse, 2011). If this occurs at the onset of a seizure in the presence of normal consciousness, is a strong indication of a contralateral frontal dorsolateral cortical onset (So, 2006). In seizures of temporal lobe origin, patients can have an initial brief ipsilateral (non-versive) head turning associated with ipsilateral automatisms (Jan & Girvin, 2008). The contralateral version occurs immediately before the secondary generalization (Foldvary-Schaefer & Unnwongse, 2011). Brodmann area six leads to contralateral version prior to secondary generalization (Loddenkemper & Kotagal, 2005).

Eye movements are another important feature of partial seizures. Seizure-related eye version is forced, sustained, and the conjugate eye deviation typically accompanies the head version. Eye version that occurs before secondary generalization usually originates from the contralateral hemisphere (Wyllie *et al.*, 1986; Foldvary-Schaefer & Unnwongse, 2011). Prominent contralateral head and eye deviation can occur with occipital seizures, which may even be accompanied by contralateral turning of the body (Jan & Girvin, 2008).

Frontal and Temporal Lobe Epilepsy Features		
Type of epilepsy	Frontal lobe	Temporal lobe
Seizures frequency	Frequent, often daily	Less frequent
Sleep activation	Characteristic	Less common
Seizure onset	Abrupt, explosive	Less abrupt
Progression	Rapid	Less abrupt
Initial motionless staring	Less common	Common
Automatisms	Less common	More common and longer
Bipedal automatism	Characteristic	Rare
Complex postures	Early, frequent and prominent	Less frequent and prominent, occurring later as seizure starts to generalize
Hypermotor (Hyperkinetic)	Common	Rare
Somatosensory symptoms	Common	Rare
Speech	Loud vocalization (grunting, screaming, moaning)	Verbalization speech in non-dominant seizures
Seizure duration	Brief	Longer
Secondary generalization	Common	Less common
Postictal confusion	Absent or less prominent and shorter	More prominent and longer
Postictal dysphasia	Rare, unless it spreads to the dominant temporal lobe	Common in dominant temporal lobe seizures

Table 2: Frontal and Temporal Lobe Epilepsy Features

Focal clonic activity is one of the most reliable lateralizing signs during epileptic seizures (Jan & Girvin, 2008). It is a sign related with activation of the primary motor cortex (Loddenkemper & Kotagal, 2005). The hand and face are most frequently involved. Clonic seizures that originate in the frontal cortex are early and before loss of awareness (So, 2006). In temporal lobe seizures, clonic movements usually occur late in the seizure when the patient is unconsciousness, and due to seizure spreading to the dorso-lateral motor cortex (Loddenkemper & Kotagal, 2005; So, 2006; Jan & Girvin, 2008).

Asymmetric tonic limb posturing is usually observed during the early tonic phase of partial seizures. Figure of four sign usually localizes to temporal lobe (So, 2006). One arm is extended at the elbow while the other is flexed at the elbow, giving the appearance of a figure of "4". Both arms are slightly raised in front of the chest. The seizure onset is contralateral to the extended limb (So, 2006). Further lateralizing and localizing aspects of partial seizure semiology are summarized in a table (see table 3).

3.6   Language

Language is important in localizing and lateralizing seizures (Loddenkemper & Kotagal, 2005; Noachtar & Peters, 2009; Foldvary-Schaefer & Unnwongse, 2011). Speech disturbances during seizures include receptive, expressive, or global dysphasia (Jan & Girvin, 2008). Ictal verbalization, consisting of under-standable names, verbal phrases or sentences, should be distinguished from guttural vocalization such as moaning, grunting, and screaming. Verbalizations are more common in non-dominant temporal lobe seizures (Gabr *et al.*, 1989). However, vocalizations are more commonly seen in frontal lobe seizures with no clear lateralizing value (Janszky *et al.*, 2000). Postictal dysphasia is a very useful lateralizing sign for the dominant hemisphere, but it may not be detected unless the epilepsy monitoring unit staffs routinely

Localizing and Lateralizing Value of Epileptic Signs			
Semiologic features	Localization	Lateralization	Lateralizing value (%)
Auras			
Abdominal	Anterior insula, frontal operculum, mesial temporal lobe, and SMA (limbic system)	NL	
Psychic (déjà vu/jamais vu)	Temporal neocortex	NL	
Olfactory	Orbitofrontal region, amygdala, and insula	NL	
Hemifield simple visual	Occipital (Brodmann areas 17-19)	Contralateral	100
Hemifield complex visual	Occipito-temporal o temporal posteromesial	Contralateral	
Simple auditory	Primary auditory cortex (areas 41)	NL	
Complex auditory	Auditory association cortex (areas 42 and 22)	NL	
Unilateral somatosensory aura	Parietal (Brodmann areas 1, 2, and 3)	Contralateral	89
Gustatory	Mesiobasal temporal cortex and parietal operculum	NL	
Vertiginous	Temporo-occipital junction	Often non-dominant	
Cephalic/whole body	Amygdala, entorhinal cortex and temporal neocortex	Often non-dominant	
Orgasmic	Temporal	Non-dominant	
Automatism			
Oral automatism	Temporal lobe, typically hippocampal	NL	
Unilateral limb automatism	Temporal	Ipsilateral	90
Automatisms with preserved responsiveness	Temporal	Non-dominant	100
Bipedal automatisms	95% Frontal and 5% temporal	NL	
Automatism followed by clonic seizure	Temporal Neocortical	Ipsilateral	
Automatism followed by dystonic hand posturing	Temporal mesial	Ipsilateral	
Unilateral eye blinks	Temporal	Ipsilateral	83
Whistling	Temporal	NL	
Language abnormalities			
Ictal panic attack	Temporal	Non-dominant	
Ictal speech arrest	Temporal	Dominant	PPV 67
Ictal speech preservation	Temporal	Non-dominant	83
Postictal dysphasia and aphasia	Temporal	Dominant	100
Vocalization	Frontal	Dominant	82
Motor abnormalities			
Early non-forced head turn	Frontal or temporal	Ipsilateral	30
Late contraversive forced head turn	Frontal (Brodmann 6 area) or temporal	Contralateral	PPV 94

Late ipsiversive forced head turn	Temporal	Ipsilateral	
Late non-forced head turn	Frontal or temporal	Ipsilateral	
Forced eye deviation	Frontal (Brodmann 8 area)	Contralateral	
Solitary eye deviation	Occipital	Contralateral	
Epileptic nystagmus	Occipital	Contralateral	100
Unilateral clonic jerking	Frontal (Brodmann 4 area) peri-rolandic	Contralateral	PPV 95
Asymmetric clonic ending	Frontal (Brodmann 4 area) peri-rolandic	Ipsilateral	83
Unilateral tonic seizure (isolated)	Frontal	Contralateral	89
Dystonic limb/hand posturing	Temporal or frontal	Contralateral	100
Fencing posture (M2E)	Frontal (SMA)	Contralateral	PPV 90
Figure of 4 sign	70% Temporal, 30% extratemporal	Contralateral to the extended limb	PPV 89
Unilateral ictal paresis or immobile limb	Frontal (FIG)	Contralateral	PPV 100
Postictal			
Postictal Todd's paresis	Frontal	Contralateral	PPV 100
Postictal nose wiping/rubbing	Temporal	Ipsilateral	97
Postictal coughing	Temporal	Non-dominant	
Postictal disorientation	Temporal	Non-dominant	85
Postictal verbal memory dysfunction	Temporal	Dominant	
Postictal visual memory dysfunction	Temporal	Non-dominant	
Tongue biting (side)	--	Ipsilateral	71
Others			
Ictal spitting	Temporal	Non-dominant	76
Ictal drinking	Temporal, hypothalamic	Non-dominant	
Ictal laughter (gelastic)	Hypothalamic, mesial temporal or frontal cingulate	NL	
Dacrystic seizures	Temporal, more hippocampal and hypothalamic	NL	
Ictus vomiting	Temporal	Non-dominant	81
Ictal urinary urge	Temporal	Non-dominant	100
Unilateral ear plugging	Temporal (STG)	Contralateral	
Piloerection (goose bumps)	Temporal	Ipsilateral*	84
Tachycardia	Temporal	NL	
Unilateral emotional facial alteration	Temporal mesial (amygdala), prefrontal bitofrontal region, hypothalamus, insula	Contralateral	PPV 86

Table 3: Abbreviations. SMA: supplementary motor area, FIG: frontal inferior gyrus, STG: superior temporal gyrus, PPV: positive predictive value. NL: no lateralization. References: (Loddenkemper & Kotagal, 2005; So, 2006; Jan & Girvin, 2008; Noachtar & Peters, 2009; Foldvary-Schaefer & Unnwongse, 2011). *Piloerection occurs mostly in left TLE (So, 2006).

checks the postictal speech function (Gabr *et al.*, 1989). Speech arrest may occur at the onset of a seizure from the dominant temporal lobe, but can also occur from involvement of inferior Rolandic cortex and the SMA (So, 2006).

3.7 Posictal Signs

Postictal nose wiping and cough are due to increased parasympathetic activity resulting in increased nasal and pharyngeal secretions. These behaviors are believed to be reflexive in nature, occurring postictally as they are inhibited during the ictal period (Leutmezer *et al.*, 1998). Postictal paresis or "Todd's paralysis" is one of the oldest described lateralizing signs corresponding to contralateral motor cortex. Postictal hemianopia is seen in the contralateral occipital seizures (Loddenkemper & Kotagal, 2005). Suspected mechanisms include neuronal exhaustion of the primary motor areas due to increased lactic acid levels, and cerebrovascular dysfunction. Additionally, active inhibition by endogenous endorphins has been proposed (Loddenkemper & Kotagal, 2005).

3.8 Other Signs

Cardiac manifestations are the most well recognized autonomic manifestations of partial seizures (Foldvary-Schaefer & Unnwongse, 2011). Ictal tachycardia, defines as a heart rate more than 100 beats per minute, is reported in more than 50% of seizures. Early and significant tachycardia is more common in TLE than in ETLE (Weil *et al.*, 2002) and is associated especially with right mesial TLE (Weil *et al.*, 2005). Pure ictal tachycardia without any other clinical symptoms is highly correlated with temporal rather than extratemporal epileptogenic activity (Weil *et al.*, 2002). Ictal bradycardia, which is one of the causes of SUDEP, is more common in TLE as opposed to ETLE (Tinuper *et al.*, 2001; Britton *et al.*, 2006; So & Sperling, 2007). The lateralizing value of ictal bradycardia is questionable. Although in some reports left temporal lobe is more commonly involved (Tinuper *et al.*, 2001), others suggest bilateral involvement (Britton *et al.*, 2006).

Seizure semiology has several potential limitations in localizing seizure onset. Although many semiologic features have high positive predictive values for localization, each feature has some potential to falsely localize seizure onset (So, 2006). Therefore, the investigators must exercise caution when using these findings during evaluation of an epileptic patient for epilepsy surgery. It is also important to keep in mind those extratemporal regions, such as orbitofrontal area, cingulum, insula, and temporo parieto occipital junction might demonstrate similar electro-clinical characteristics to those of the temporal lobe (Loddenkemper & Kotagal, 2005; Ryvlin & Kahane, 2005; So, 2006; Jan & Girvin, 2008; Noachtar & Peters, 2009; Foldvary-Schaefer & Unnwongse, 2011).

4   EEG and Video-EEG

EEG is the most useful diagnostic test for epilepsy (Noachtar & Rémi, 2009). Activation procedures such as hyperventilation, photic stimulation, and sleep deprivation enhance the diagnostic sensitivity of EEG and should be a routine practice (Foldvary *et al.*, 2001). Although surface EEG recordings are less sensitive than invasive studies, they provide the best overview and, therefore, the most efficient way to define the approximate localization of the epileptogenic zone (Noachtar & Rémi, 2009). Video-EEG allows increasing the likelihood of detecting interictal epileptiform activity, as well as allowing visual analysis of the seizures and simultaneous clinical and electrographic correlation helpful in presurgical evaluation (Binnie *et al.*, 1981; Chen *et al.*, 1995).

4.1   Interictal Findings

Surface interictal EEG changes occur more commonly in TLE than in other kind of seizure locations (Noachtar & Rémi, 2009). Lateralized arrhythmic (irregular) delta activity may be found in up to 66% of patients with TLE and is highly concordant with temporal spiking (Koutroumanidis *et al.*, 2004). Temporal intermittent rhythmic delta activity (TIRDA) is a more specific and accurate interictal indicator of TLE (Geyer *et al.*, 1999; Jan *et al.*, 2010). TIRDA consists of trains of rhythmic delta activity lasting 4-20 seconds (Javidan, 2012). It is related with epilepsy in 80% of cases (Geyer *et al.*, 1999).

The classic interictal EEG abnormality of mesial TLE is a spike or sharp wave, which usually are electronegative waves over the anterior temporal region (F7/F8) (Javidan, 2012). Mid temporal (T3/T4) and posterior temporal (T5/T6) spikes or sharp waves are more likely to originate from the temporal neocortex (Williamson *et al.*, 1993; Jan *et al.*, 2010). Interictal spikes predict the epileptogenic focus with a probability greater than 95% (Holmes *et al.*, 1996). Patients with TLE frequently have interictal epileptiform discharges independently in both temporal lobes (Serles *et al.*, 1998; Noachtar & Rémi, 2009). The TLE is commonly a bilateral disease even though a unilateral focus is likely to predominate in the great majority of cases. According to different studies (Blume *et al.*, 1993; Williamson *et al.*, 1993; Chee *et al.*, 1993; Ergene *et al.*, 2000) independent bitemporal spikes (IBS) are present in 13% to 73% of patients with TLE and the incidence is higher when longer recordings are obtained (Ergene *et al.*, 2000). The incidence of IBSs has been reported in 13-17% of patients with TLE and routine EEGs of 30 to 40 min duration (Williamson *et al.*, 1993; Chee *et al.*, 1993). The incidence is higher (61%) using 24-hour continuous recordings (Ergene *et al.*, 2000), and (73%) with four or more consecutive EEGs recorded (Blume *et al.*, 2000). Furthermore, there is a correlation between a successful outcome after surgery for TLE and a high degree of lateralization of interictal epileptiform discharges (IEDs) before surgery. Epileptiform activity has often been considered "lateralized" in TLE by many investigators if more than 80-90% of the discharges originated from one temporal lobe (Ergene *et al.*, 2000).

4.2   Ictal Findings

The ictal EEG recording is the main component of the presurgical evaluation (Engel, 1993). Ictal EEGs are more localizing in TLE versus ETLE (Foldvary *et al.*, 2001). Different temporal lobe ictal patterns have been described through history. In 1978 Geiger et al (Geiger & Harner, 1978) pointed out that focal hypersynchrony on the scalp EEG was an accurate localizing indicator of cortical irritability. In 1996 Ebersole et al (Ebersole & Pacia, 1996) described three different ictal rhythms in TLE. The Type I is characterized by rhythmic 5-9 Hz theta activity that slowly evolves and remains localized to the temporal or sub-temporal regions. It is the most specific pattern for seizures originating from the hippocampal areas. The Ebersole type II is characterized by rhythmic slow activity (2-5 Hz) with widespread temporal distribution. It is frequently associated with neocortical seizures. The Ebersole type III is characterized by diffuse ictal EEG changes or attenuation without clear lateralization. This pattern can be seen in hippocampal and temporal neocortical seizures (Ebersole & Pacia, 1996). Other Ictal rhythms include background attenuation and start-stop-start (SSS) phenomenon (Jan *et al.*, 2010).

4.2.1 Start-Stop-Start Phenomenon

Defined as a pair of sequential ictal potentials separated by complete or almost complete cessation of seizure activity, the SSS phenomenon was initially identified in 1993 by Blume et al on subdural recordings in 23% patients (Blume & Kaibara, 1993). Three years later, Atalla et al described the same ictal pattern in 13% of patients with TLE using scalp-sphenoidal electrodes. The first "start" usually has a narrow field, typically in the sphenoidal electrodes. The mean duration of the "start" is eleven seconds and usually the clinical onset correlates with these changes. The stop last eight seconds and the restart often had a different morphology, frequency, and a wider field (Atalla *et al.*, 1996). A simple hypothesis for the unknown physiological mechanism underlying the SSS phenomenon in the same region may be that seizure-terminating factors act ineffectively, producing only a pause – then resumption. Theories for restart at a distance include those of seizure propagation, and an alternative mechanism might be a long-loop reverberating circuit. The stop phase may simply represent unrecorded continuing distant seizure activity located away from electrode placements, or masked due to muscle and movement artifact (Blume & Kaibara, 1993). The SSS phenomenon is a clinical electroencephalographic pattern that should be considered and recognized at seizure onset in some patients. If this phenomenon is missed, the restart may be misinterpreted as the actual seizure onset, and some seizures may be considered non-localized (Atalla *et al.*, 1996).

A lateralized ictal change characterized by irregular polymorphic theta and delta (2-5 Hz) is most often associated with TLE originating from the neocortex. A lateralized ictal change of rhythmic 5-10Hz sharp activities, maximally at F7/F8 or sphenoidal electrode is most commonly seen in hippocampal onset (Jan *et al.*, 2010). The ictal EEG manifestation of limbic seizures also could have a nonspecific beginning of low-voltage fast (electro-decrement) activity, with focal or regional background attenuation (Javidan, 2012). Some postictal patterns are described in TLE including polymorphic delta activity and regional attenuation of focal spikes (Jan *et al.*, 2010). Postictal lateralized slowing is present in 67% of TLE patient (Williamson *et al.*, 1993).

Another abnormality of possible significance is the potential bradycardia or tachycardia before the onset of ictal EEG discharges. This phenomenon is associated with EEG pattern of TLE originating from the mesial structures, suggesting activation of the neuronal circuits involved in sympathetic regulation (Jan *et al.*, 2010).

Several "non-standard" electrodes can be used to further evaluate the EEG abnormalities including sphenoidal, nasopharyngeal, anterior temporal (T1/T2), foramen oval (FO) electrodes, and surface electrodes applied over the mandibular notch (MN) or zygoma (Jan *et al.*, 2010). Sphenoidal electrodes especially have been suggested to be helpful in identifying the irritative and seizure onset zones in patients with TLE (Hamaneh *et al.*, 2011). These electrodes are inserted bilaterally through the skin below the zygomatic arch, two to three centimeters anterior to the tragus and directed postero-superiorly towards foramen ovale. A qualified physician should perform this procedure with local anesthesia (Jan *et al.*, 2010). T1, T2, and MN electrodes are able to record all the sphenoidal detected spikes, are not invasive, more confortable, and easy to adjust (Sadler & Goodwin, 1989; Krauss *et al.*, 1992; Blume, 2003). Although sphenoidal electrodes detect spikes from seizures rising from the mesial temporal region, they could also be present with seizures originating in the neocortical temporal or orbitofrontal area. Therefore, although sensitive, sphenoidal spikes are not very specific (Wilkus *et al.*, 1991).

4.3   Foramen Oval Electrodes

In thirty percent of mesial TLE patients, scalp-sphenoidal EEG recordings fail to demonstrate a unilateral ictal onset; also showing contralateral, bitemporal independent, and non-lateralized ictal onsets. In addition, the surface EEG recordings may not be interpretable because of movement artifacts. Foramen ovale (FO) evaluation provides accurate neurophysiologic data about lateralization of seizures that were not clearly lateralized by surface EEGs (Velasco *et al.*, 2006). FO electrodes are used to record from mesial temporal structures without requiring penetration of the skull; a multi-contact flexible electrode is placed in the ambient cistern with the aid of a needle inserted through the foramen ovale (Jan *et al.*, 2010). This procedure is safe and can be an alternative to invasive implantation of depth electrodes in mesial TLE patients who are candidates for temporal lobectomy (Velasco *et al.*, 2006). These electrodes are not as close to hipocampal structures as intracerebral electrodes and do not allow as large a recording field as grids and strips. However, they detect mesial temporal EEG discharges as well as sphenoidal electrodes (Jan *et al.*, 2010); and the signal-to-noise ratio of FO is better than that in the scalp-sphenoidal electrode recordings (Velasco *et al.*, 2006).

Alarcón *et al,* have used FO electrodes successfully in presurgical evaluation of TLE patients. As the FO is a natural hole, the implantation of FO electrodes does not involve disruption of the cranium (Alarcón *et al.*, 2012). They introduce six electrodes through the FO, with the deepest contacts recording from mesial temporal structures. Such deep contacts usually show interictal and ictal patterns, which are not seen on the scalp and are considered as semi-invasive electrodes that provide significantly more information than scalp recordings (Kissani *et al.*, 2001).

Figure 1 demonstrates a 36 years old right-handed male with an unremarkable past medical history, which began having daily complex partial seizures three years ago. The patient experienced an aura described as "feeling anxious, uneasy, and dreadful", followed by loss of awareness lasting 60 seconds. He had mild postictal confusion and rare secondary generalization. Seizure control could not be achieved with a combination of levetiracetam, Lamotrigine and Clobazam. Brain MRI revealed atrophy of the left hippocampus, with an increased T2 (weighted) signal.

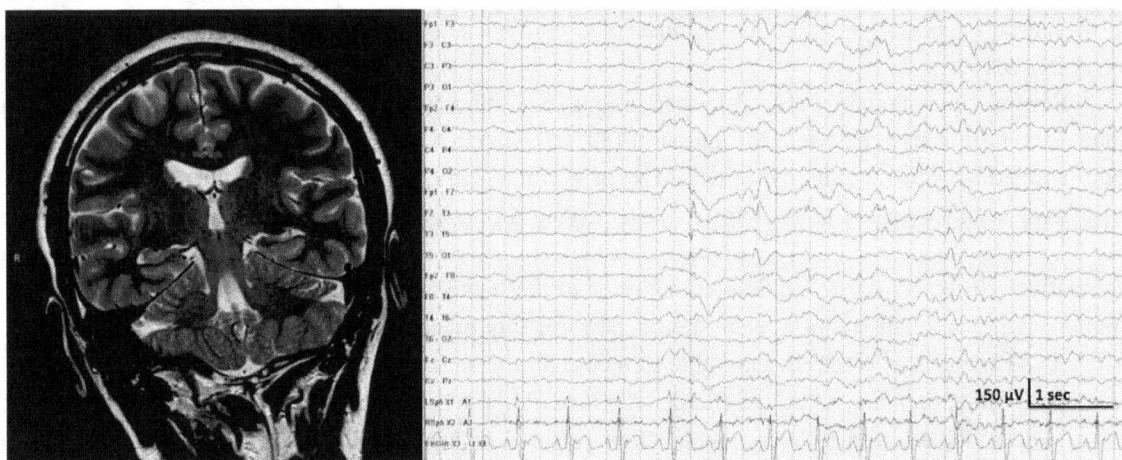

Figure 1: On the left: A coronal T2-weighted 3T MRI section shows reduced hippocampal volume and increased signal, consistent with left mesial temporal sclerosis. On the right: scalp EEG recording shows interictal epileptiform activity on the left anterior temporal region (maximum at F7 electrode).

Scalp video-EEG monitoring revealed abundant spikes over the left temporal region, maximum at F7-T3 with spread to T5 electrode. See figure 1. Three seizures were recorded during video-EEG monitoring; all of them had a clear left temporal onset (maximum at F7 electrode). See figure 2. His neuropsychological evaluation reported low average vocabulary skills, phonemic fluency, and verbal memory consistent with left temporal functional impairment. He underwent left temporal lobectomy. Histopathology revealed severe neuronal loss and gliosis involving predominantly hippocampal sector CA1 and the dentate gyrus, consistent with MTS. After resection his seizures resolved with no memory complaints. After 5-6 months of postoperative follow up he remains seizure free.

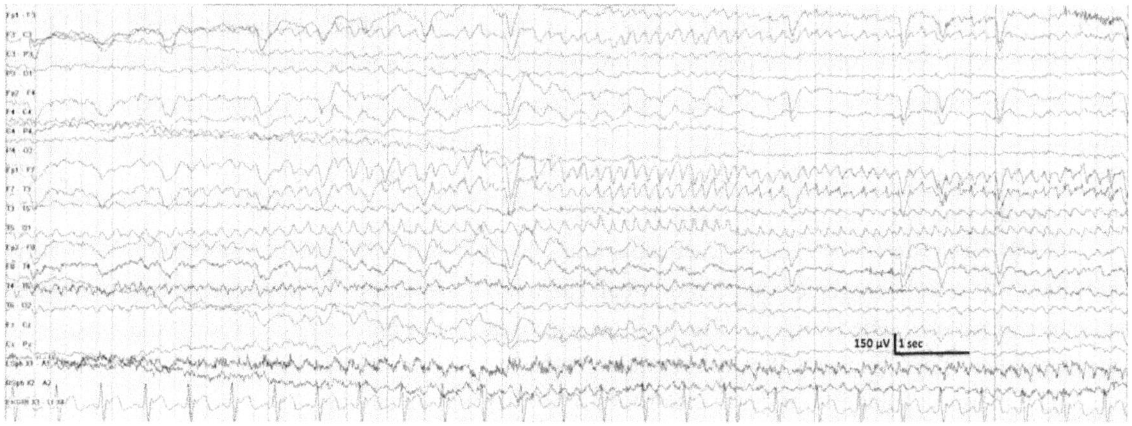

Figure 2: Scalp EEG recording showing lateralized ictal rhythmic 7 Hz activity, maximally at F7 with involvement of the ipsilateral scalp sphenoidal electrode.

5 Intracranial Recording

Non-invasive methods are sufficient to evaluate 60 to 85% of patients before surgical resection (Engel, 1993; Holmes *et al.*, 1996). The main purpose of intracranial recording is to delineate the area of onset and early propagation of a seizure. It is therefore important to cover the suspected zone by placing electrodes in strategic areas. The idea is to confirm that seizures all arise in one area and not in another (Dubeau & McLachlan, 2000; Pondal-Sordo *et al.*, 2007). Ultimately, the localization is achieved by combining the data from invasive monitoring with a detailed analysis of the clinical semiology, and the information obtained from the video-EEG monitoring and other tests such as MRI, SPECT or PET.

There are six main reasons for invasive recordings: 1) seizures lateralized, but not localized; 2) seizures localized, but not lateralized; 3) seizures neither localized, nor lateralized; 4) discrepancy between electrographic seizure location and the rest of the data (e.g. location of lesion on imaging); 5) seizures localized in eloquent cortical areas; and 6) relation of seizure localization to lesion (Dubeau & McLachlan, 2000).

Scalp electrodes detect activity generated from a large cortical surface (6 cm^2) give reference, whereas subdural or depth electrodes will detect changes over only a few millimeters of cortex. Therefore, some interictal spikes that are not otherwise visible on scalp EEG can be easily identified with invasive electrodes. While invasive electrodes are more sensitive in detecting spikes and seizures from a localized area, they may miss epileptiform activity in other regions due to covering a limited surface (Jan *et al.*, 2010).

Intracranial recordings have several advantages compared to surface EEG. These advantages include better spatial resolution and increased sensitivity, no attenuation from scalp and skull, reduced ictal electromyographic artifacts, and providing the option of cortical stimulation (Dubeau & McLachlan, 2000; Javidan, 2012). The disadvantages of invasive monitoring include: limited cortical sampling or risk for sampling error (tunnel vision), and risk of significant complications such as hemorrhage and infection (2-3%).

Subdural electrodes are inserted surgically to record over the cerebral cortex. Electrode grids are square or rectangular in shape with small platinum or stainless steel disks embedded into a soft silastic sheet with several contact points. Electrode strips, which come in various sizes, consist of a row of contacts and are usually inserted through a burr hole (Dubeau & McLachlan, 2000; Gonzalez-Martinez *et al.*, 2012). Currently, subdural electrodes are the most common invasive method used in the United States. Despite the high spatial resolution provided by the subdural methodology, relatively deep epileptogenic foci cannot be sampled (Gonzalez-Martinez *et al.*, 2012).

Depth electrodes or stereo-electroencephalography is a safe and accurate procedure for invasive assessment of the epileptogenic zone. Traditional Talairach's methodology, implemented by multimodal planning and robot assisted surgery, allows direct electrical recording from superficial and deep-seated brain structures, providing essential information in the most complex cases of DRE (Cardinale *et al.*, 2012). The main advantage from depth electrodes over subdural electrodes is that the former allow sampling from deep zones such as, amygdala, hippocampus, entorhinal cortex, and insular cortex (Dubeau & McLachlan, 2000).

Selection between subdural electrodes and depth electrodes depends on the experience of each epilepsy center. Several studies (Eisenschenk *et al.*, 2001; Gonzalez-Martinez *et al.*, 2012; Wellmer *et al.*, 2012) comparing the two techniques have shown no superiority of one over the other.

Hader (Hader *et al.*, 2013) published a systematic review about complications of invasive EEG monitoring. They described minor complications as those that resolved completely within three months. Major neurological complications persisted beyond that time frame. According to these definitions, minor neurological complications occurred in 10.9% of patients, whereas major complications were identified in 4.7% of patients. The overall frequency of minor complications associated with invasive monitoring was higher in the pediatric population than in adults (11.2% vs. 5.5%), possibly because in the pediatric population subdural grid implantation via craniotomy was more commonly utilized in the investigations. Major neurological complications were more common after extratemporal resections than temporal resections (6.5% vs. 4.1% respectively) (Hader *et al.*, 2013).

Arya (Arya *et al.*, 2013) published a systematic review about adverse effects of subdural electrodes. The most common adverse effects found were as follows: neurological infections (2.3%), superficial infections (3%), intracranial hemorrhage (4%), and elevated intracranial pressure (2.4%). The mean number of electrodes per patient varied from 52 to 95 and the mean number of electrodes placement duration varied from five to 17 days. Increased number of electrodes (>67) was found to be associated with increased incidence of adverse effects.

Figure 3 shows a case of a 49-years-old right-handed male with eight years of epilepsy history. His only epilepsy risk factor was head trauma at the age of 25 years. He suffered a closed brain injury secondary to a grenade explosion. His seizures were charazterized by staring followed by oroalimentary and bimanual automatisms and mild postictal confusion. Secondary generalization was rare. Complex

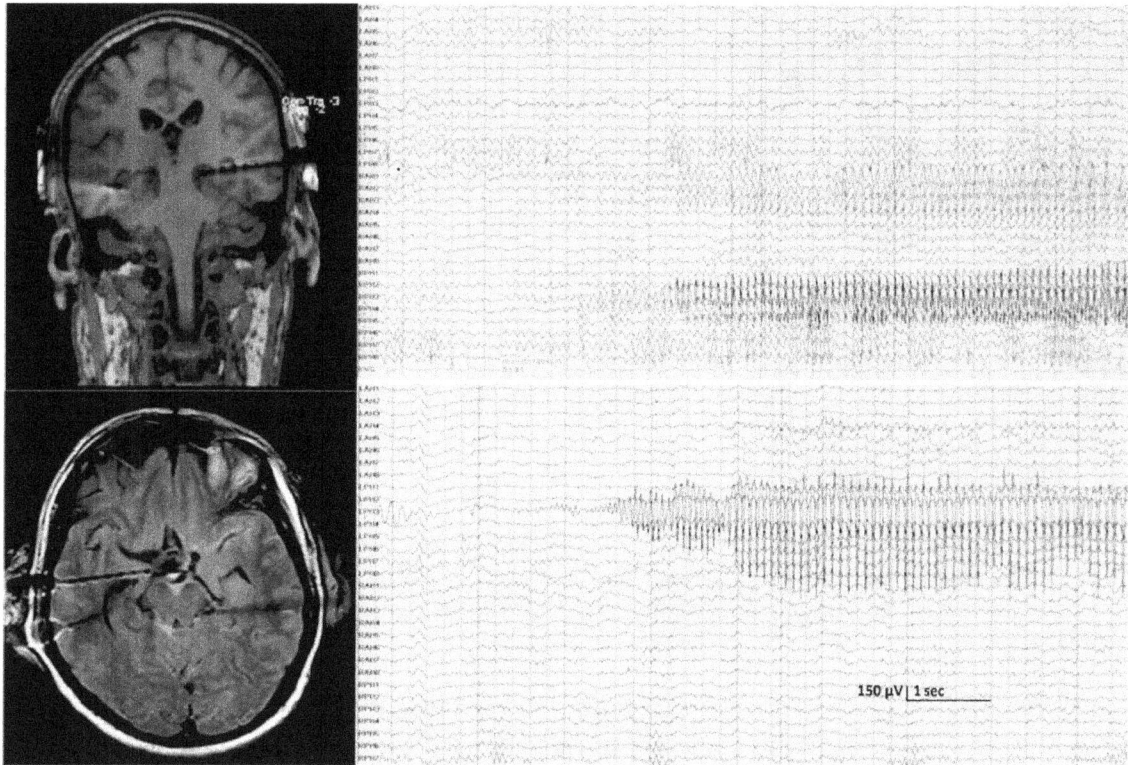

Figure 3: On the left: at the top coronal Fluid-attenuated inversion recovery (FLAIR) 3T MR, at the bottom axial FLAIR 3T MRI. Both sequences showing bilateral implanted depth electrodes. On the right: at the top intracranial EEG recording showing ictal lateralized fast activity (12Hz), maximally at RPH3-4 (Right Posterior Hippocampus), at the bottom there is ictal lateralized fast activity (16Hz), maximally at LPH3 (Left Posterior Hippocampus).

partial seizures occured daily, and at times in clusters. Patient had failed treatment with Phenytoin, Carbamazepine, Levetiracetam, Clobazam; and he was taking Lamotrigine with no improvement. MRI was normal. Video-EEG showed equal number of electrographic seizures from each temporal lobe as well as independent bitemporal inter-ictal epileptiform discharges. An interictal PET showed right temporal hypometabolism. The intracranial recording with depth electrodes confirmed an equal independent bitemporal onset for seizures (see figure 3). Based on the PET findings a right temporal lobectomy was done. Twelve months after surgery, the patient has only had three complex partial seizures, always related with stressful situations or lack of compliance. In this case the intracranial recording did not help to lateralize the seizure onset and the PET scan was the key test for making the decision to offer a right temporal lobecotmy.

Figure 4 demonstrates the case of a 33-year-old right-handed male with a long history of seizures. He had a head concussion at the age of 17 months secondary to falling out of his stroller. Seizures started after this event with two types of spells. The most common were complex partial seizures characterized by the lack of aura, staring, bimanual and oral automatisms and postictal confusion. The patient had ictal speech in many of the seizures. These events occurred daily for the last two years. The patient also had complex partial seizures with secondary generalization (one per month). He received treatment

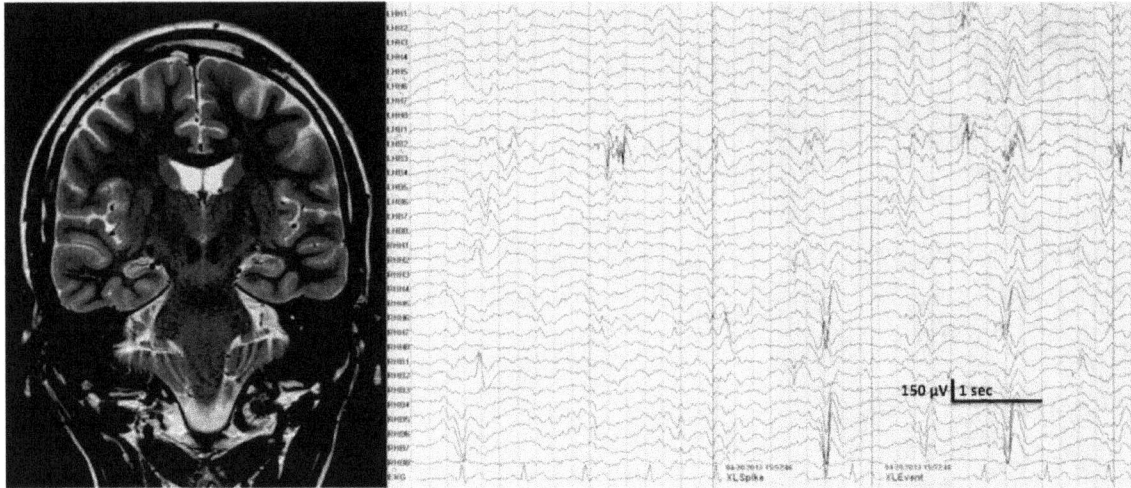

Figure 4: On the left: coronal T2-weighted 3T MRI showing signs of right mesial temporal sclerosis (atrophy of the head of the hippocampus with loss of digitations) On the right: intracranial EEG recording showing independent interictal activity on both temporal regions.

with Lamotrigine and Levetiracetam. He had failed in the past to Phenytoin, Carbamazepine, Clobazam. Several interictal EEGs showed right temporal spikes, and brain MRI showed right MTS.

Video-EEG telemetry was performed, showing independent bitemporal spikes. Ten seizures were recorded with a potential bitemporal onset, but no clear ictal activity in the right temporal region. Neuropsychological test reported a lower average cognitive function, with bilateral impairment on tasks of visual and verbal memory. The intracranial investigation showed frequent independet bitemporal spikes (see Figure 4). Five seizures were recorded with depth electrodes, all of them with clear onset over the head of right hippocampus (mesial electrodes), the left side was sileen at the onset of the seizures (see Figure 5). In this case the depth electrodes helped to corroborate that the seizures were coming from the same side as the structural lesion.

6   MRI

After a careful evaluation of the clinical semiology and EEG findings, the next step in presurgical evaluation of epilepsy is the detection of structural abnormalities. MRI is the most sensitive and useful examination for identifying structural abnormalities in patients with partial epilepsy. Most partial epilepsies arise from the temporal lobe and HS is the most common underlying pathological substrate (Wehner & Lüders, 2008). MRI has been the single most important test to document and diagnose HS, as it is a non-invasive test with a high yield in localizing the abnormalities in patients with TLE (Spencer, 1994).

Although patients with normal MRIs have a less possibility to render seizure free after epilepsy surgery than patients with an obvious MRI lesion, the use of invasive monitoring can improve the outcomes and still a large percentage of patients with epilepsy (50 to 70%) can render seizure free after surgery (Téllez-Zenteno et al., 2005).

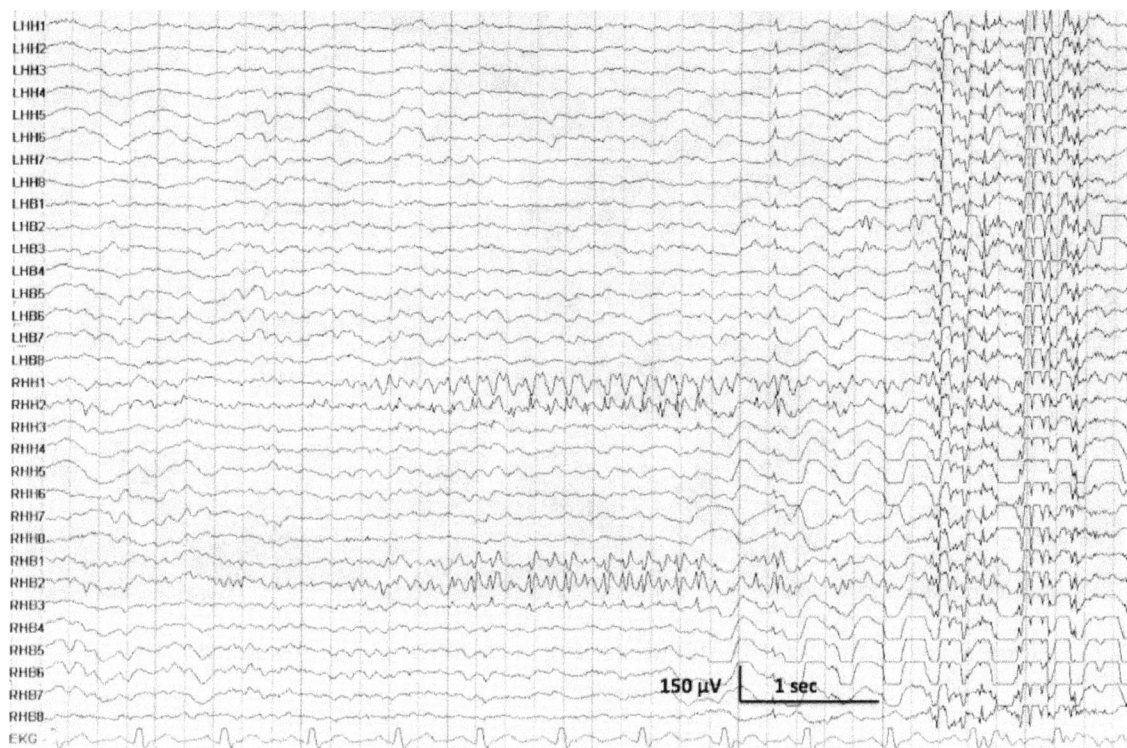

Figure 5: Intracranial EEG recording with depth electrodes showed a clear onset over the mesial electrodes in the right temporal region (RHH1-2 (Right hippocampus head) and RHB1-2 (right hippocampus body).

In patients with TLE, the mesial temporal structures should be carefully evaluated, (hippocampus, parahipocampal gyrus and amygdala) (Wehner & Lüders, 2008). The suggested sequences are FLAIR, T2-weighted and T1-weighted, with coronal sections perpendicular to the long axis of the hippocampus. Contrast medium is not necessary if there is no suspicion of a tumor (Woermann & Vollmar, 2009). Classic findings of HS are atrophy of the hippocampus (95%) with increased signal intensity on T2-weighted (85%) or FLAIR sequences; these changes are better appreciated when both sides are compared in the same subject. In addition, minor findings may be seen in TLE such as loss of hippocampal surface and internal structure (60-95%), enlargement of the cerebrospinal fluid (CSF) space in the temporal horn of the lateral ventricle, atrophy of ipsilateral temporal structures (temporal lobe, fornix, mammillary body, white matter of the parahipocampal gyrus), and decreased signal intensity on T1-weighted (10-95%). The minor findings are less consistent and their diagnostic value is limited (Woermann & Vollmar, 2009).

Cavernous angiomas are the most frequent forms of vascular malformation related with seizures. They are benign vascular lesions with thin-walled endothelium lined spaces that contain blood products in different stages of evolution. On MRI, they have a characteristic "popcorn" appearance with a core of mixed signal intensities, reflecting various stages of blood degradation, and a hypointense rim, reflecting hemosiderin deposition (see Figure 6). Gradient echo sequences increases the sensitivity of MRI by demonstrating punctuate micro hemorrhages (Wehner & Lüders, 2008).

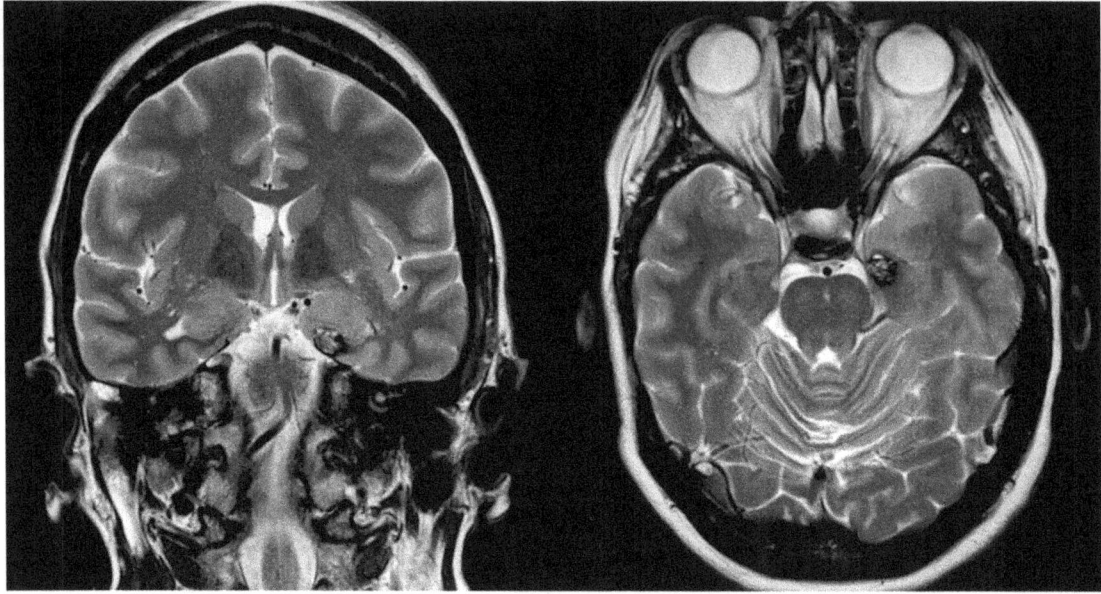

Figure 6: Coronal T2-weighted 3T MRI (on the left), and axial T2-weighted (on the right) showing a cavernous angioma in the left mesial temporal region.

The hemorrhages associated with cavernous angiomas are considered a major factor in their epileptogenicity. In the setting of a single cavernous angioma and consistent electro-clinical seizures, further testing is not required; even pure lesionectomy achieves seizure freedom in two-thirds of patients (Ferroli *et al.*, 2006).

It is important to bear in mind the possibility of dual pathology that occurs in up to 15% of adult cases and 67% of pediatric cases (Alvarez-Linera Prado, 2007). Dual pathology refers to patients who have two (or more) distinct lesions on MRI, classically the combination of HS with another epileptogenic lesion. The most frequent clinical scenario is the coexistence of HS with a malformation of cortical development, most commonly focal cortical dysplasia, particularly type I (Bautista *et al.*, 2003).

Figure 7 shows the case of a 29-year-old right-handed female. She began having complex partial seizures six years ago, and after one year they became intractable. Video-EEG showed three seizures, all with a clear onset over the right mesial temporal region. MRI shows dual pathology, HS and a focal region of heterotopic grey matter.

7   Functional Imaging

Functional imaging detects changes in cerebral metabolism or cerebral perfusion in the interictal or ictal state. It is important to obtain a strong correlation between clinical findings, EEG and the different imaging techniques. Ictal perfusion single photon emission computed tomography (SPECT) and interictal fluorodeoxyglucose (FDG) positron emission tomography (PET) are important imaging tools in the presurgical evaluation of patients with partial DRE. In SPECT scan, the largest and most intense ictal hyperperfusion cluster is assumed to represent the ictal onset zone; however, in PET scan, the region of predominant hypometabolism contains the epileptogenic zone (Van Paesschen *et al.*, 2007).

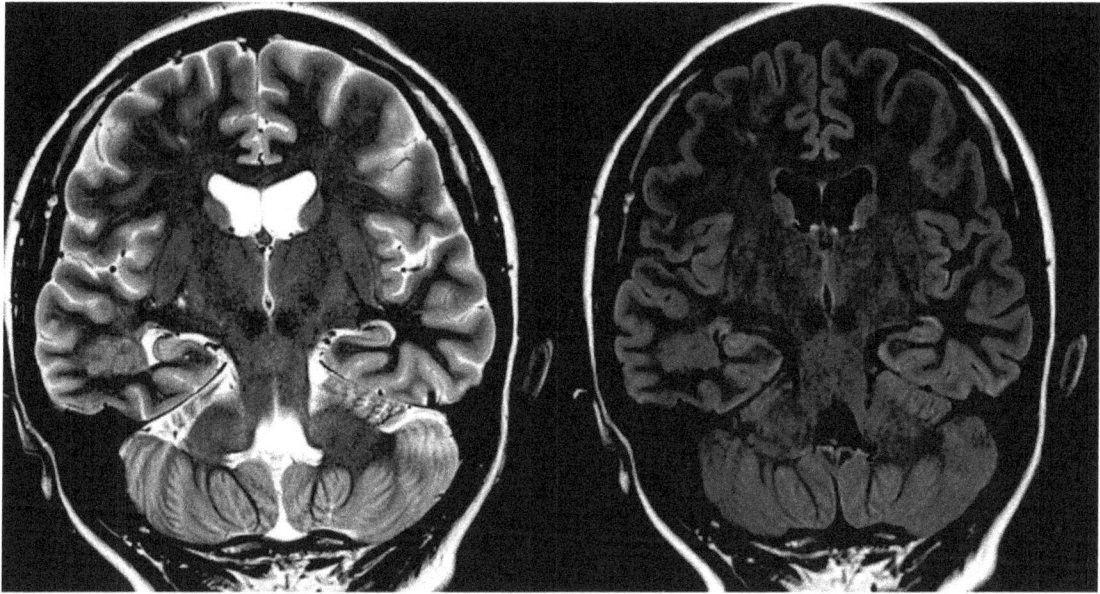

Figure 7: Coronal T2-weighted 3T MRI (on the left), and coronal FLAIR (on the right) showing het-erotopic grey matter nodules in the right temporal region, and atrophy of the ipsilateral hippocampus with loss of surface and internal structure, and enlargement of the CSF space in the respective temporal horn.

7.1 SPECT

Its application is based on the assumption that the increased ictal neuronal activity during epileptic sei-zures is associated with increased metabolism and regional cerebral blood flow (rCBF) (La fougère *et al.*, 2009). Ictal SPECT has a high sensitivity to localize the epileptic focus (Lee *et al.*, 2011). Ictal SPECT is performed by injecting radiotracer intravenously during seizures. It utilizes 99m Tc-hexamethyl-propyleneamine oxime (99m Tc-HMPAO) or 99m Tc-ethylcysteinate dimer (99m Tc-ECD) to study cer-ebral perfusion in the ictal state. Both of these tracers have a rapid first pass uptake and a relatively long half-life (Van Paesschen *et al.*, 2007). This allows storing them at the bedside for ictal injection as well as a generous time window of up to six hours post-injection to acquire the images (Wehner & Lüders, 2008).

Cortical and subcortical rCBF changes during seizures may begin with hyperperfusion in the epi-leptic zone followed by rapid extension to other regions due to seizure spread and generalization. Thus, a SPECT hyperperfusion pattern often contains both the ictal onset zone and the propagation pathways (La fougère *et al.*, 2009). This phenomenon is followed by postictal hypoperfusion within one to two minutes in TLE (Richardson, 2010). It has been estimated that the seizure should last at least ten seconds after the injection in order to obtain localizing information (Wehner & Lüders, 2008). Ictal SPECT may result in a false localization or lateralization because of a delay between seizure onset and tracer injection, which is called "posictal switch" phenomenon (Newton *et al.*, 1992).

7.2 SISCOM (Substraction Ictal SPECT Coregistered to MRI)

This multimodality imaging, combines the structural and functional imaging information, improves the ability to detect and define the extent of epileptogenic lesions and to regionalize potentially epileptogenic foci in patients who have normal MRI scans (La fougère *et al.*, 2009). The protocol was introduce by O`Brien and colleagues at Mayo Clinic.

SISCOM technique compares an ictal SPECT image with the same patient's interictal SPECT image, and produces a difference image between the two SPECTs. Theoretically SISCOM is expected to reveal cerebral perfusion changes during seizure more accurately than the visual inspection of ictal SPECT. SISCOM significantly increased the sensitivity of ictal SPECT and provides a more accurate anatomic localization of seizures by also using MRI (Lee *et al.*, 2011).

7.3   PET

The glucose analog FDG is the tracer most widely used. It is an indirect marker of neuronal activity. The epileptogenic focus in the interictal phase usually appears as a hypometabolic area on FDG-PET (La fougère *et al.*, 2009). Although the underlying neurobiology of hypometabolism is not well understood, it has been ascribed to factors such as neuronal loss, diaschisis, inhibitory processes and reduction in synaptic density (Van Paesschen *et al.*, 2007).

The area of decreased glucose utilization in TLE is typically more extensive than the epileptogenic zone and may extend into the adjacent inferior frontal or parietal lobe cortex, as well as the ipsilateral thalamus. The extent of cortical glucose metabolism on PET scan represents a dynamic process related to the frequency of seizures. Most patients with persistent or increased seizure frequency show enlargement in the area of hypometabolism on the second PET scan. In patients with improved seizure control, a decrease in the size of the hypometabolic cortex is observed (Van Paesschen *et al.*, 2007). Additionally there is a direct relationship between severity of FDG-PET hypometabolism and interictal regional delta slowing in TLE, suggesting related underlying pathophysiological mechanisms for metabolic and electrical dysfunction in TLE (Van Paesschen *et al.*, 2007; Richardson, 2010).

Thus FDG-PET has lateralizing value rather than localizing significance in TLE, mainly by confirming hypometabolism in the area considered for surgical resection (Wehner & Lüders, 2008). FDG-PET may offer localizing value in patients with TLE who do not have a structural abnormality on MRI, which led to coin the term "MRI-negative PET-positive TLE" (Carne *et al.*, 2007). The patients with non-lesional epilepsy usually demonstrate more widespread PET abnormalities than those with HS.

As a rule, PET and SPECT scans must be used only as an adjunct test in surgical planning of patients with epilepsy.

8   Language and Memory Tests

8.1   Neuropsychological Evaluation

The assessment of the presurgical cognitive functioning can provide key information about seizure lateralization and localization and help to identify patients who are at risk of cognitive decline following surgical treatment (Sheth, 2002). Patients with TLE often show deficits of memory, particularly if the seizures are arising from the dominant temporal lobe. Patients with dominant TLE typically display deficits in verbal memory, whereas those with epilepsy arising from the non-dominant TLE show deficits in visuospatial memory (Giovagnoli & Avanzini, 1999). In addition to memory dysfunction, patient with mesial TLE in the dominant hemisphere often demonstrate confrontation-naming problems, marked by word-finding difficulties.

8.2   The Wada Test

The intracarotid amobarbital procedure (IAP) was first reported by Wada in 1949 and was used for language lateralization. Since the early 60s the Wada test also has been used to predict postoperative amnesia, memory decline and language disability in the presurgical evaluation of TLE. This test uses the functional inactivation of a single hemisphere by injection of sodium amobarbital into the ipsilateral internal carotid artery. During this temporary deficit, the language and memory abilities of the active contralateral hemisphere can be assessed in isolation. Both hemispheres are tested consecutively with about 30 minutes between injections. There is a general consensus that over 90% of right-handed individuals show left hemispheric language dominance. Thus, language can often be reliably lateralized by the Wada test (Dinner & Loddenkemper, 2008).

Because of its invasiveness, IAP carries risks and therefore should be performed only in selected patients. The IAP is still valid in evaluating epilepsy surgery candidates with atypical or bilateral language representation and when functional MRI (fMRI) is inconclusive regarding language lateralization. When EEG or neuropsychological testing provides evidence of significant bitemporal dysfunction, the IAP can provide information regarding the risk for postoperative amnesia (Sharan et al., 2011).

8.3   fMRI

Changes in brain blood flow are accompanied by changes in blood oxygenation, which can be detected with fMRI through the so-called blood oxygenation-level-dependent (BOLD) response. If blood flow changes can be deliberately manipulated by controlling a subject's activity, the brain regions responsible for that activity may be detected (Richardson, 2010). fMRI using BOLD techniques is increasingly used in patients with TLE, mainly in the presurgical evaluation, to determine the hemispheric dominance for language. Numerous studies have demonstrated a very good correlation between fMRI and the Wada test (Sabbah et al., 2003, Rabin et al., 2004). The fMRI has several advantages over Wada test, which include being a non-invasive risk-free technique, lower cost, repeatability, and generating continuous measure of language lateralization. The main limitations of the fMRI are the presence of artifacts mainly generated by movement and patients' high cooperation demand in order to perform the tasks (Alvarez-Linera Prado, 2007).

Expressive language function is assessed with verbal fluency and verb generation tests, while receptive language function is tested with a reading comprehension task. The symmetry of activation can be calculated, allowing hemispheric language dominance to be estimated as a continuous variable. Considerable heterogeneity exists with regard to the degree of language reorganization in patients with epilepsy. This heterogeneity is related to the underlying pathology, and must be taken into account when planning surgical treatment adjacent to language areas (Duncan, 2010).

9   Treatment

9.1   Antiepileptic Drugs and Education

Antiepileptic drugs (AEDs) provide satisfactory control of seizures in most patients with epilepsy. About 60% of patients with TLE respond to AEDs, and 40% have DRE epilepsy (Kwan & Sander, 2004). If two or three drug regimens have not brought seizure control, the diagnosis of TLE should be reevaluated, and if DRE epilepsy is confirmed, surgical or palliative options should be considered (Elger & Schmidt, 2008). To improve patient care and facilitate clinical research, the ILAE appointed a Task Force to formulate a consensus definition of DRE. This definition outlines DRE as failure of adequate trials of two tolerated and appropriately chosen and used AED schedules (whether as monotherapies or in combination) to achieve sustained seizure freedom (Kwan *et al.*, 2010).

The choice of the AED needs to be individualized taking into account the patient profile, tolerability, safety, ease of use, pharmacokinetics, including the current or likely future need for concomitant medication for comorbidity, and cost (Elger & Schmidt, 2008). The drug is started at the lowest effective dose. If seizures continue, the daily dose is increased by small increments to the average effective dose (Elger & Schmidt, 2008). When single-drug therapy is not able to control seizures, adding a second drug and substitution monotherapy are common options. When the initially prescribed AED fails to produce seizure freedom, transfer to monotherapy with an alternative agent (substitution) will lead to seizure control in as many as 15–30% of cases (Schmidt & Gram, 1995; Kwan & Brodie, 2001).

The new AEDs are generally similar in efficacy; none of the modern AEDs evaluated in the SANAD trials was more efficacious than carbamazepine or valproate in their respective comparison groups (Marson *et al.*, 2007). Carbamazepine leads to complete seizure control in about 50% of patients; subsequent regimens with combination or substitution achieve control in up to 10-15% (Marson *et al.*, 2007). In general, treatment with modern AEDs results in fewer adverse drug interactions and in fewer hypersensitivity reactions (Elger & Schmidt, 2008). Recently, Bolin & Forsgren evaluated the cost-effectiveness of newer AEDs as treatment for partial-onset seizures. Bolin concluded that some newer AEDs are cost effective and when used as adjunctive treatment they generate significant clinical effects (Bolin & Forsgren 2012). Although reviewed studies report the cost effectiveness of several new (second-generation) AEDs, the cost effectiveness for most drug-setting combinations is unknown.

Non-pharmacological measures play an important supporting role in treating patients with TLE. There is a broad and extensive literature documenting the psychiatric, behavioral, and psychosocial comorbidities of epilepsy. However, research evaluating formal psychosocial interventions to ameliorate these comorbidities is rare. Mittan described a tremendous lack of psychosocial support programs in epilepsy centers; low participation by patients was an unexpected barrier (Mittan, 2009). Undoubtedly, epilepsy targeted psychosocial treatments need to be integrated into the treatment flow of specialty clinics. Specific therapies such as cognitive behavioral therapy have demonstrated to be useful patients with epilepsy and comorbid depression and anxiety symptoms. A pilot study results demonstrated improvements in depression, anxiety, negative automatic thoughts, and cognitive therapy knowledge and skills (Macrodimitris *et al.*, 2011b).

In general, patients with TLE need to know that continued treatment with AEDs is necessary. Family members must be taught a commonsense attitude toward the patient. Overprotection should be replaced with sympathetic support in order to reduce feelings of inferiority and self-consciousness and other emotional handicaps. Exercise is recommended; even such sports as swimming and horseback riding can be permitted when seizures are controlled. A normal life with social activities should be encouraged including challenges that healthy persons face. A seizure provoking life style should be avoided; in particular excessive alcohol intake and sleep deprivation. Cocaine and several other illicit drugs can trigger seizures (Elger & Schmidt, 2008). DRE is associated with significant risks for death, physical injury, cognitive impairment, and psychosocial problems. Early referral for epilepsy surgery is advisable in selected cases.

9.2   Surgical Treatment

Forty percent of patients with partial epilepsy will eventually become refractory to medical treatment and could be potential candidates for epilepsy surgery (Kwan & Sander, 2004). In this population successful surgery improves quality of life and reduces health care costs by minimizing hospitalization and use of AEDs (Unnwongse et al., 2010). Predictors of DRE are high frequency of seizures, presence of a structural lesion, neurological abnormalities, duration of epilepsy, early onset, previous history if FS, previous occurrence of status epilepticus and multifocal EEG findings (Spencer, 2002a). Mesial TLE is one of the most intractable partial epilepsies achieving seizure control with medical therapy in only 25-40% of patients (Spencer, 2002a).

The safety and efficacy of surgery for TLE was well established in a randomized clinical trial by Wiebe (Wiebe et al., 2001). In this study, patients with TLE were randomized to receive medical treatment versus surgical treatment. At the end of the first year of follow-up 58% of patients in the surgical group were seizure-free compared with only 8% of those receiving medical treatment ($P < 0.0001$). Recently Engel (Engel et al., 2012) conducted a multicenter randomized controlled trial in patients with mesial TLE, comparing a group of patients who underwent early surgery for epilepsy with another group who only used AEDs, with a minimum follow-up of two years. Seizure freedom was established as the primary outcome. Quality of life, cognitive function and social adaptability were the secondary outcomes. The calculated sample was 200 patients, but only 38 were included. The authors conclude that surgical intervention group has more probability of being seizure free at two years follow-up compared with the control group (Engel et al., 2012). The recruitment failure was due to patients with TLE not accepting to be operated in the early stages. This finding indicates that patients require a certain number of years with intractable epilepsy and a significant impairment in their quality of life to feel the need to be operated.

The most common epilepsy surgery procedure is temporal lobe resection. Hader (Hader et al., 2013) published a systematic review about epilepsy surgery complications. They found that the majority of postsurgical complications are trivial or temporary, and tend to resolve completely. Minor medical complications are reported in 5.1% of patients, whereas major medical complications occur in 1.5% of cases. The most common minor medical complication is CSF leak noted in 8.5% of patients followed by aseptic meningitis 3.6%, bacterial infection 3.0%, and intracranial hematomas 2.5%. Minor neurologic complications occur in 10.9% of patients, whereas major complications are identified in 4.7% of patients. Minor neurologic complications are twice as frequent in children. Major neurologic complications are also more common in children and they are usually seen after extratemporal resections. The most common neurologic complication after resective epilepsy surgery is a minor visual field deficit (one quadrant or less) seen in 12.9% of patients, and the majority of cases are asymptomatic (Hader et al., 2013).

Other studies have shown that despite effectiveness and safety of TLE surgery, it carries risks to memory and naming functions. The evidence shows that after left temporal lobectomy, 44% of patients exhibit verbal memory decline, and 34% show naming difficulties (Sherman et al., 2011). Underlying mood and psychiatric disorders may also worsen in up to 18% of patients (Macrodimitris et al., 2011a).

The procedures more frequently practiced are standard anterior temporal resection and amygdalohippocampectomy. Several studies report similar success rate with both techniques achieving seizure freedom between 60 and 70% (Lutz et al., 2004). It is believed that memory is better preserved in patients who undergo amygdalohippocampectomy compared with patients who receive anterior temporal resection (Wieser & Hane, 2003; Wieser et al., 2003; Lutz et al., 2004), however no randomized study exists to corroborate the information.

Téllez-Zenteno *et al* performed a systematic review evaluating long-term outcomes in epilepsy surgery. On average, 14% of the patients with temporal lobe surgery achieved long-term AED discontinuation, 50% achieved monotherapy, and 33% remained on polytherapy. Long-term seizure freedom was consistently lower after extratemporal surgery and palliative procedures. Children achieved better AED outcomes than adults. Seizure freedom after surgery was associated with lower mortality. Intelligence was unchanged by surgery. Additionally, successful epilepsy surgery can halt or improve the cognitive decline seen in chronic epilepsy, and that left temporal resections have a higher risk of additional postoperative verbal memory impairment (Téllez-Zenteno *et al.*, 2007).

9.3   Vagal Nerve Stimulation

Vagal nerve stimulation (VNS) is a procedure that has been used in recent years (Cramer *et al.*, 2001). The device produces intermittent electrical current to the cervical vagus nerve; it desynchronizes the cerebral cortical activity, thereby attenuating seizure frequency (Connor *et al.*, 2012). When patients feel an aura, they can activate the stimulator and likely stop the seizure by swiping a magnet over the device (Cramer *et al.*, 2001). VNS has been shown to reduce the frequency and intensity of seizures, but it has failed to produce any visible electroencephalographic changes (Hammond *et al.*, 1992).

The stimulator is implanted around the left vagus nerve. The left side is chosen, as the stimulation of the right vagus nerve is more likely to cause bradycardia (Bingmann, 2008). Sometimes Left VNS implantation can be hindered because of the presence of acute side effects associated with its placement (wound infection, left vocal cord palsy, lower facial palsy, bradycardia or asystole), or intraoperative complications (severe bleeding during cervicotomy). Right side VNS placement may be considered in these cases. Navas et al described two patients with intractable epilepsy who underwent a Right VNS procedure due to complicated or failed previous Left VNS. In both patients, Right VNS therapy successfully reduced seizure activity without causing cardiac side effects. It seems that Right VNS placement is an optional therapy for children and adults with refractory epilepsy who are not candidates for Left VNS implantation. However, close follow-up and frequent electrocardiographic monitoring is required to detect the presence of cardiac side effects (Navas *et al.*, 2010).

In 1997, The US Food and Drug Administration approved VNS as an adjunctive therapy in the reduction of seizures in adults and in adolescents older than 12 years with partial onset seizures, who are refractory to antiepileptic medications, and are not candidates for potentially curative surgical resections, such as lesionectomies or mesial temporal lobectomies (Fisher & Handforth, 1999). Since 1997, VNS has been an alternative treatment for intractable epilepsy worldwide (Burakgazi *et al.*, 2011). Recently, a controlled clinical trial has reported a 50% seizure control rate in about 30% of patients (The Vagus Nerve Stimulation Study Group, 1995). However, VNS efficacy seems to vary among teams and the type of patients. For example, according to Burakgazi (Burakgazi *et al.*, 2011) VNS is more effective in treatment of partial seizures originating from frontal lobe with 65% satisfactory response rather than in temporal lobe seizure with 15% satisfactory response.

Common adverse effects include coughing, hoarseness of voice, dyspnea, and headache. These effects are seen during stimulation and tend to habituate with time. Serious adverse effects have been reported and include vocal cord paralysis, infection, Horner's syndrome, lower facial muscles paresis, and cardiac arrest (Bingmann, 2008).

García-Navarrete et al. performed a prospective study to assess the long-term outcome of VNS treatment in adults with DRE (García-Navarrete *et al.*, 2013). They published 18-months follow-up data from a sample of patients treated with VNS and stable AEDs, they found that 62.8% of their series of

43 medication-resistant epileptic patients experienced a significant (similar or greater than 50% reduction in their seizure frequency) long-term seizure reduction after VNS, even in a situation of an unchanged medical therapy, concluding that VNS is an effective therapy in the long-term control of medication-resistant seizures (García-Navarrete *et al.*, 2012). This finding is completely in line with the great number of reports on VNS from the last 15 years. Hoppe (Hoppe, 2013) commented in an editorial that the recommendation of VNS in patients with DRE is currently not supported by appropriate evidence, inquiring that the studies on therapeutic superiority are still missing and the clinical effectiveness of add-on VNS over best drug therapy has not been shown so far (Hoppe, 2013).

9.4   Electrical Brain Stimulation

Virtually all open-label electrical stimulation studies in epilepsy report beneficial effects, regardless of the stimulation target (thalamus, subthalamus, neocortex, hippocampus and cerebellum). These procedures hold the promise of an intervention that is nonresective, minimally invasive, dose adjustable, largely reversible, and presumably safe (Téllez-Zenteno & Wiebe, 2011).

The anterior thalamus is known to play a role in seizure propagation. Thalamic deep brain stimulation is a novel treatment for patients with generalized seizures, who are not typically candidates for resective surgery. Recently, a multicenter randomized blinded study explored the effect of electrical brain stimulation of the anterior nuclei of the thalamus for localization-related epilepsy. Half of 110 patients were randomized to receive stimulation and the other half received no stimulation during a three month blinded phase, followed by unblinded stimulation for all patients in the study. The mean seizure frequency decreased by 14.5% in the control group as opposed to 40% in the stimulation group during the first three months (blinded phase) of the study. By two years, 54% of patients had a seizure reduction of at least 50%, and 14 patients were seizure free for at least six months (Fisher *et al.*, 2010).

The available evidence for Hippocampal stimulation (HS) is weak. The limited evidence suggests that the effects of HS appear to be cumulative and accrue with time, and the procedure seems to be safe. Neither the optimum target (amygdala, hippocampus, pes hippocampus, parahippocampal gyrus) nor the optimum stimulation parameters are known. However the reversibility of HS, supported partly by histopathological integrity of the stimulated tissue and lack of overt clinical or EEG changes on short-term studies, is also alluring. However, almost nothing is known about the late or long-lasting effects of electrical stimulation on synaptic physiology, connectivity, function, and epileptogenicity. Therefore, the HS may be considered for patients with contraindications for a resective procedure due to risks to memory and naming functions or because of bitemporal epilepsy. In addition, it could be an option for patients with a strong preference for a nonresective, minimally invasive procedure (Téllez-Zenteno & Wiebe, 2011).

9.4.1   Trigeminal Nerve Stimulation

Trigeminal nerve stimulation (TNS) is an emerging neuromodulation therapy with unique advantages: it can be delivered externally or subcutaneously, bilaterally, and at low cost. Initial experiments showed that TNS was effective at reducing pentylenetetrazole-induced seizures in awake-animals. Additionally, these studies showed that bilateral trigeminal stimulation was more effective than unilateral stimulation, and that TNS was effective when delivered in a closed-loop, seizure-triggered paradigm (DeGiorgio *et al.*, 2011). The safety and preliminary efficacy of TNS for epilepsy was evaluated in a pilot feasibility study of transcutaneous stimulation of the infraorbital and supraorbital branches of the trigeminal nerve. Four (57%) of seven subjects who completed three months or more experienced a more than 50% reduction in seizure frequency (DeGiorgio *et al.*, 2006). On the other hand, external TNS of the supraorbital or infraorbital nerve is safe and well tolerated. No adverse hemodynamic effects have been observed (Pop *et al.*, 2011). Results from early studies provide important data on effectiveness and safety. Future studies will be required to demonstrate the real efficacy of this therapy.

9.5   Radiosurgical Treatment

Radiosurgery is the precise application of focused radiation to a targeted volume area within the brain identified on MRI. Radiosurgery allows the neurosurgeon to deliver precise and accurate radiation to a smaller volume without effecting large portions of normal parenchyma allowing for a powerful radiobiologic effect on the chosen targeted volume (Nguyen & Spencer, 2003).

TLE is particularly amenable to radiosurgery because 80–90% of these cases show changes on MRI (Dillon & Barbaro, 1999). A prospective multicenter European study evaluating Gamma Knife(R) surgery for MTS showed comparable efficacy rates (65%) for seizure reduction by conventional surgery or radiosurgery, after two years of follow up (Régis *et al.*, 2004). Although radiosurgery has proven effective and safe in ameliorating MTS associated seizures, the beneficial effects of radiosurgery are not displayed immediately. Most patients achieve seizure reduction at 9–12 months and complete cessation of seizures between 18–24 months after radiosurgical treatment (Yang & Barbaro, 2008). This procedure is an attractive option for TLE treatment because of its low morbidity and mortality, however prospective trials with larger numbers of patients will be required to establish radiosurgery as a standard therapy for mesial TLE.

9.6   Future Directions in the Management of TLE

Epilepsy is a disorder characterized by a diffuse brain dysfunction, not just a disorder that produces seizures. After some years of investigation finally we understand that there is a strong relationship between TLE and other comorbidities such as cognitive, behavioral, and psychiatric disorders (Linehan *et al.*, 2011). This complex scenery will determine future directions in the management of patients. In the last years, there have had technological outbreaks in electrophysiological techniques, neuroimaging, and genetic testing. Integrated approaches, such as imaging and electrophysiology will be central to progress in predicting epileptogenic zone in people with epilepsy (Jacobs *et al.*, 2001). At the same time, the range of available pharmacological and non-pharmacological treatments, including use of surgery, has greatly expanded.

Research directions for the future include determination of mechanisms of epilepsy development, identification of genes for common epilepsy syndromes through linkage analysis and gene chip technology, and validation of new models of epilepsy and epileptogenesis. Directions for therapeutics include identification of new molecular targets, focal methods of drug delivery tied to EEG activity, gene and cell therapy, and surgical and non-ablative therapies (Jacobs *et al.*, 2001). The evaluation of patients with refractory epilepsy should use studies that better characterize the epilepsy network (specifically PET, functional MRI) in addition to studies that are aimed to localize the "seizure onset" like EEG (Spencer, 2002b).

Acknowledgement

Dr. Téllez-Zenteno receives grants from the University of Saskatchewan, UCB Canada and the Royal University Hospital Foundation in Saskatoon, Saskatchewan, through the Mudjadik Thyssen Mining Professorship in Neurosciences.

References

A randomized controlled trial of chronic vagus nerve stimulation for treatment of medically intractable seizures. The Vagus Nerve Simulation Study Group. (1995). Neurology, 45(2), 224–30.

Acharya, V., Acharya, J., & Lüders, H. (1998). Olfactory epileptic auras. Neurology, 51(1), 56–61.

Alarcón, G., Muthinji, P., Kissani, N., Polkey, C.E., & Valentín, A. (2012). Value of scalp delayed rhythmic ictal transformation (DRIT) in presurgical assessment of temporal lobe epilepsy. Clin Neurophysiol, 123(7), 1269–1274.

Alvarez-Linera Prado, J. (2007). 3-Tesla MRI and temporal lobe epilepsy. Semin Ultrasound CT MRI, 28(6), 451–461.

Arya, R., Mangano, F.T., Horn, P.S., Holland, K.D., Rose, D.F., & Glauser, T.A. (2013). Adverse events related to extraoperative invasive EEG monitoring with subdural grid electrodes: A systematic review and meta-analysis. Epilepsia, 54(5), 828–839.

Atalla, N., Abou-Khalil, B., & Fakhoury, T. (1996). The star-stop-star phenomenon in scalp-sphenoidal recordings. Electroencephalogr Clin Neurophysiol, 98(1), 9–13.

Bautista, J.F., Foldvary-Schaefer, N., Bingaman, W.E., & Lüders, H.O. (2003). Focal cortical dysplasia and intractable epilepsy in adults: Clinical, EEG, imaging, and surgical features. Epilepsy Res, 55(1-2), 131–136.

Bercovici, E., Kumar, B.S., & Mirsattari, S.M. (2012). Neocortical temporal lobe epilepsy. Epilepsy Res Treat, 103160, 1–15.

Bingmann, W.E. (2008). Vagal nerve stimulation: surgical technique and complications. In H.O. Lüders (Ed.), Textbook of epilepsy surgery (pp. 1184-1187). London, UK: Informa Healthcare.

Binnie, C.D., Rowan, A.J., Overweg, J., Meinardi, H., Wisman, T., Kamp, A., & Lopes da Silva, F. (1981). Telemetric EEG and video monitoring in epilepsy. Neurology, 31(3), 298–303.

Blair, R.D. (2012). Temporal lobe epilepsy semiology. Epilepsy Res Treat, 751510, 1–10.

Blume, W.T. (2003). The necessity for sphenoidal electrodes in the presurgical evaluation of temporal lobe epilepsy: con position. J Clin Neurophysiol, 20(5), 305–310.

Blume, W., Borghesi, J.L., & Lemieux, J.F. (1993) Interictal indices of temporal seizure origin. Ann Neurol, 34(5), 703–709.

Blume, W.T & Kaibara, M. (1993). The start-stop-start phenomenon recorded seizures of subdurally. Electroencephalogr Clin Neurophysiol, 86(2), 94–99.

Blümcke, I. (2008). Neuropathology of mesial temporal sclerosis. In H.O. Lüders (Ed.), Textbook of epilepsy surgery (pp. 1331–1337). London, UK: Informa Healthcare.

Bolin, K., & Forsgren, L. (2012). The cost effectiveness of newer epilepsy treatments: a review of the literature on partial-onset seizures. Pharmacoeconomics, 30(10), 903–923.

Britton, J.W., Ghearing, G.R., Benarroch, E.E., & Cascino, G.D. (2006). The ictal bradycardia syndrome: localization and lateralization. Epilepsia, 47(4), 737–744.

Burakgazi, A.Z., Burakgazi-Dalkilic, E., Caputy, A.J., & Potolicchio, S.J. (2011). The correlation between vagus nerve stimulation efficacy and partial onset epilepsies. J Clin Neurophysiol, 28(4), 380–383.

Cardinale, F., Cossu, M., Castana, L., Casaceli, G., Schiariti, M.P., Miserocchi, A., (...), & Lo Russo, G. (2012). Stereoelectroencephalography: surgical methodology, safety and stereotactic application accuracy in five hundred procedures. Neurosurgery, 72(3), 353–366.

Carne, R.P., O'Brien, T.J., Kilpatrick, C.J., Macgregor, L.R., Litewka, L., Hicks, R.J., & Cook, M.J. (2007). MRI-negative PET-positive temporal lobe epilepsy (TLE) and mesial TLE differ with quantitative MRI and PET: a case control study. BMC Neurol, 24(7), 16.

Cendes, F. (2004). Febrile seizures and mesial temporal sclerosis. Curr Opin Neurol, 17(2), 161–164.

Cendes, F. (2005). Mesial temporal lobe epilepsy syndrome: an updated overview. J Epilepsy Clin Neurophysiol, 11(3), 141–144.

Cendes, F., Cook, M.J., Watson, C., Andermann, F., Fish, D.R., Shorvon, S.D., (...), & Arnold, D.L. (1995). Frequency and characteristics of dual pathology in patients with lesional epilepsy. Neurology, 45(11), 2058–2064.

Chee, M.W., Morris, H.H. 3rd., Antar, M.A., Van Ness, P.C., Dinner, D.S., Rehm, P., & Salanova, V. (1993). Presurgical evaluation of temporal lobe epilepsy using interictal temporal spikes and positron emission tomography. Arch Neurol, 50(1), 45–48.

Chen, C., Shih, Y.H., Yen, D.J., Lirng, J.F., Guo, Y.C., Yu, H.Y., & Yiu, C.H. (2003). Olfactory auras in patients with temporal lobe epilepsy. Epilepsia, 44(2), 257–260.

Chen, L.S., Mitchell, W.G., Horton, E.J., & Snead, O.C. 3rd. (1995). Clinical utility of video-EEG monitoring. Pediatr Neurol, 12(3), 220–224.

Connor, D.E. Jr., Nixon, M., Nanda, A, & Guthikonda, B. (2012). Vagal nerve stimulation for the treatment of medically refractory epilepsy: a review of the current literature. Neurosurg Focus, 32(3), E12.

Cramer, J.A., Ben Menachem, E., & French, J. (2001). Review of treatment options for refractory epilepsy: new medications and vagal nerve stimulation. Epilepsy Res, 47(1-2), 17–25.

DeGiorgio, C.M., Fanselow, E.E., Schrader, L.M., & Cook, I.A. (2011). Trigeminal nerve stimulation: seminal animal and human studies for epilepsy and depression. Neurosurg Clin N Am, 22(4), 449–456.

DeGiorgio, C.M., Shewmon, A., Murray, D., & Whitehurst, T. (2006). Pilot study of trigeminal nerve stimulation (TNS) for epilepsy: a proof-of-concept trial. Epilepsia, 47(7), 1213–1215.

Dillon, W.P. & Barbaro, N. (1999). Noninvasive surgery for epilepsy: the era of image guidance. AJNR Am J Neuroradiol, 20(2), 185.

Dinner, D.S. & Loddenkemper, T. (2008). Wada test and epileptogenic zone. In H.O. Lüders (Ed.), Textbook of epilepsy surgery (pp. 844–857). London, UK: Informa Healthcare.

Dubeau, F. & McLachlan, R.S. (2000). Invasive electrographic recording techniques in temporal lobe epilepsy. Can J Neurol Sci, 27(1), 29–34.

Duncan, J.S. (2010). Imaging in the surgical treatment of epilepsy. Nat Rev Neurol, 6(10), 537–550.

Dupont, S., Semah, F., Boon, P., Saint-Hilaire, J.M., Adam, C., Broglin, D., & Baulac, M. (1999). Association of ipsilateral motor automatisms and contralateral dystonic posturing: a clinical feature differentiating medial from neocortical temporal lobe epilepsy. Arch Neurol, 56(8), 927–932.

Ebersole, J.S., & Pacia, S.V. (1996). Localization of temporal lobe foci by ictal EEG patterns. Epilepsia, 37(4), 386–399.

Ebner, A. (1994). Lateral (neocortical) temporal lobe epilepsy. In: P. Wolf (Ed.), Epileptic seizures and syndromes (pp. 375–382). London: John Libbey.

Ebner, A., Dinner, D.S., Noachtar, S., & Lüders, H. (1995). Automatisms with preserved responsiveness: a lateralizing sign in psychomotor seizures. Neurology, 45(1), 61–64.

Eisenschenk, S., Gilmore, R.L., Cibula, J.E., & Roper, S.N. (2001). Lateralization of temporal lobe foci: depth versus subdural electrodes. Clin Neurophysiol, 112(5), 836–844.

Elger, C.E., & Schmidt, D. (2008). *Modern management of epilepsy: a practical approach. Epilepsy Behav, 12(4), 501–539.*

Elliott, B., Joyce, E., & Shorvon, S. (2009a). *Delusions, illusions and hallucinations in epilepsy: 1. Elementary phenomena. Epilepsy Res, 85(2-3), 162–171.*

Elliott, B., Joyce, E., & Shorvon, S. (2009b). *Delusions, illusions and hallucinations in epilepsy: 2. Complex phenomena and psychosis. Epilepsy Res, 85(2-3), 172–186.*

Engel, J. Jr. (1993). *Update on surgical treatment of the epilepsies. Summary of the Second International Palm Desert Conference on the surgical treatment of the epilepsies (1992). Neurology, 43(8), 1612–1617.*

Engel, J. Jr., McDermott, M.P., Wiebe, S., Langfitt, J.T., Stern, J.M., Dewar, S., (...), Kieburtz, K. (2012). *Early surgical therapy for drug-resistant temporal lobe epilepsy a randomized trial. JAMA, 307(9), 922–930.*

Ergene, E., Shih, J.J., Blum, D.E., & So, N.K. (2000). *Frequency of bitemporal independent interictal epileptiform discharges in temporal lobe epilepsy. Epilepsia, 41(2), 213–218.*

Ferroli, P., Casazza, M., Marras, C., Mendola, C., Franzini, A., & Broggi, G. (2006). *Cerebral cavernomas and seizures: A retrospective study on 163 patients who underwent pure lesionectomy. Neurol Sci, 26(6), 390–394.*

Fisher, R.S. & Handforth, A. (1999). *Reassessment: vagus nerve stimulation for epilepsy: a report of the therapeutics and technology assessment subcommittee of the American Academy of Neurology. Neurology, 53(4), 666–669.*

Fisher, R., Salanova, V., Witt, T., Worth, R., Henry, T. Gross, R., (...), & Graves, N. (2010). *Electrical stimulation of the anterior nucleus of thalamus for treatment of refractory epilepsy. Epilepsia, 51(5), 899–908.*

Foldvary, N., Klem, G., Hammel, J., Bingaman, W., Najm, I., & Lüders, H. (2001). *The localizing value of ictal EEG in focal epilepsy. Neurology, 57(11), 2022–2028.*

Foldvary-Schaefer, N. & Unnwongse, K. (2011). *Localizing and lateralizing features of auras and seizures. Epilepsy Behav, 20(2), 160–166.*

French, J.A., Williamson, P.D., Thadani, V.M., Darcey, T.M., Mattson, R.H., Spencer, S.S., & Spencer, D.D. (1993). *Characteristics of medial temporal lobe epilepsy: I. Results of history and physical examination. Ann Neurol, 34(6), 774–780.*

Gabr, M., Lüders, H., Dinner, D., Morris, H., & Wyllie, E. (1989). *Speech manifestations in lateralization of temporal lobe seizures. Ann Neurol, 25(1), 82–87.*

García-Navarrete, E., Torres, C.V., Gallego, I., Navas, M., Pastor, J., & Sola, R.G. (2012) *Long-term results of vagal nerve stimulation for adults with medication-resistant epilepsy, on unchanged antiepileptic medication. Seizure, 22(1), 9–13.*

García-Navarrete, E., Torres, C.V., Gallego, I., Navas, M., Pastor, J., & Sola, R.G. (2013). *Response to "Vagus nerve stimulation: Urgent need for the critical reappraisal of clinical effectiveness". Seizure, 22(6), 490–491.*

Geiger, L.R., & Harner, R.N. (1978). *EEG patterns at the time of focal seizure onset. Arch Neurol, 35(5), 276–286.*

Geyer, J.D., Bilir, E., Faught, R.E., Kuzniecky, R., & Gilliam, F. (1999). *Significance of interictal temporal lobe delta activity for localization of the primary epileptogenic region. Neurology, 52(1), 202–205.*

Gil-Nagel, A. & Risinger, M.W. (1997). *Ictal semiology in hippocampal versus extrahipocampal temporal lobe epilepsy. Brain, 120(1), 183–192.*

Giovagnoli, A.R. & Avanzini, G. (1999). *Learning and memory impairment in patients with temporal lobe epilepsy: relation to the presence, type, and location of brain lesion. Epilepsia, 40(7), 904–911.*

Gonzalez-Martinez, J., Bulacio, J., Alexopoulos, A., Jehi, L., Bingaman, W., & Najm, I. (2012). *Stereoelectroencephalography in the "difficult to localize" refractory focal epilepsy: early experience from a North American epilepsy center. Epilepsia, 54(2), 323–330.*

Hader, W.J., Téllez-Zenteno, J., Metcalfe, A., Hernández-Ronquillo, L., Wiebe, S., Churl-So, K., & Jette, N. (2013). *Complications of epilepsy surgery a systematic review of focal surgical resections and invasive EEG monitoring. Epilep-*

sia, 54(5), 840–847.

Hamaneh, M.B., Limotai, C., & Lüders, H.O. (2011). Sphenoidal electrodes significantly change the results of source localization of interictal spikes for a large percentage of patients with temporal lobe epilepsy. J Clin Neurophysiol, 28(4), 373–379.

Hammond, E.J., Uthman, B.M., Reid, S.A., & Wilder, B.J. (1992). Electrophysiological studies of cervical vagus nerve stimulation in humans: I. EEG effects. Epilepsia, 33(6), 1013–1020.

Hauser, W.A. & Kurland, L.T. (1975). The epidemiology of epilepsy in Rochester, Minnesota, 1935 through 1967. Epilepsia, 16(1), 1–66.

Holmes, M.D., Dodrill, C.B., Wilensky, A.J., Ojemann, L.M., & Ojemann, G.A. (1996). Unilateral focal preponderance of interictal epileptiform discharges as a predictor of seizure origin. Arch Neurol, 53(3), 228–232.

Hoppe, C. (2013). Vagus nerve stimulation: urgent need for the critical reappraisal of clinical effectiveness. Seizure, 22(1), 83–84.

Jacobs, M.P., Fischbach, G.D., Davis, M.R., Dichter, M.A., Dingledine, R,. Lowenstein, D.H., (...), & Theodore, W.H. (2001). Future directions for epilepsy research. Neurology, 57(1),1536–1542.

Jan, M.M. & Girvin, J.P. (2008). Seizure semiology: value in identifying seizure origin. Can J Neurol Sci, 35(1), 22–30.

Jan, M.M., Sadler, M., & Rahey, S.R. (2010). Electroencephalographic features of temporal lobe epilepsy. Can J Neurol Sci, 37(4), 439–448.

Janszky, J., Fogarasi, A., Jokeit, H., & Ebner, A. (2000). Are ictal vocalisations related to the lateralisation of frontal lobe epilepsy? J Neurol Neurosurg Psychiatry, 69(2), 244–247.

Janszky, J., Schulz, R., & Ebner, A. (2004). Simple partial seizures (isolated auras) in medial temporal lobe epilepsy. Seizure, 13(4), 247–249.

Javidan, M. (2012). Electroencephalography in mesial temporal lobe epilepsy: a review. Epilepsy Res Treat, 637430, 1–17.

Kissani, N., Alarcon, G., Dad, M., Binnie, C.D., & Polkey, C.E. (2001). Sensitivity of recordings at sphenoidal electrode site for detecting seizure onset: evidence from scalp, superficial and deep foramen ovale recordings. Clin Neurophysiol, 112(2), 232–240.

Krauss, G.L., Lesser, R.P., Fisher, R.S., & Arroyo, S. (1992). Anterior "cheek" electrodes are comparable to sphenoidal electrodes for the identification of ictal activity. Electroencephalogr Clin Neurophysiol, 83(6), 333–338.

Kwan, P. & Brodie, M.J. (2001). Effectiveness of first antiepileptic drug. Epilepsia, 42(10), 1255–1260.

Kwan, P. & Sander, J.W. (2004). The natural history of epilepsy: an epidemiological view. J Neurol Neurosurg Psychiatry, 75(10), 1376–1381.

Kwan, P., Arzimanoglou, A., Berg, A.T., Brodie, M.J., Hauser, W.A., Mathern, G., (...), & French, J. (2010). Definition of drug resistant epilepsy: consensus proposal by the ad hoc Task Force of the ILAE Commission on Therapeutic Strategies. Epilepsia, 51(6), 1069–1077.

Kennedy, J.D. & Schuele, S.U. (2012). Neocortical temporal lobe epilepsy. J Clin Neurophysiol, 29(5), 366–370.

Kotagal, P. (1991). Seizure symptomatology of temporal lobe epilepsy. In: H.O. Lüders (Ed.), Epilepsy surgery (pp. 143–156). New York: Raven Press.

Koutroumanidis, M., Martin-Miguel, C., Hennessy, M.J., Akanuma, N., Valentin, A., Alarcón, G., (...), & Polkey, C. (2004). Interictal temporal delta activity in temporal lobe epilepsy: correlations with pathology and outcome. Epilepsia, 45(11), 11351–11367.

La Fougère, C., Rominger, A., Förster, S., Geisler, J., & Bartenstein, P. (2009). PET and SPECT in epilepsy: a critical review. Epilepsy Behav, 15(1), 50–55.

Lee, J.Y., Joo, E.Y., Park, H.S., Song, P., Young-Byun, S., Seo, D.W., & Hong, S.B. (2011). Repeated ictal SPECT in partial epilepsy patients: SISCOM analysis. Epilepsia, 52(12), 2249–2256.

Leutmezer, F., Serles, W., Lehrner, J., Pataraia, E., Zeiler, K., & Baumgartner, C. (1998). Postictal nose wiping: a lateralizing sign in temporal lobe complex partial seizures. Neurology, 51, 1175–1177.

Linehan, C., Téllez-Zenteno, J.F., Burneo, J.G., & Berg, A.T. (2011). Future directions for epidemiology in epilepsy. Epilep Behav, 22(1), 112–117.

Loddenkemper, T. & Kotagal, P. (2005). Lateralizing signs during seizures in focal epilepsy. Epilepsy Behav, 7(1), 1–17.

Lutz, M.T., Clusmann, H., Elger, C.E., Schramm, J., & Helmstaedter, C. (2004). Neuropsychological outcome after selective amygdalohippocampectomy with transsylvian versus transcortical approach: a randomized prospective clinical trial of surgery for temporal lobe epilepsy. Epilepsia, 45(7), 809–816.

Macrodimitris, S., Sherman, E.M., Forde, S., Téllez-Zenteno, J.F., Metcalfe, A., Hernández-Ronquillo, L., (...), & Jetté N. (2011a). Psychiatric outcomes of epilepsy surgery: a systematic review. Epilepsia, 52(5), 880–890.

Macrodimitris, S., Wershler, J., Hatfield, M., Hamilton, K., Backs-Dermott, B., Mothersill, K.,(...), & Wiebe, S. (2011b). Group cognitive-behavioral therapy for patients with epilepsy and comorbid depression and anxiety. Epilepsy Behav, 20(1), 83–88.

Maillard, L., Vignal, J.P., Gavaret, M., Guye, M., Biraben, A., McGonigal, A., (...), & Bartolomei, F. (2004). Semiologic and electrophysiologic correlations in temporal lobe seizure subtypes. Epilepsia, 45(12), 1590–1599.

Manford, M., Fish, D.R., & Shorvon, S.D. (1996). An analysis of clinical seizure patterns and their localizing value in frontal and temporal lobe epilepsies. Brain, 119(1), 17–40.

Manford, M., Hart, Y.M., Sander, J.W., & Shorvon, S.D. (1992). National General Practice Study of Epilepsy (NGPSE): partial seizure patterns in a general population. Neurology, 42(10), 1911–1917.

Marson, A.G., Al-Kharusi, A.M., Alwaidh, M., Appleton, R., Baker, G.A., Chadwick, D.W., (...), & Williamson, P.R. (2007). The SANAD study of effectiveness of carbamazepine, gabapentin, lamotrigine, oxcarbazepine, or topiramate for treatment of partial epilepsy: an unblended randomised controlled trial. Lancet, 369(9566), 1000–1015.

Mittan, R.J. (2009). Psychosocial treatment programs in epilepsy: a review. Epilepsy Behav, 16(3), 371–380.

Navas, M., Navarrete EG, Pascual JM, Carrasco R, Núñez JA, Shakur SF,(...), & Sola, R.G. (2010). Treatment of refractory epilepsy in adult patients with right-sided vagus nerve stimulation. Epilepsy Res, 90(1–2), 1–7.

Newton, M.R., Berkovic, S.F., Austin, M.C., Rowe, C.C., McKay, W.J., & Bladin, P.F. (1992). Postictal switch in blood flow distribution and temporal lobe seizures. J Neurol Neurosurg Psychiatry, 55(10), 891–894.

Nguyen, D.K. & Spencer, S.S. (2003). Recent advances in the treatment of epilepsy. Arch Neurol, 60(7), 929–935.

Noachtar, S. & Peters, A.S. (2009). Semiology of epileptic seizures: A critical review. Epilepsy Behav, 15(1), 2–9.

Noachtar, S. & Rémi, J. (2009). The role of EEG in epilepsy: A critical review. Epilepsy Behav, 15(1), 22–33.

O'Brien, T.J., Kilpatrick, C., Murrie, V., Vogrin, S., Morris, K., & Cook, M.J. (1996). Temporal lobe epilepsy caused by mesial temporal sclerosis and temporal neocortical lesions: a clinical and electroencephalographic study of 46 pathologically proven cases. Brain, 119(6), 2133–2141.

Oun, A., Haldre, S., & Mägi, M. (2003). Prevalence of adult epilepsy in Estonia. Epilepsy Res, 52(3), 233–242.

Palmigiano, A., Pastor, J., García de Sola, R., Ortega, G.J. (2012). Stability of Synchronization Clusters and Seizurability in temporal lobe epilepsy. PLoS One, 7(7), e41799.

Palmini, A. & Gloor, P. (1992). The localizing value of auras in partial seizures: a prospective and retrospective study. Neurology, 42(4), 801–808.

Pondal-Sordo, M., Diosy, D., Téllez-Zenteno, J.F., Sahjpaul, R., & Wiebe, S. (2007). Usefulness of intracranial EEG in the decision process for epilepsy surgery. Epilepsy Res, 74(2-3), 176–182.

Pop, J., Murray, D., Markovic, D., & DeGiorgio, C.M. (2011). Acute and long-term safety of external trigeminal nerve stimulation for drug-resistant epilepsy. Epilepsy Behav, 22(3), 574–576.

Proposal for classification of epilepsies and epileptic syndromes. Commission on classification and terminology of the International League against Epilepsy. (1989). Epilepsia, 30(4), 389–399.

Rabin, M.L., Narayan, V.M., Kimberg, D.Y., Casasanto, D.J., Glosser, G., Tracy, J.I., (...), & Detre, J.A. (2004). Functional MRI predicts post-surgical memory following temporal lobectomy. Brain, 127(10), 2286–2298.

Régis, J., Rey, M., Bartolomei, F., Vladkya, V., Liscak, R., Schrottner, O., & Pendl, G. (2004). Gamma knife surgery in mesial temporal lobe epilepsy: a prospective multicenter study. Epilepsia, 45(5), 504–515.

Richardson, M. (2010). Update on neuroimaging in epilepsy. Expert Rev Neurother, 10(6): 961–973.

Rona, S. (2008). Auras: localizing and lateralizing value. In H.O. Lüders (Ed.), Textbook of epilepsy surgery (pp. 432-442). London, UK: Informa Healthcare.

Ryvlin, P. & Kahane, P. (2005). The hidden causes of surgery-resistant temporal lobe epilepsy: extratemporal or temporal plus? Curr Opin Neurol, 18(2), 125–127.

Sabbah, P., Chassoux, F., Leveque, C., Landre, E., Baudoin-Chial, S., Devaux, B., (...), & Cordoliani, Y.S. (2003). Functional MR imaging in assessment of language dominance in epileptic patients. Neuroimage, 18(2), 460–467.

Sadler, R.M. & Goodwin, J. (1989). Multiple electrodes for detecting spikes in partial complex seizures. Can J Neurol Sci, 16(3), 326–329.

Schmidt, D. & Gram, L. (1995). Monotherapy versus polytherapy in epilepsy. CNS Drugs, 3, 194–208.

Semah, F., Picot, M.C., Adam, C., Broglin, D., Arzimanoglou, A., Bazin, B., (...), & Baulac, M. (1998). Is the underlying cause of epilepsy a major prognostic factor for recurrence? Neurology, 51(5), 1256–1262.

Sharan, A., Ooi, Y.C., Langfitt, J., & Sperling, M.R. (2011). Intracarotid amobarbital procedure for epilepsy surgery. Epilepsy Behav, 20(2), 209–213.

Sherman, E.M., Wiebe, S., Fay-McClymont, T.B., Téllez-Zenteno, J., Metcalfe, A., Hernandez-Ronquillo, L., (...), & Jetté, N. (2011). Neuropsychological outcomes after epilepsy surgery: systematic review and pooled estimates. Epilepsia, 52(5), 857–869.

Sheth, R.D. (2002). Epilepsy surgery. Presurgical evaluation. Neurol Clin, 20(4), 1195–1215.

So, E.L. (2006). Value and limitations of seizure semiology in localizing seizure onset. J Clin Neurophysiol, 23(4), 353–357.

So, N.K. & Sperling, M.R. (2007). Ictal asystole and SUDEP. Neurology, 69(5), 423–424.

Spencer, D.D. & Spencer, S.S. (1985). Surgery for epilepsy. Neurol Clin, 3(2), 313–330.

Spencer, S.S. (1994). The relative contributions of MRI, SPECT, and PET in epilepsy. Epilepsia, 35 (S6), S72–89.

Spencer, S. (2002a). When should temporal-lobe epilepsy be treated surgically?. Lancet Neurol, 1(6), 375–382.

Spencer, S.S. (2002b). Neural networks in human epilepsy: Evidence of and implications for treatment. Epilepsia, 43(3), 219-227.

Tatum, W.O. 4th. (2012). Mesial temporal lobe epilepsy. J Clin Neurophysiol, 29(5), 356–365.

Téllez-Zenteno, J.F., Dhar, R., & Wiebe, S. (2005). Long-term seizure outcomes following epilepsy surgery: a systematic review and meta-analysis. Brain, 128(5), 1188–1198.

Téllez-Zenteno, J.F. & Hernández-Ronquillo, L. (2012). A review of the epidemiology of temporal lobe epilepsy. Epilepsy Res Treat, 630853, 1–5.

Téllez-Zenteno, J.F., Hernández-Ronquillo, L., Moien-Afshari, F., & Wiebe, S. (2010). Surgical outcomes in lesional and non-lesional epilepsy: a systematic review and meta-analysis. Epilepsy Res, 89(2–3), 310–318.

Téllez-Zenteno, J.F. & Wiebe, S. (2011). Hippocampal stimulation in the treatment of epilepsy. Neurosurg Clin N Am, 22(4), 465–475.

Téllez-Zenteno, J.F., Dhar, R., Hernandez-Ronquillo, L., & Wiebe, S. (2007). Long-term outcomes in epilepsy surgery:

antiepileptic drugs, mortality, cognitive and psychosocial aspects. Brain, 130(2), 334–345.

Thompson, S.A., Duncan, J.S., & Smith, S.J. (2000). *Partial seizures presenting as panic attacks. BMJ, 321(7267), 1002–1003.*

Tinuper, P., Bisulli, F., Cerullo, A., Carcangiu, R., Marini, C., Pierangeli, G., & Cortelli, P. (2001). *Ictal bradycardia in partial epileptic seizures: Autonomic investigation in three cases and literature review. Brain, 124(12), 2361–2371.*

Unnwongse, K., Wehner, T., & Foldvary-Schaefer, N. (2010). *Selecting patients for epilepsy surgery. Curr Neurol Neurosci Rep, 10(4), 299–307.*

Van Paesschen, W., Dupont, P., Sunaert, S., Goffin, K., & Van Laere, K. (2007). *The use of SPECT and PET in routine clinical practice in epilepsy. Curr Opin Neurol, 20(2), 194–202.*

Velasco, T.R., Sakamoto, A.C., Alexandre, V. Jr., Walz, R., Dalmagro, C.L., Bianchin, M.M., & Carlotti, C. Jr. (2006). *Foramen ovale electrodes can identify a focal seizure onset when surface EEG fails in mesial temporal lobe epilepsy. Epilepsia, 47(8), 1300–1307.*

Wehner, T. & Lüders, H. (2008). *Role of neuroimaging in the presurgical evaluation of epilepsy. J Clin Neurol, 4(1), 1–16.*

Weil, S., Arnold, S., Eisensehr, I., & Noachtar, S. (2005). *Heart rate increase in otherwise subclinical seizures is different in temporal versus extratemporal seizure onset: support for temporal lobe autonomic influence. Epileptic Disord, 7(3), 199–204.*

Weil, S., Arnold, S., & Noachtar, S. (2002). *Heart rate increase in otherwise subclinical seizures is different in temporal versus extratemporal EEG seizure pattern. Epilepsia, 43(7), 244.*

Wellmer, J., Von der Groeben, F., Klarmann, U., Weber, C., Elger, C.E., Urbach, H., (...), & Von Lehe, M. (2012). *Risks and benefits of invasive epilepsy surgery workup with implanted subdural and depth electrodes. Epilepsia, 53(8), 1322–1332.*

Wiebe, S., Blume, W.T., Girvin, J.P., & Eliasziw, M. (2001). *Effectiveness and efficiency of surgery for temporal lobe epilepsy study group. A randomized, controlled trial of surgery for temporal-lobe epilepsy. N Engl J Med, 345, 311–318.*

Wieser, H.G. (1983). *Electroclinical features of psychomotor seizure. London, UK: Butterworths.*

Wieser, H.G., & Häne, A. (2003). *Antiepileptic drug treatment before and after selective amygdalohippocampectomy. Epilepsy Res, 55(3), 211–223.*

Wieser, H.G., Ortega, M., Friedman, A., & Yonekawa, Y. (2003). *Long-term seizure outcomes following amygdalohippocampectomy. J Neurosurg, 98(4), 751–763.*

Wilkus, R.J., Thompson, P.M., & Vossler, D.G. (1991). *Quantitative comparison of ictal EEG from sphenoidal, minisphenoidal, anterior temporal, and midtemporal electrodes. Epilepsia, 32(13), 100–101.*

Williamson, P.D., French, J.A., Thadani, V.M., Kim, J.H., Novelly, R.A., Spencer, S.S., (...), & Mattson, R.H. (1993). *Characteristics of medial temporal lobe epilepsy: Interictal and ictal scalp electroencephalography, neuropsychological testing, neuroimaging, surgical results, and pathology. Ann Neurol, 34(6), 781–787.*

Woermann, F.G. & Vollmar, C. (2009). *Clinical MRI in children and adults with focal epilepsy: a critical review. Epilepsy Behav, 15(1), 40–49.*

Wyllie, E., Lüders, H., Morris, H.H., Lesser, R.P., & Dinner, D.S. (1986). *The lateralizing significance of versive head and eye movements during epileptic seizures. Neurology, 36(5), 606–611.*

Yang, I. & Barbaro, N.M. (2008) *Radiosurgical treatment of epilepsy. In H.O. Lüders (Ed.), Textbook of epilepsy surgery (pp. 1173–1178). London, UK: Informa Healthcare.*

New Advances in the Understanding of the Current Sources of Epileptic Activity in Mesial Areas

Lorena Vega-Zelaya, Oscar Garnés-Camarena
Clinical Neurophysiology
Hospital Universitario La Princesa, Madrid, Spain

Guillermo Ortega, Rafael Garcia de Sola
Neurosurgery, National Unit for the Treatment of Refractory Epilepsy
Hospital Universitario La Princesa, Madrid, Spain

Jesús Pastor
Clinical Neurophysiology
Hospital Universitario La Princesa, Madrid, Spain

1   Introduction

Epilepsy is one of the most common neurological conditions, with an estimated prevalence of approximately 0.4%-1.0%. Most patients with epilepsy experience seizures that are well controlled with antiepileptic drugs. Medical intractability, also known as drug-resistant epilepsy, occurs in 40% of patients with focal epilepsy (Téllez-Zenteno & Ladino, 2013), of which temporal lobe epilepsy (TLE) is the most frequent and most difficult to treat using antiepileptic drugs. Surgical treatment for these patients is typically a safe, effective and well-established option, with a success rate between 70 and 90% (Sola *et al.*, 2005). The best surgical outcomes are obtained when the epileptic zone (EZ) (Luders & Awad, 1991) is accurately localised through a presurgical evaluation, where patients are subjected to a number of noninvasive ancillary tests: video-electroencephalography (v-EEG), magnetic resonance imaging (MRI), single photon emission-computed tomography (SPECT) and positron emission tomography (PET). When the results from these tests are not functionally and anatomically consistent, invasive recordings are required, such as foramen ovale, subdural or depth electrodes. Activation through drugs that induce or increase interictal activity is often used as a complementary method together with v-EEG (Schmitt *et al.*, 1999; Brockhaus *et al.*, 1997; Krieger *et al.*, 1995; Pastor *et al.*, 2010). Etomidate, a selective modulator of the g-aminobutyric acid receptor A (GABA$_A$), is a hypnotic agent with a rapid speed of onset, a short duration of action, and minor side effects associated with intravenous perfusion. Etomidate might activate seizure foci, manifesting as a selective increase in the spiking activity on the EEG. In recent studies, we described the many benefits of etomidate-induced activation during the presurgical evaluation of patients with TLE, as this drug facilitates the reliable identification of the ictal onset zone (IOZ) and could be used to diagnose patients who do not experience seizures during v-EEG recordings or to influence decisions regarding the placement of intracranial electrodes. Moreover, the regional cerebral blood flow (CBF), assessed using SPECT with ^{99m}Tc-HmPAO, changed after perfusion with etomidate (Pastor *et al.*, 2010; Herrera-Peco *et al.*, 2010). Thus, it is necessary analyse the electrophysiological properties of the etomidate-induced irritative activity to ensure that this effect is generated through the same cortical regions observed at basal conditions. Therefore, the accuracy of this model to the biological system must be determined before drawing conclusions about its application.

Recently, we described a method to localise and evaluate current sources in mesial regions, combining the classical electrostatic approach with pharmacological activation through etomidate (Herrera-Peco *et al.*, 2010). However, several questions still remain. In this study, we specifically address the theoretical and topographical aspects of current sources.

2   Methods

2.1   Patients

A total of 13 patients (6 men and 7 women) were included in this study. The mean age and time of intractable epilepsy were 37.5 ± 4.3 and 30.6 ± 5.8 years for men and 39.8 ± 5.6 and 29.8 ± 4.4 years for women, respectively. Two patients had seizures during etomidate perfusion and were not included in the analysis.

The Ethical Committee of the Hospital de la Princesa approved this research. Informed consent was obtained from all patients. The patients were evaluated pre-surgically in accordance with the protocol of the Hospital de La Princesa (Pastor *et al.*, 2005; Sola *et al.*, 2005). Briefly, all patients were studied through scalp electroencephalography (EEG), interictal SPECT, MRI 1.5 T and v-EEG, using 19 scalp electrodes according to the international 10-20 system. Six-contact platinum foramen ovale (FO) electrodes, with 1-cm centre-to-centre spacing (AD-Tech, Racine, USA), were inserted bilaterally under general anaesthesia (Wieser & Moser, 1988; Pastor et al., 2008). In all cases, the correct implantation was assured using fluoroscopic imaging in the operating room. The most rostral electrode in the foramen ovale was referred to as FO#0, and the most occipital electrode was referred to as FO#5. During the v-EEG recording, antiepileptic drugs were progressively removed from the second to the fourth day, at approximately one-third of the dose per day. The digital EEG (NeuroWorks, XLTEK®, San Carlos, USA) and FO electrodes data were sampled at 256 Hz and filtered at 0.5-50 Hz for scalp and 1-100 Hz for FO electrodes recording. The IOZ was defined as the region where the seizures originated according to the v-EEG + FO recording. An expert neurophysiologist (JP), blinded to the results of the etomidate injection, identified this area.

2.2   Etomidate Administration

Under the continuous supervision of an experienced anaesthesiologist, etomidate (Janssen-Cilag, Spain) was intravenously applied (0.1 mg/kg) under inactive conditions, with the patient lying in the supine position (Herrera-Peco et al., 2009; Pastor et al., 2010). Supplementary oxygen was administered through nasal prongs at a 5-L/min rate. The electrocardiogram (EKG), capillary oxygen saturation (SaO_2) and respiratory rate (RR) were continuously monitored during the entire process, although these variables were not analysed in this study. The analysis with intravenous etomidate was performed between the third and fourth days in the v-EEG unit, except in one case performed on the fifth day. Discrete measurements of all variables were obtained at 30-s intervals at 5 min before (basal level) and 15 min after etomidate application.

The kinetics of the etomidate-induced activity was assessed using an expression equivalent to the first derivative for the discrete time-series of the frequency of spikes:

$$\frac{\Delta f}{\Delta t} = \frac{f(t+\Delta t) - f(t)}{\Delta t}, \tag{1}$$

where Δf is the change in frequency (spikes/min), and Δt represents the time increment (min).

Lateralisation induced through etomidate perfusion was assessed, comparing the frequency in the left and right areas and the frequency in the mesial and lateral areas. We defined the lateralisation coefficient (lc) using the following expression:

$$lc = \frac{1}{15} \sum_{i=1}^{15} \frac{v_{li} - v_{ri}}{v_{li} + v_{ri}}, \tag{2}$$

where v_{li} signifies the left frequency (either from the mesial or lateral areas) and v_{ri} represents the right frequency for $i = 1, 2 ...13$ on the time-series of spike instantaneous frequencies. According to this method, etomidate activity lateralises to the left if $0 < lc < 1$ and to the right if $1 < lc < 0$. A bolus of ^{99m}Tc-HmPAO (740 MBq) was intravenously injected immediately after etomidate administration.

2.3   Measure of Cerebral Perfusion

The regional cerebral blood flow (CBF) was determined using SPECT imaging. The analyses were performed using ^{99m}Tc- HmPAO, with a low-energy high-resolution collimator, a simple-head camera

(Starcam 3200, General Electric®, Milwaukee, WI, U.S.A.), and 96 projections of 22 s each, with a 64 x 64 matrix. The slices were reconstructed through filtered back-projection using a Butterworth filter (order 10 with a 0.6 cut-off). The brain SPECT images were acquired in the 30 min following the complete recovery of the patient.

The quantitative analysis of the brain perfusion was performed using NeuroGam software (General Electric®) to compare several areas of interest, including the frontal, temporal, parietal, and occipital lobes, and the putamen, globus pallidus, and thalamus, as defined using the software. Moreover, we defined the following areas according to the Talairach and Tournaux atlas (1998): the laterobasal temporal cortex, amygdaloid body, anterior hippocampus, and posterior hippocampus.

To evaluate changes in CBF, we defined the next variable using the following equation:

$$\Delta = CBF_{etom} - CBF_{basal},\qquad(3)$$

where CBF_{etom} and CBF_{basal} are measures of the regional CBF after etomidate administration and under basal conditions, respectively.

2.4   Monopole Model

We applied a classical electrostatic theory to derive mathematical expressions for interictal epileptiform discharges (IED, i.e., spikes and sharp waves) recorded using FO (Malmivuo & Plonsey, 1995). We assumed an infinite and homogenous volume conductor and an isotropic medium, according to the following equation:

$$V = \frac{i_{equiv}}{4\pi\sigma r}.\qquad(4)$$

(See Pastor et al., 2006 for further details). However, we modified our theoretical framework, replacing the equivalent charge (q_{equiv}) with the equivalent current (I_{equiv}) at coordinates (z0, r0) responsible for a particular spiking activity (V). This voltage was recorded from two consecutive FOs, n and $n + 1$ (bipolar linkage), and is given by the following expression:

$$i_{equiv} = k\frac{\sqrt{\left[(n+1)L-z_0\right]^2+r_0^2}\sqrt{\left(nL-z_0\right)^2+r_0^2}}{\sqrt{\left(nL-z_0\right)^2+r_0^2}-\sqrt{\left[(n+1)L-z_0\right]^2+r_0^2}},\qquad(5)$$

where r_0 is the radial distance to the charge, $k = \frac{1}{4}\pi\sigma$, s is the conductivity tensor and L is the interelectrode distance in mm. In all cases, the z=0 corresponds with the position of FO#0, placed at the inner face of the foramen ovale.

The three-equation system (r_0, z_0 and i_{equiv}) was solved numerically using the IED amplitude data from three consecutive channels. For this purpose, we first identified IED simultaneously recorded using three consecutive differentially arranged electrodes, namely V_1 (posterior by definition), V_2 and V_3 (anterior). The spikes were identified according to the IFSECN criteria (Chatrian et al., 1974) and were only included when a phase reversal between two consecutive channels was observed (Pastor et al., 2006; Herrera-Peco et al., 2009). The spike amplitude was measured from the base line to either the positive or negative peak. Some bioelectrical activity, representing $40 \pm 4.3\%$ of the recorded activity, did not fit with our criteria (spikes with multiple peaks, asynchronous spikes, etc.) and were not included in the analysis. For the rest of the activity, under the conditions specified, a single source approximation was reliably applied, and the most common spike profile is included in the study.

Typically, more than fifty spikes per patient were collected for analysis in each state (awake, sleep and after etomidate). Non-REM sleep was scored according to the conventional rules for sleep staging (Rechtschaffen & Kales, 1968). For each patient, the following variables for interictal, ictal and pharmacologically induced activity were examined:

1. The relative position (z_0, r_0) in the zr-plane defined by the FO.

2. The equivalent current (i_{equiv})

3. The mean scattering of the current sources in the zr plane. This measure is an estimate of the scattering of current sources from all spikes examined. We estimated the mean scattering using a centre-of-mass approach.

4. The relative frequency of activity (% of spikes) along the z-axis.

5. Relative topography of the different states: wakefulness, sleep, ictal and pharmacologically induced activities. See below.

6. The CBF immediately after etomidate administration.

2.5   Topographical Analysis of Current Sources

It is important to establish the degree of superposition among sources obtained from interictal, ictal and pharmacologically induced activity. Thus, the zr-plane, or configuration space, was divided into small non-overlapping patches of:

$$\Delta x \times \Delta y, \tag{6}$$

where $\Delta x = 1$ mm, $\Delta y = 1$ mm and area = 1 mm^2). This tessellation covers the entire theoretical surface. We have defined the active area (where current-source appears, irrespective of the functional state) in two steps: (i) patches where spiking activity 1 spike/mm^2; and (ii) spikes less than a minimum distance (d_{min}) from other spikes. We have chosen:

$$d_{min} = \sqrt{\Delta x^2 + \Delta y^2} = 1.4 \text{ mm.} \tag{7}$$

In this way, spurious spikes were excluded from the active area. Therefore, for each pair of activities, e.g., interictal and etomidate induced, we obtain the total area where the current sources appear for each type of activity and the superposition between them. Moreover, the degree of superposition for the number of sources was also computed. This analysis was performed using a homemade script in MATLAB^{TM} (R2008b).

2.6   Numerical Model

To address the behaviour of different source configurations, we implemented a simple numerical model. We assumed a simplistic approach, according to the following hypotheses:

1. A current source is placed in a model of the cortex.

2. The dynamics of the spike (whose mechanism is negligible) are generated in the source and scaled at different points according to the voltage generated for each source configuration.

3. The medium is considered homogeneous and isotropic. Real values for conductance are consciously ignored because we are only interested in relative, not real, magnitudes.

We have assessed three different configurations:

1. Monopolar, with a current i placed 3 mm below the cortical surface.

2. Dipolar, with two currents (i and $-i$), oriented vertically and located 6 mm apart (d).

3. Quadripolar source, with a current i placed at the same point as the dipole, but with a negative source ($-i$), divided into three currents, $-i_j$, j = 1, 2, 3, where:

$$i + \sum_{j=1}^{3} -i_j = 0 \qquad (8)$$

According to the cable theory (see below), the relationship between these currents is $-i_1 < -i_2 < -i_3$.

This model was implemented in Matlab(R) 9.0 and run using a personal computer. Briefly, the dynamics for the interictal epileptiform discharge was simulated from a model of spike obtained from two opposite and partially overlapped Gaussian curves, with different constants. We considered that the spike dynamics did not change with position, but amplitude should be scaled for every position according to the voltage induced for every configuration, e.g. equation 10 for monopolar and modified accordingly for quadripolar, and equation 11 for dipolar configurations.

2.7   Statistical Analysis

Statistical comparisons between groups were performed using Student's t-test or Mann-Whitney's rank sum test if normality failed. Groups that did not fit to normality were subjected to the Kruskal-Wallis one-way ANOVA on ranks. In cases of more than two records per patient, Dunn's multiple pair-wise comparison was used.

Significant changes in regional CBF (Δ) were assessed using the z-score, according to the following (null and alternative) hypotheses:

$$H0: \mu1 = 0 \; ; H1: \mu1 \neq 0.$$

Pearson's correlation coefficient was used to study dependence between variables. Linear regression was calculated using the least square sum. A contrast hypothesis against the null hypothesis $r = 0$ used the following statistic:

$$t = \frac{r\sqrt{N-2}}{\sqrt{1-r^2}}. \qquad (9)$$

This statistic describes a Student's t-distribution with N - 2 degrees of freedom (Spiegel, 1991). SigmaStat 3.5 software (SigmaStat, Point Richmond, CA, USA) was used for the statistical analysis. The significance level was set at p = 0.05. The results are shown as the means ±SEM, except where otherwise indicated.

3 Results

All the patients were operated by anterior medial temporal resection. The main clinical features of the patients are shown in Table 1.

Patients	Age	Sex	vEEG	RM	SPECT	lc. mesial	lc. laternal	Surgery / Engel
1	43	M	L-TM	TMS-L	AMT-L	0.96	1	L/I
2	55	F	L-TM	TMS-L	AMT-L	0.92	1	L/I
3	48	F	R-TM	TMS-R	Mes-R	- 1	- 0.97	R/II
4	57	F	R-TM	Normal	Bi-T (L>R)	- 0.42	- 0.27	R/I
5	38	M	R-TM	TMS-R	Bi-T (R>L)	-0.69	-0.47	R/I
6	28	M	R-TM	TMS-R	AMT-R	- 0.97	- 0.29	R/I
7	16	F	R-TM	TMS-R	AMT-R	-0.91	-0.80	R/I
8	39	F	L-TM	Normal	Mes-L	1	1	L/I
9	23	M	L-TM	TMS-L	AMT-R	0.81	1	L/I
10	36	F	R-TM	TMS-R	AMT-R	-0.91	-0.80	R/I
11	52	M	L-TM	Normal	AMT-L	1	1	L/I
12	41	M	L-TM	TMS-L	AMT-L	1	1	L/I
13	28	F	L-TM	TMS-L	AMT-L	1	1	L/I

Table 1: Clinical features of analysed patients. AMT: anterior mesial temporal. L, left; R, right. TMS: temporal mesial sclerosis. Mes: mesial. ATR, anterior temporal resection. lc, lateralisation coefficient.

3.1 Bioelectrical Activity Induced Through Etomidate

The changes observed in the scalp EEG after etomidate administration were characterised by small increases in the amplitude and frequency of the activity recorded (stage 1), followed by generalised, large-amplitude delta activity (stage 2) (Figure 1). In terms of irritative activity, the frequency (spikes/min) of high-voltage spikes and sharp-waves increased in temporal areas, particularly in the mesial areas. These activities only appeared in areas included among the ictal zone (IZ), i.e., etomidate induced this activity only in areas where spikes were recorded under basal conditions (Figure 2).

3.2 Effects Of Etomidate During Cerebral Perfusion

We observed a significant increase in the regional CBF with respect to basal state in the thalamus ($p < 0.05$, z-score, $n = 13$), the posterior hippocampus ($p < 0.05$, z-score), and putamen ($p < 0.05$, z-score), and these changes occurred bilaterally. However, the only brain structure in which the regional CBF differed between epileptic and nonepileptic hemispheres was the posterior hippocampus (Figure 3). In this area, a CBF was significantly increased in the nonepileptic lobe compared with the epileptic lobe ($p < 0.05$, paired Student's t-test).

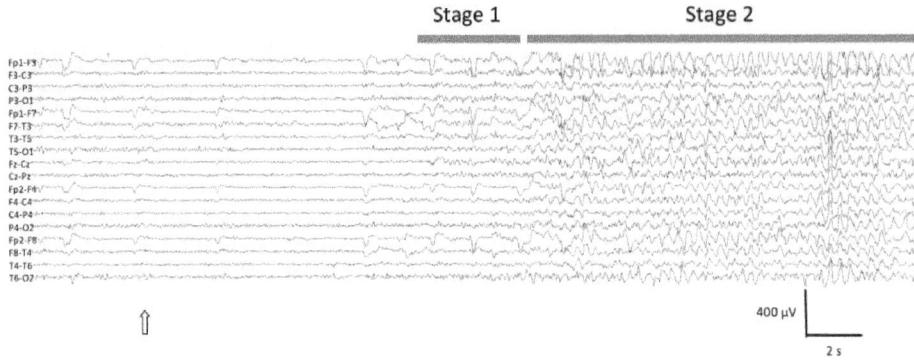

Figure 1: Shortly after completion of etomidate administration, (arrow) increases in the amplitude and frequency (stage 1), followed by generalized large amplitude delta activity (stage 2) is observed in the bioelectrical activity recorded on scalp EEG.

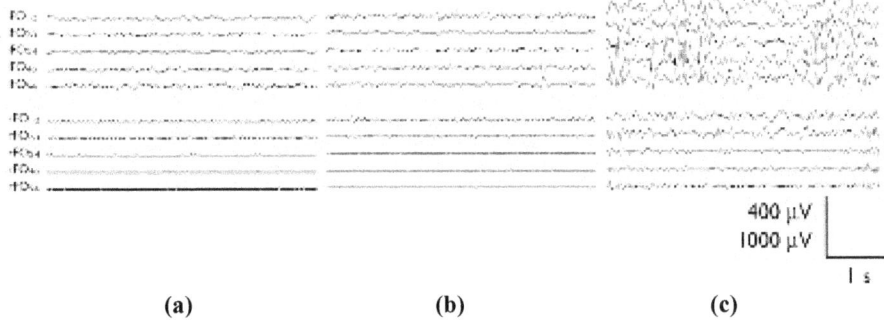

(a)   **(b)**   **(c)**

Figure 2: Activity recorded using FO electrodes after administration of etomidate. A) Basal activity. B) Activity at 30 s and C) 2 min after etomidate administration.

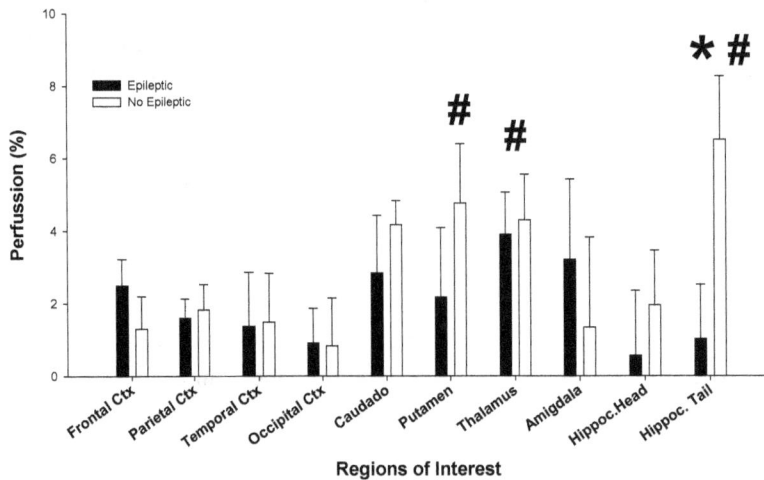

Figure 3: Effects of etomidate on CBF. The graph summarizing the CBF changes by etomidate in regions pertaining to the epileptic hemisphere (black box) and nonepileptic hemisphere (empty box). # $p < 0.05$, z-score test (n = 13);*$p < 0.05$, paired Student's-t-test. Ctx: cortex. Hippoc: hippocampus.

3.3   Fitting The Data To The Monopole Model

To analyse the proper fit of our data to the single source model, we calculated the percentage of spikes recorded in three consecutive channels, with fitting errors >5%. The spikes observed showing an error greater than 5% during interictal (awake and sleep states) and ictal activities, representing approximately 10% of the cases. However, the scattering and the i_{equiv} were similar for interictal and pharmacologically induced activities (Figure 4), suggesting that the single source model could reliably explain interictal and etomidate-induced spiking recorded using FO electrodes in MTLE. No differences were observed between the characteristics of the interictal activity recorded from either wakefulness or sleep with respect to the interictal activity in the presence of etomidate. Therefore, both physiological states can be used for the study of basal interictal activity.

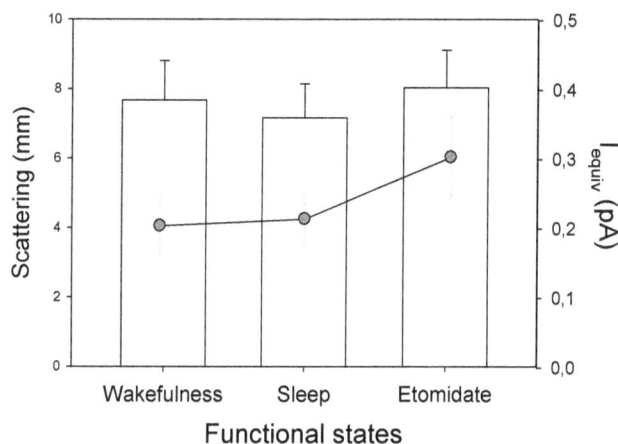

Figure 4: Biophysical properties of current sources from the mesial temporal lobe. The scattering, iequiv, was similar during both interictal and pharmacological induction.

3.4   Voltage Source Distribution And Scattering

We analysed the anterior-to-posterior distribution in the z-axis for the entire group compared with the distribution obtained for etomidate. The spatial distribution of the voltage sources responsible for interictal baseline activity was similar to that obtained for etomidate-induced activity. Moreover, there was a close correlation between areas where irritative activity occurred under basal conditions and those induced through etomidate (Figure 5). We attempted to determine whether there were interindividual differences in the irritative activity distribution in the patients sampled. The analysis of the normalised sources showed that 76,9% of the patients did not show the localised distribution of voltage sources at either the interictal baseline or in the presence of etomidate. A more scattered distribution along the axis z, with $IP_{20-75} > 20$ mm (Rank: 21,5-28,3 mm), was observed in 22,1% of the patients.

We compared the antero-posterior current source distribution for different pairs of functional states, e.g., interictal vs ictal, interictal vs etomidate and ictal vs etomidate. Therefore, we plotted the percentage of frequency of spikes for each segment along the z-axis. The results were fitted to a linear regression using the least square method. We observed a linear relationship among the three functional states.

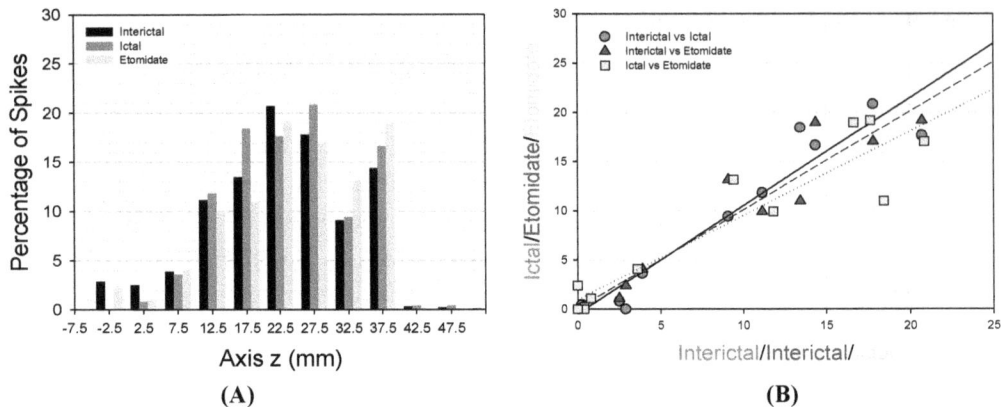

Figure 5: Biophysical properties for current-sources induced through different functional states. (A) Scattering along the antero-posterior theoretical axis. (B) Linear regression for the location of current-sources for pairs of functional states, shown in the same colours. The linear regression for inter-ictal/ictal is y = 1.09x-0.50, r = 0.930, for interictal/etomidate y = 1.01x+0.01, r = 0.922 and for ictal/interictal y = 0.856x+0.952, r = 0.867.

3.5   Current Topography Sources

Considering the importance of the specificity of activation using etomidate, we analysed the topographical relationship between pharmacologically induced activity and the IOZ in 6 patients. We previously demonstrated that current sources obtained during wakefulness and sleep share common biophysical properties; hence, both types of activities can be considered as similar from a biophysical point of view. However, it remains unknown whether these activities are generated from the same cortical structures. To address this question, we analysed the topographical distribution of current-sources in the configuration space.

The active area (mm2), where the current-sources appears for each of the functional states (interictal, ictal and etomidate induces), was 33.3 ± 5.8; 4.0 ± 0.6 and 10.7 ± 1.4, respectively. Similarly, the occurrence of spikes (spikes/mm2) was 63.3 ± 11.5; 16.7 ± 3.1; and 20.0 ± 3.3, respectively. For each pair of activities, the area and the spikes of superposition were interictal-ictal: 10.0 ± 1.5 mm2. (31%) and 74.7 ± 12.6 spikes/ mm2 (12%); interictal-etomidate induced: 7.3 ± 1.4 mm2 (24%) and 74.7 spikes/ mm2 (12%) and ictal-etomidate induced: 4.7 ± 1.0 mm2 (24%) and 30.0 spikes/mm2(45%), respectively.

Thus, there is a great degree of superposition for the current-source topography for interictal, ictal and pharmacologically induced activity.

3.6   Theoretical Approach To Mesial Sources

An electric field (**E**) is a vectorial magnitude, whose calculation, even in a simple system, is laborious and usually difficult. To overcome these problems, physicists and, subsequently, neurophysiologists have extensively used the following potential approach.

Briefly, the electric field generated through an electrical charge (q, in coulombs -C) can be theoretically related to a scalar potential (f) using the following expression:

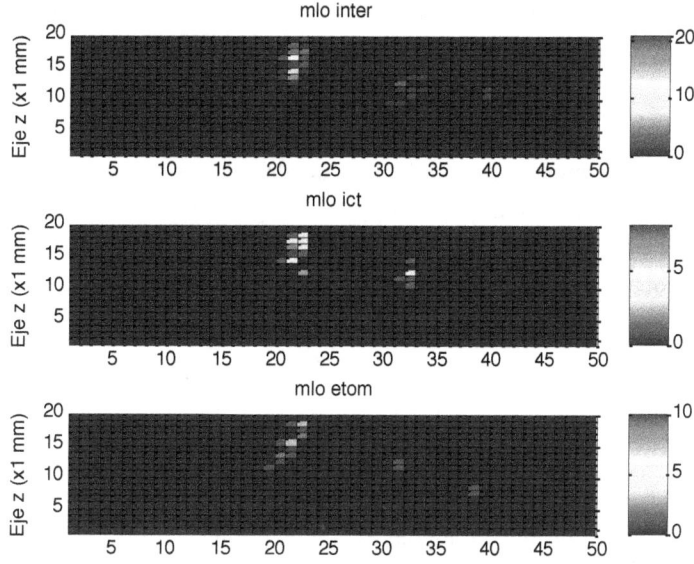

Figure 6: Example of topography for current source density locations in different states. A) Interictal epileptiform discharge, B) ictal onset and C) pharmacologically induced activity.

$$\vec{E}(r) = -\frac{\partial}{\partial x}\left(\frac{q}{4\pi\varepsilon_0 R}\right) \qquad (10)$$

where e_0 represents the permittivity in a vacuum (in F/m), and R is the magnitude of the relative position between the source (r') and the field point (r), typically measured in centimetres (cm) for the central nervous system (CNS). For simplicity, we have reduced this problem to a monodimensional problem, assuming that the charge is placed in the vacuum. While this situation does not actually occur in the central nervous system (CNS), this formalism is still frequently used.

As discussed above, this expression is vectorial. However, the expression between brackets, which represents the potential, is scalar. Thus, several charges placed at different points can be defined using the following equation:

$$\phi(r) = \sum_i \frac{q}{4\pi\varepsilon_0 R_i} \qquad (11)$$

This magnitude represents the potential generated through several charges q_i placed (at vacuum) at r_i' and measured in r. This theoretical magnitude is relative; thus, we can only measure differences in the potential between pairs of points, and there is not any point where we can define an absolute value. To overcome these flaws, we define a value of zero as infinity. The main advantage of potential is the scalar character, as we can perform easier calculations and subsequently convert these results to the real physical magnitude E using Equation 10.

There is a powerful approach in electromagnetism called multipolar potential development. Using this approach, we can decompose the potential generated from any source in different polar components, which retain the main features of source distribution and the distance to the point of the field. Therefore, using the most adequate polar component of our system, we can simplify the (usually) extremely tedious and difficult calculations.

The formal features of the multipolar approach are out of the scope of this study, but these features can be represented using this general expression (Wangness 1986; Pastor *et al.*, 2002):

$$\phi(r) = \phi_M(r) + \phi_D(r) + \phi_Q(r) + \cdots \tag{12}$$

where *M, D* and *Q* represent monopole, dipolar and quadripolar components, respectively. For systems, such as those studied by Clinical Neurophysiology, orders greater than dipolar are not of interest. Therefore, we can focus on the first two simpler components of this approach.

The following equations show the formal expressions for both terms.

$$\phi_M(r) = \frac{q}{4\pi\varepsilon_0 r}, \tag{13}$$

$$\phi_D(r) = \frac{\vec{p}\vec{r}}{4\pi\varepsilon_0 r^2}. \tag{14}$$

In these expressions, *Q* represents the monopolar moment, defined (for discrete sources) as:

$$Q = \sum_i q_i, \tag{15}$$

and *p* is the dipolar moment, defined as:

$$\vec{p} = \sum_i q_i \vec{r}_i, \tag{16}$$

where r_i' represent the places for charges q_i. As shown in Equation 14, there is a dot product for $p \cdot r$. Therefore, we can simplify this equation:

$$\phi_D(r) = \frac{p\cos\theta}{4\pi\varepsilon_0 r^2}, \tag{17}$$

where *q* represents the angle between the dipolar moment *p* and the radio-vector of the field. When two charges are equal in magnitude (*q*) and opposite in sign and placed at *d* cm apart, the dipolar moment is *p* = *qd*, oriented from -*q* to +*q*.

Traditionally, theoretical considerations and some empirical facts have favoured the dipolar approach in neurophysiological recordings in humans. It is assumed that there is a charge conservation strictly applied to the CNS; therefore, where a charge source appears, a sink of the same magnitude must counterbalance the appearance of the charge. This model has been empirically corroborated in several models on both microscopic and macroscopic levels (Ramon *et al.*, 2009; Plummer *et al.*, 2010; Campi *et al.*, 2011; Lelic *et al.*, 2012). A dipolar model has been proposed between the upper and lower layers of the cortex (Dümpelman *et al.*, 2012). This model assumes that a source (sink) in a distal location from an apical dendrite of a pyramidal neuron must have a sink (source) of the same magnitude in the soma. Nevertheless, recent data have shown that cortical sources cannot be precisely represented through a single equivalent dipole, and the existence of monopolar components must also be considered at the mesoscopic level (Riera *et al.*, 2012).

Thus, there are several considerations about this model. First, this approach captures only a portion of the actual definition of potential (equation 11) and cannot be considered as true potential. Secondly, although there is a charge counterbalance in a real system in the CNS, the simple soma-dendrite dipolar model (SDDM) is not completely true.

To approach to the SDDM, we have to implement the core-conductor theory and the related cable theory of current propagation. The application of Kirchhoff's laws to the core-conductor model network generates the *cable equations*. These equations are the basic mathematical relationships used to study the electrical response of a uniform fibre to subthreshold stimuli (Plonsey & Barr, 2007).
The model is represented in the next figure.

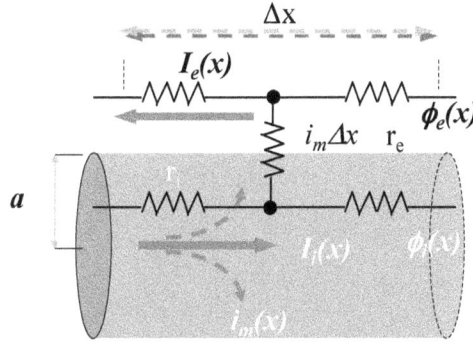

Figure 7: Linear core-conductor model for a single fibre of radius a. A schematic electrical circuit of membrane is superimposed. Ie and Ii are extra and intracellular currents, respectively, while fe and fi represent potentials for the same compartments, im means transmembrane current density and Dx refers to a length unit. The intracellular and extracellular resistances are given as ri and re, respectively.

The extra and intracellular axial currents are associated with the potentials through the following expressions:

$$\frac{\partial \phi_e}{\partial x} = -r_e I_e \ , \quad \frac{\partial \phi_i}{\partial x} = -r_i I_i \tag{18}$$

The intracellular axial current decreases along the axis path because there is a current flowing from the fibre through the membrane (im, in A/cm). Thus, the relationship between intracellular and transmembrane current is expressed as:

$$\frac{\partial I_e}{\partial x} = -i_m \tag{19}$$

The transmembrane potential (Vm) is the difference among intra and extracellular potential; therefore, from Equation 18, we obtain the following equation:

$$\frac{\partial V_m}{\partial x} = \frac{\partial \phi_i}{\partial x} - \frac{\partial \phi_c}{\partial x} = -r_i I_i + r_e I_e \tag{20}$$

However, from Kirchhoff's first law, we know that $I_i + I_e = =0$; therefore, the above equation can be written as:

$$\frac{\partial V_m}{\partial x} = -(r_i + r_e) I_i \tag{21}$$

Assuming that $r_i \gg r_e$ and using equation 21, we obtain the equation:

$$\frac{1}{r_i}\frac{\partial^2 V_m}{\partial x^2} = -i_m \tag{22}$$

This important equation relates the transmembrane current density along the axial path (typically not measured) with the transmembrane voltage (the magnitude is typically measured). Transmembrane voltage can be obtained from the cable equation (Davis & Lorente, 1947):

$$v_m(X,T) = \frac{r_i I_0 \lambda}{4}\left[e^{-X}erfc\left(\frac{X}{2\sqrt{T}} - \sqrt{T}\right) - e^{-X}erfc\left(\frac{X}{2\sqrt{T}} + \sqrt{T}\right)\right]. \tag{23}$$

Equation 23 is an extraordinary equation whose meaning we will try to clarify. Notably, this equation is dimensionless, as the dimensions of space (x) and time (t) have been replaced with the dimensionless variables:

$$X = \frac{x}{\lambda}; \quad T = \frac{t}{\tau_m}. \tag{24}$$

The constant λ (cm) or length constant and τ_m space (s), the time constant of the membrane can be determined using these expressions. The magnitudes observed in the first fraction are axial resistance ($[r_i]$ = Ω/cm), the injected current ($[I_0]$ = A) and the constant τ_m and λ view. The expression *erfc* (x) is the complementary error function. This equation can be solved easily for simple theoretical situations stationary, yielding the potential along the dendrite ($V_m(x)$), in response to a current injection, resulting in a maximum potential at the injection site (V_0):

$$V_m(x) = V_0 e^{-x/\lambda} \tag{25}$$

This expression shows a single exponential decay for the voltage, as the injected current flows from the dendrite at a constant rate. Therefore, we can use this expression, obtained from an extremely simplified (and not real) situation, in Equation 23 to obtain the transmembrane current density along the fibre path. The numerical model demonstrates that the amplitudes of the spikes for dipolar and monopolar sources are similar for points close to the source. However, when the distance increases, the difference between dipolar and monopolar spikes increases and the dipolar spike becomes more similar to the quadripolar source.

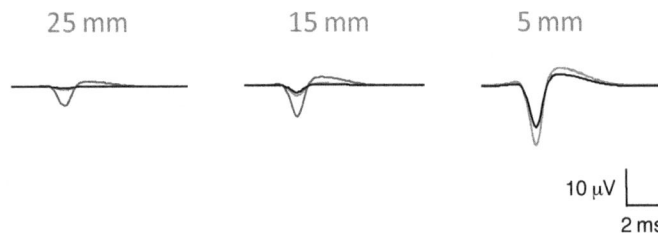

Figure 8: Spikes generated using different current sources configurations at different distances from the source, indicated above the traces. Blue: monopolar source; red: dipolar source; and black: quadripolar source.

Another important fact obtained from this model is that we cannot resolve Equation 11 with an error < 5% when using spikes generated from a dipolar or a quadripolar current source. Thus, the important point of this analysis is that the current density along the fibre cannot be strictly considered as a dipole, with an equal source and sink located far apart, and a current (and voltage, consequently) that exponentially decays along the fibre. This analysis particularly applies to the cell soma and dendrites, which are not myelinated, and the sources generated in the cerebral cortex. Therefore, this monopolar approach could be used in some cases, which remain to be accurately determined.

4   Discussion

In previous studies (Pastor *et al.*, 2010; Herrera-Peco *et al.*, 2010), we showed that the administration of etomidate is a safe and efficient pharmacological method for patients suffering from TLE during pre-surgical evaluation. However, the changes observed in regional CBF, specifically in areas associated with the EZ, are more difficult to explain.

Traditionally, several different drugs are used to induce brain activity. As previously discussed, it is clinically important that the patient tolerate the drug side effects (Herrera-Peco *et al.*, 2009). For etomidate, the primary side effects observed were myoclonus and moderate pain. Etomidate is a very fast acting agent, inducing a loss of consciousness within 10 s and a state of anesthesia in 3-5 min and is rapidly eliminated due to hepatic extraction (Van Hamme *et al.*, 1978). Therefore, etomidate has optimal pharmacokinetics characteristics to induce the EEG activity. Moreover, it has been described as a safe hypnotic (Vanlersberghe & Camu, 2008). Indeed, no significant hemodynamic effects have been observed (Gooding *et al.*, 1979), although higher doses (0.35 ± 0.17 mg/kg) induce tachycardia and increase the mean arterial pressure (Arden *et al.*, 1986).

In contrast to other anaesthetics, etomidate has a specific target at clinical concentrations (Voss *et al.*, 2008). Indeed, etomidate almost exclusively acts on the the β_2 and β_3 subunits of the GABA$_A$ receptor. This specificity might be important for diagnosis in pre-surgical evaluation. The exact mechanism by which etomidate activates the irritative area is not completely understood. However, several lines of evidence might explain this effect. Studies in cultured astrocytes have shown that etomidate inhibits glutamate uptake, increasing the extracellular glutamate concentration to a level that can escape the synaptic cleft and activate extra-synaptic receptors. As a consequence, irritative activity would be increased (Räth *et al.*, 2008). However, an examination of slices obtained from epileptic patients revealed a decrease in the reversal potential for Cl$^-$ anions (Cohen *et al.*, 2002). This change could induce depolarisation, not hyperpolarisation, following GABA release, thereby driving irritative activity.

Several biophysical properties of spontaneous and pharmacologically induced activities are similar, including the i_{equiv}, scattering and rate-to-monopolar fitting. However, in this study, we addressed two important questions concerning topography and theoretical considerations about the current-source model. First, we showed that interictal, ictal and etomidate-induced activities greatly overlap, indicating that the biophysical mechanisms are similar, and the cortical areas where all types of activity appear are likely the same or closely related. This fact suggests that this technique can be used to better define the region resected during surgery. Theoretically, the current-source model demonstrates that monopolar and dipolar sources are similar in the vicinity of the source; therefore, we can consider this monopolar model as a good approach to a dipolar source. However, when the distance from the source increases, the potential induced through both configurations clearly differs, suggesting that a dipolar source cannot be fitted to a set of potentials obtained from a monopolar source at a certain distance. However, neither monopolar nor dipolar theoretical sources can be fitted to real current sources from the cortex (Riera *et al.*, 2012). Cortical macro-columns are a complex set of current sources (Nunez & Srinivasan, 2009), and the best theoretical model will likely be different for different configurations. Notably, there is a high degree of accuracy (> 95%) for most of the sources concerning the monopolar model in current sources from the mesial temporal lobe. Thus, we cannot consider this fact as a demonstration, as this empirical fact emphasises the use of a monopolar approach to bioelectrical sources in humans. Indeed, much more work remains, both theoretical and empirical, before completely elucidating this aspect.

Etomidate perfusion induces a brief increase in the amplitude and frequency of brain activity, recorded using scalp EEG, followed by generalised high-voltage delta activity. The latter activity resembles that observed during non-rapid eye movement (NREM) delta sleep. Etomidate is a potent GABA agonist, and GABA plays an important role in NREM delta sleep (Gottesmann, 2002). These results might explain the increased thalamic regional CBF induced by etomidate. Although we cannot exclude the fact that increases in CBF in the basal ganglia might be associated with ictal patterns in epileptic patients (Norden & Blumenfeld, 2002). Traditionally, an intense increase in regional CBF is a hallmark of partial-onset seizures, potentially reflecting the increase in regional synaptic activity and changes in neurotransmission. During the ictal SPECT, the ^{99m}Tc-HMPAO infusion is performed briefly after the seizure starts, and a delay must be overcome before the radiotracer reaches the brain. Thus, ictal SPECT, likely shows an increase in regional cerebral perfusion associated with the seizure (Van Paesschen, 2004), and almost certainly indicates propagation from the area of ictal onset. Indeed, a true ictal SPECT recording has corroborated the increase in CBF induced through epileptic activity (Pastor *et al.*, 2008)

Considering the significant increase in the IED induced through etomidate, we expected an increase in the regional CBF in the IOZ. Surprisingly, however, we observed a relative decrease in the regional CBF in the posterior hippocampus of the EZ. Recently, we showed that there is a consistent and highly significant reduction of micro-blood vessels, particularly in the CA1 field in the sclerotic hippocampus (Kastanauskaite *et al.*, 2009). This reduction might be associated with the relative inability of the epileptic posterior hippocampus to increase CBF locally in response to etomidate. However, it is also reasonable to conclude that etomidate increases the CBF more significantly in the structures spared through epileptic discharges. Although further experiments are needed to fully elucidate the mechanisms underlying etomidate-induced increases in CBF and brain activity, from a clinical point of view, these findings demonstrate significant methods of pre-surgical evaluation. Indeed, differential SPECT perfusion could be used to identify the EZ in TLE patients with a dubious lateralisation.

To conclude, etomidate-induced bioelectrical activity in mesial structures of patients under presurgical evaluation is a powerful and confident technique to validate hypotheses concerning the location of the epileptic zone. Moreover, this activity facilitates the identification of different patients regarding the activity topography, and we can use this technique for new surgical approaches, e.g., high-definition radiosurgery, in patients with well-localised sources.

Acknowledgment

This work was supported through a grant from the Plan Nacional de Investigación Científica, Desarrollo e Innovación Tecnológica (I+D+I), Instituto de Salud Carlos III, Subdirección General de Evaluación y Fomento de la Investigación PI12/02839.

References

Arden, J. R., Holley, F. O. & Stanski, D.R. (1986). *Increased sensitivity to etomidate in the elderly: initial distribution versus altered brain response. Anesthesiology, 65(1):19-27.*

Brockhaus, A., Lehnertz, K., Wienbruch, C., Kowalik, A., Burr, W., Elbert, T., et al. (1997). *Possibilities and limitations of magnetic source imaging of methohexital-induced epileptiform patterns in temporal lobe epilepsy patients. Electroencephalogr Clin Neurophysiol, 102:423-36.*

Campi, C., Pascarella, A., Sorrentino, A., & Piana, M. (2011). *Highly Automated Dipole Estimation (HADES). Comput Intell Neurosci, 982185, Epub 20011.*

Chatrian, G. E., Bergamini, L., Dondey, M., Klass, D.W., Lennox-Buchtal, M., & Petersen, I. (1974). *A glossary of terms most commonly used by clinical electroencephalographers. Electroenceph Clin Neurophysiol, 37:538-48.*

Cohen, I., Navarro, V., Clemenceau, S., Baulac, M., & Miles, R. (2002). *On the origin of interictal activity in human temporal lobe epilepsy in vitro. Science, 298:1418-21.*

Davis, L. Jr., & Lorente, de No. (1947). *Contribution to the mathematical theory of the electrotonus. Stud Rockefeller Inst Med Res Repr., 131:442-496.*

Dümpelmann, M., Ball, T., & Schulze-Bonhage, A. (2012). *sLORETA allows reliable distributed source reconstruction based on subdural strip and grid recordings. Hum Brain Mapp, May;33(5):1172-88.*

Gancher, S., Laxer, KD., & Krieger, W. (1984). *Activation of epileptogenic activity by etomidate. Anesthesiology, 61(5):616-618.*

Gooding, J. M., Weng, J. T., Smith, R. A., Berninger, G. T., & Kirby, R. R. (1979). *Cardiovascular and pulmonary responses following etomidate induction of anesthesia in patients with demonstrated cardiac disease. Anesth Analg, 58:40-41.*

Gottesmann, C. (2002). *GABA mechanisms and sleep. Neuroscience, 111(2):231-239.*

Herrera-Peco, I., Wix-Ramos, R., Domínguez-Gadea, L., Meilán- Paz, M. L., Martínez-Chacón, J. L., De Dios, E., et al. (2009). *Cambios en la perfusión cerebral inducidos por etomidato en pacientes con epilepsia del lóbulo temporal. Rev Neurol, 49: 561-565.*

Herrera-Peco, I., Ortega, G. J., Hernando-Requejo, V., Sola, R. G., & Pastor, J. (2010). *Fuentes de voltaje en la región temporal mesial inducidas por etomidato. Rev Neurol, 51:263-70.*

Herrera-Peco, I., Wix, R., Domínguez-Gadea, L., Meilán, M. L., Martínez Chacón, J. L., De Dios, E., Sola, R. G., & Pastor, J. (2010). *What changes in brain perfusión induced by etomidate suggest about epilepsy in human patients? Epilepsy Research and Treatment, 1-7.*

Kastanauskaite, A., Alonso-Nanclares, L., Blazquez-Llorca, L., Sola, R. G., & de Felipe, J. (2009). *Alterations of the microvascular network in the sclerotic hippocampus from epileptic patients. Neuropathol Exp Neurol, 68(8):939-950.*

Krieger, W., Copperman, J., & Laxer, K. D. (1985). *Seizures with etomidate anesthesia. Anesth Analg, 64:1226-7.*

Lelic D., Mørch, C. D., Hennings, K., Andersen, O. K., & Drewes, A. M. (2012). *Differences in perception and brain activation following stimulation by large versus small area cutaneous surface electrodes. Eur J Pain., 16(6):827-37.*

Lüders, H. O., & Awad, I. (1991). *Conceptual considerations. In Lüders HO, ed. Epilepsy surgery. New York: Raven Press, 51-56.*

Malmivuo, J., & Plonsey, R. (1995). *Bioelectromagnetism: principles and applications of bioelectric and biomagnetic fields. New York: Oxford University Press.*

Meinck, H. M., Moehlenhof, O., & Kettler, D. (1980). *Neurophysiological effects of etomidate, a new short-acting hypnotic. Electroencephalography and Clinical Neurophysiology, 50(5-6):515-522.*

Norden, A. D., & Blumenfeld, H. (2002). *The role of subcortical structures in human epilepsy. Epilepsy Behav, 3:219-231.*

Nunez, P. L., & Srinivasan, R. (2009). *Electric fields of the brain, 2nd Ed. New York:Oxford University Press.*

Pastor, J., & Sola, R. G. (2002). Fundamentos biofísicos de la magnetoencefalografía. Rev. Neurol, 34(9):843-850.

Pastor, J., Hernando-Requejo, V., Domínguez-Gadea, L., De Llano, I., Meilán-Paz, M. L., Martínez-Chacón, J. L., et al. (2005). Impacto de la experiencia sobre los resultados quirúrgicos en la epilepsia del lóbulo temporal. Rev Neurol, 41:709-16.

Pastor, J., Menéndez de la Prida, L., Hernando, V., & Sola, R. G. (2006). Voltage sources in mesial temporal lobe epilepsy recorded with foramen ovale electrodes. Clin Neurophysiol, 117:2604-14.

Pastor, J., Sola, R. G., Hernando-Requejo, V., Navarrete, E. G., & Pulido, P. (2008). Morbidity associated with the use of foramen ovale electrodes. Epilepsia, 49:464-469.

Pastor, J., Domínguez-Gadea, L., Sola, R. G., Hernando, V., Meilán, M. L., de Dios, E. et al. (2008). First true initial ictal SPECT in partial epilepsy verified by electroencephalography. Neuropsychiatr. Dis. Treat, 4(1):305-309.

Pastor, J., Sola, R. G., & de Felipe, J. (2009). Alterations of the microvascular network in sclerotic hippocampi from patients with epilepsy. Journal of Neuropathology and Experimental Neurology, 68(8):939-950.

Pastor, J., Wix, R., Meilán, M. L., Martínez-Chacón, J. L., de Dios, E., Domínguez-Gadea, L., Herrera-Peco, I., & Sola, R. G. (2010). Etomidate accurately localizes the epileptic area in patients with temporal lobe epilepsy. Epilepsia, 51(4):602-609.

Plonsey, R., & Barr, R. C. (2017). Impulse propagation. Bioelectricity. A quantitative approach. 3rd ed. New York:Springer.

Plummer, C., Wagner, M., Fuchs, M., & Harvey, A. (2010). S. Cook MJ. Dipole versus distributed EEG source localization for single versus averaged spikes in focal epilepsy. J Clin Neurophysiol, 27(3):141-62.

Ramon, C., Freeman, W. J., Holmes, M., Ishimaru, A., Haueisen, J., Schimpf, P. H., & Rezvanian, E. (2009). Similarities between simulated spatial spectra of scalp EEG, MEG and structural MRI. Brain Topogr, 22(3):191-6.

Räth, M., Föhr, K. J., Weigt, H. U., Gauss, A., Engele, J., Georgieff, M., et al. (2008). Etomidate reduces glutamate uptake in rat cultures glial cells: involvement of PKA. Br J Pharmacol., 155(6):925-33.

Rechtschaffen, A., & Kales, A. (1968). A manual of standardized terminology, techniques and scoring system for sleep stages of human subjects. Los Angeles: UCLA: Brain Information Service.

Riera, J. J., Ogawa, T., Goto, T., Sumiyoshi, A., Nonaka, H., Evans, A., Miyakawa, H., & Kawashima, R. (2012). Pitfalls in the dipolar model for the neocortical EEG sources. J Neurophysiol., 108(4):956-75.

Schmitt, H., Druschky, K., Hummel, C., & Stefan, H. (1999). Detection of an epileptic mirror focus after oral application of clonidine. Br J Anaesth, 83:349-51.

Sola, R. G., Hernando-Requejo, V., Pastor, J., García-Navarrete, E., De Felipe, J., Alijarde, M. T., Sánchez, A., Domínguez-Gadea, L., Martín-Plasencia, P., Maestú, F., Ramón-Cajal, S., & Pulido-Rivas, P. (2005). Epilepsia farmacorresistente del lóbulo temporal. Exploración con electrodos del foramen oval y resultados quirúrgicos. Rev Neurol, 41(1):4-16

Téllez-Zenteno, J. F., & Ladino, L. D. (2013). Epilepsia temporal: aspectos clínicos, diagnósticos y de tratamiento. Rev Neurol, 56:229-42.

Van Hamme, M. J., Ghoneim, M. M., & Ambre, J. J. (1978). Pharmacokinetics of etomidate, a new intravenous anesthetic. Anesthesiology, 49: 274-277.

Van Paesschen, W. (2004). Ictal SPECT. Epilepsia, 45(4):35-40.

Vanlersberghe, C., & Camu, F. (2008). Etomidate and other non-barbiturates. Handb Exp Pharmacol., (182):267-82.

Voss, L. J., Sleigh, J. W., Barnard, J. P. M., & Kirsch, H. E. (2008). The howling cortex: Seizures and general anesthetic drugs. Anesth. Analg, 107(5):1689-1703.

Wansgness, R. K. (1986). Electromagnetic fields. Wiley.

Wieser, H. G., & Moser, S. (1988). Improved multipolar foramen ovale electrode monitoring. J Epilepsy, 1:13-22.

Coexistence of Two Rare Genetic Disorders: Cornelia de Lange Syndrome and Turner Syndrome

María Concepción Gil-Rodríguez, Carolina Baquero-Montoya
Unit of Clinical Genetics and Functional Genomics, Department of Pharmacology-Physiology
Medical School, University of Zaragoza, Spain

Jolanta Wierzba
Dept. of Pediatrics, Hematology, Oncology and Endocrinology and Dept. of General Nursery
Medical University of Gdańsk, Poland

Beatriz Puisac, María Esperanza Teresa-Rodrigo, María Hernández-Marcos
Unit of Clinical Genetics and Functional Genomics, Department of Pharmacology-Physiology
Medical School, University of Zaragoza, Spain

Anna Polucha, Dorota Winnicka
Department of Pediatrics, Hematology and Oncology
Children University Hospital, Lublin, Poland

Alicia Vicente-Gabás
Unit of Clinical Genetics and Functional Genomics, Department of Pharmacology-Physiology
Medical School, University of Zaragoza, Spain

Oscar Flórez-Gómez
Department of Pediatric
Hospital Pablo Tobon Uribe, Medellín, Colombia

Gloria Bueno-Lozano
Department of Pediatrics
Medical School, University of Zaragoza, Spain

Janusz Limon
Department of Biology and Genetics
Medical University of Gdańsk, Poland

Feliciano J. Ramos
Department of Pediatrics
Medical School, University of Zaragoza, Spain

Juan Pié
Unit of Clinical Genetics and Functional Genomics, Department of Pharmacology-Physiology
Medical School, University of Zaragoza, Spain

1   Introduction

In this chapter, we aim to highlight the atypical co-occurrence of these two genetic disorders, Cornelia de Lange syndrome and Turner syndrome, in the same individual. Each syndrome has characteristic physical features, although the neurological involvement in a lesser or greater extent is common in both syndromes.

Cornelia de Lange syndrome (CdLS; OMIM 1227470, 300590, 610759, 614701, 300882) is a genetic developmental disorder characterized by distinctive craniofacial features, severe growth retardation (pre- and postnatal), cognitive impairment, limb defects and hirsutism (Kline *et al.*, 2007b). Multisystem involvement is the norm with gastrointestinal, cardiovascular, neurological, visual or hearing disorders (Kline *et al.*, 2007b). The prevalence of CdLS is 1:62.000 to 1:45.000 (Barisic *et al.*, 2008).

To date, mutations in five genes, encoding components of the cohesion complex (*SMC1A*, *SMC3* and *RAD21*) and its regulators (*NIPBL* and *HDAC8*) have been found in CdLS patients. Approximately 70% of patients with CdLS carry an identifiable mutation in the *NIPBL* gene (5p13) (Krantz *et al.*, 2004; Pié *et al.*, 2010; Tonkin *et al.*, 2004; Wierzba *et al.*, 2012). A smaller percentage of patients (~ 4-6%) have mutations in *SMC1A* gene (Xp11.22) (Deardorff *et al.*, 2007; Musio *et al.*, 2006; Pié *et al.*, 2010) and a single male patient has been identified with a mutation in *SMC3* (10q25) (Deardorff *et al.*, 2007; Pié *et al.*, 2010). Recently, mutations in another cohesin gene, *RAD21* (<1%) (8q24.11) (Deardorff *et al.*, 2012b) and in one encoding gene from a cohesin deactylase, *HDAC8* (Xp13.1) (Deardorff *et al.*, 2012a), have been recognized as a cause of CdLS.

The cohesin complex is essential for many biological processes including chromosome segregation, DNA repair, gene expression, and chromatin structure formation (Liu & Krantz, 2008, 2009; Liu *et al.*, 2009; Remeseiro & Losada, 2013). The complex has a highly conserved ring-shaped structure that encircles chromatin and consists of the core components: SMC1A, SMC3, RAD21 and stromal antigens, and has many associated factors such as stromalin, PDS5A/B, WAPL, MAU2 and NIPBL. NIPBL directly interacts with MAU2 to form a heterodimeric complex called kollerin (Braunholz *et al.*, 2012; Nasmyth, 2011), which regulates the loading and unloading of cohesin onto chromatin (Braunholz *et al.*, 2012; Nasmyth, 2011; Seitan *et al.*, 2006; Watrin *et al.*, 2006).

Turner syndrome (TS) is a common chromosomal disorder associated with short stature, skeletal anomalies, gonadal dysgenesis, cardiovascular defects, deafness, neck webbing and lymphedema and a propensity for autoimmune diseases; although many systems and tissues may also be affected to a lesser or greater extent (Chacko *et al.*, 2012; Gravholt, 2005; Pinsker, 2012; Saenger *et al.*, 2001). TS affects about one in 2000 newborn females and results from complete or partial absence of the second sex chromosome, with or without cell line mosaicism (Bondy, 2007; Ranke & Saenger, 2001).

The nondisjunction of the sex chromosome, which results in a 45,X female with TS can occur at either meiotic division in either spermatogenesis or oogenesis. Though, more than half of all patients with TS have a mosaic chromosomal complement (e.g., 45,X/46,XX) (Ranke & Saenger, 2001; Sybert & McCauley, 2004). Because of this, some researchers claim that the pure 45,X karyotype does not exist and suggest the necessity of mosaicism for foetus survival, and thus, a mitotic origin for this syndrome (Saenger, 1996). Nonetheless, the reasons for postzygotic X chromosome loss remain unclear.

Which chromosomal regions and genes account for the physical characteristics of TS remains uncertain. It has been hypothesized that the physical manifestations of TS are due either to the absence of two normal sex chromosomes before X-chromosome inactivation or to haploinsufficiency of genes in the pseudoautosomal regions of the X or Y chromosome, as well as to aneuploidy itself. Both the short arm and the long arm of the X chromosome contain genes important for ovarian function, and aneuploidy alone may lead to a reduction in the number and survival of oocytes (Sybert & McCauley, 2004).

To date, only five CdLS patients with chromosomal rearrangements with involvement of sex chromosomes have been reported, one male with 45,X/46,XY mosaicism (Calo *et al.*, 1968), one female with 45,X karyotype (Beck & Mikkelsen, 1981) and three females with mosaic 45,X/46,XX karyotypes (Hoppman-Chaney *et al.*, 2011; Klosovskii *et al.*, 1968; Wierzba *et al.*, 2012). But unfortunately, detailed clinical information and molecular characterization has only been reported in one of them (Wierzba *et al.*, 2012). Therefore, we are going to take as a diagnostic model the patient with the most complete description (Wierzba *et al.*, 2012), in order to focus on the clinical methods used to explain each feature, with special emphasis on neurological findings.

2   Case Presentation of the Model Patient with Co-existence of Both Syndromes

The patient is the first child of a 35-year-old father and a 37-year-old mother at the time of her birth; the parents are healthy and unrelated. The child is 5-year 6-month-old, born at 35 weeks of gestation by cesarean section due to fetal distress secondary to chronic intrauterine growth restriction. There was no family history of congenital defects but her mother had recurrent miscarriages. She also has a healthy younger brother. Her birth weight was 1.350 kg, length was 43 cm and the head circumference was 25 cm (all below the 3rd centile for gestational age). Apgar score was 7 in the first minute and 9 at five minutes. Craniofacial dysmorphism showed: synophrys, arched eyebrows, long and irregularly placed eyelashes, hypertelorism, depressed nasal bridge, anteverted nares, long and flat philtrum, thin upper lip, downslanting corners of the mouth, microretrognathia, high arched and vaulted palate, low-set and posteriorly rotated ears, low posterior hairline, short and webbed neck, microbrachycephaly and narrow bitemporal diameter (Figure 1 a-b, Table 1). Small hands and feet, 5th finger clinodactyly, proximally placed thumbs, single palmar crease and hip dysplasia were also noted. Other features apparent in the newborn period were hirsutism, slight feet lymphedema, *cutis marmorata* and lack of the sucking reflex (Figure 1 a-b, Table 1). Ophthalmological examination revealed congenital bilateral glaucoma and retinopathy. Echocardiogram showed an atrial and ventricular septal defect (ASD, VSD) with pulmonary stenosis (PS) that did not require surgery. The transfontanelar and abdominal ultrasonographies were normal. At two years of age, the gastroscopy revealed a gastritis antral I/II grade, but pH-metry was normal. The constipation, which responded poorly to the therapy, was noted from infancy, but Hirschsprung disease was excluded (Table 1).

At the last examination, at the age of 5 years and 3 months (Figure 1 c-d), her weight was 9.8 kg, height was 89 cm (both below 50th centile on CdLS growth charts), and head circumference was 43 cm (near 50th centile on CdLS growth charts). Additional findings included: broad chest with widely spaced nipples, short sternum, bilateral *cubitus valgus*, limited elbow extension, small and hypoplastic nails and myopia (Table 1). PS and VSD seen at birth, had resolved without therapy but a hemodynamically insignificant ASD still persists. Abdominal ultrasonography (USG) showed no abnormalities. Mild bilateral sensorineural hypoacusia was detected by auditory brainstem response (ABR), but good response to sounds was demonstrated (Table 1).

	Clinical features of Turner Syndrome	Clinical features of Cornelia de Lange Syndrome
Craniofacial features	Dental abnormalities **High and arched palate** **Micrognathia** **Low-set ears** **Low posterior hairline** **Short neck** Webbed neck	Synophrys Arched eyebrows Thick and long eyelashes Depressed nasal bridge Anteverted nares Long philtrum Thin upper lip Downturned corners Dental abnormalities **High and arched palate** **Micrognathia** Retrognathia **Low-set** and posteriorly rotated ears **Low posterior hairline** **Short neck** Microbrachycephaly Narrow bitemporal diameter
Neurologic findings and Cognitive profile	Most normal intelligence Learning disabilities Hyperactivity **Attention deficit disorder** **Anxiety** Social isolation Immaturity	CNS anomalies Seizures Hypertonia/ Hypotonia Intellectual disability and developmental delay Learning disabilities Emotional instability Hyperactivity **Attention deficit disorder** Autistic-like features Aggression and self-injurious behaviour Obsessive-compulsive characteristics High pain threshold Extreme shyness Perseveration Constant roaming Stereotype movements Depression **Anxiety**
Musculoskeletal system	Abnormal upper-to-lower segment ratio *Cubitus valgus* Short 4th metacarpal Short sternum Broad chest with widely-spaced nipples **Hip dysplasia** *Genu valgum* Patellae dislocation Scoliosis Bone age retardation Low bone mineral density	Absent arms or forearms/ Oligodactyly Radial head dislocation Abnormal elbow extension Small hands and/or feet Single palmar crease Proximally placed thumb 5th finger clinodactyly Short 1st metacarpal *Pectus excavatum* **Hip dysplasia** Syndactyly 3rd-4rd toes

ENT	**Hearing loss** Chronic otitis media	**Hearing loss** Otitis media/Sinusitis
Ophthalmic systems	**Ptosis** Epicanthus Strabismus Amblyopia Cataracts Nystagmus Hyperopia	**Ptosis** Telecanthus Hypertelorism Tear duct malformation Blepharitis Major eye malformation Peripapillary pigmentation Myopia
Skin & nails	Lymphoedema of hands and/or feet Multiple pigmented/Melanocytic nevi Hypoplastic nails	Hirsutism *Cutis marmorata*
Cardiac system	Bicuspid aortic valves (BAV) Coarctation of the aorta (COA) Aortic dilation/aneurysm and dissection Partial anomalous pulmonary connection (PAPVC) Conduction or repolarization abnormalities Systemic hypertension	Ventricular septal defect (VSD) Atrial septal defect (ASD) Pulmonar stenosis (PS)
Gastrointestinal system	**Feeding problems** **GERD during infancy** Vascular malformations of the gastrointestinal tract Inflammatory bowel disease (IBD) Celiac disease	**Feeding problems** **GERD** Gastrointestinal malformation/malrotation Constipation Diaphragmatic hernia Pyloric stenosis
Genitourinary systems	Horseshoe kidney Rotational abnormalities Double collecting systems Urinary tract infections Hydronephrosis Gonadal dysgenesis No pubertal development Premature ovarian failure Infertility Chronic estrogen deficiency /Elevated levels of FSH	Vesiculoureteral reflux Pelvic dilatation Renal dysplasia Hypoplastic genitalia
Endocrine involvement	Glucose intolerance/ Insulin resistance/ Type 2 diabetes Hypothyroidism / Thyroid antibody formation Elevated hepatic enzymes Dyslipidaemia Obesity	Develop obesity with age

Table 1: Typical clinical features of CdLS and TS[1] related to the proband's clinical findings, which are marked in black. Features highlighted in bold are those shared by both syndromes. Notes.- ENT: Ear-Nose-Throat; GERD: Gastroesophageal Reflux Disease. [1]These clinical features are compiled from different sources (CdLS: Gillis *et al.*, 2004; Kline *et al.*, 2007a; Kline *et al.*, 2007b; Oliveira *et al.*, 2010; Pie *et al.*, 2010; Rohatgi *et al.*, 2010; Yan *et al.*, 2006; and TS: Bondy, 2007; Chacko *et al.*, 2012; Gravholt, 2004, 2005; Hjerrild *et al.*, 2008; Pinsker, 2012; Ranke & Saenger, 2001; Saenger *et al.*, 2001; Sybert & McCauley, 2004).

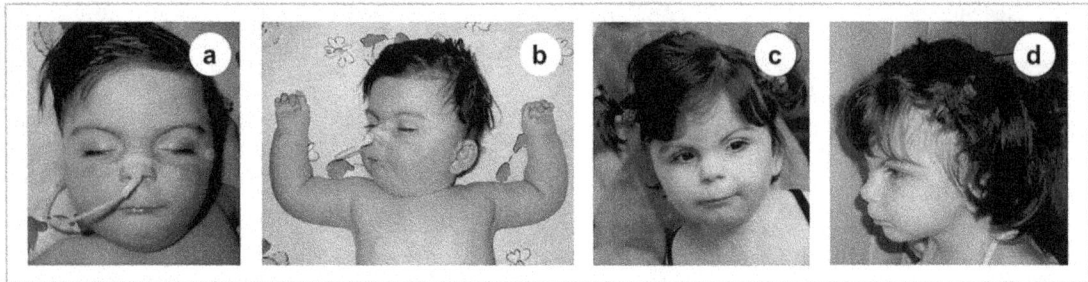

Figure 1: Phenotype of the patient. (a-b) Frontal and side-views and upper limb of the patient at the age of 2 years and 10 months. (c-d) Frontal and side-views at 5 years. Note typical CdLS facial features included synophrys, arched eyebrows, long eyelashes, depressed nasal bridge and anteverted nares, long and flat philtrum, thin upper lip, downslanting corners of the mouth, low set and posteriorly rotated ears and microretrognathia. She also showed some TS findings like the peripheral lymphedema and broad chest with widely-spaced nipples.

Biochemical, endocrine and metabolic features were also examined. Mean serum FSH concentration was close to normal. Thyroid function tests (T3, T4, TSH) and celiac screening (IgA-TTG and IgA-EmA antibodies) showed no abnormalities. Routine lipid profile was normal except for high TG (triglycerides) levels (232 mg/dL; normal value range for TG levels is <98 mg/dL).

Brain computed tomography (CT) revealed a slight focal cerebral atrophy (Figure 2). At the age of 4 years and 3 months, nystagmus was observed and the subsequent electroencephalography (EEG) was abnormal. Background rhythm in the parietal-occipital region contained beta and theta waves. There was a mild attenuation and slowing of the background rhythm. There was noted the presence of rhythmic sharp discharge and variable sharp discharge – slow discharge in the centro-temporal region. Those changes showed a tendency to left lateralization and generalization. Epilepsy was effectively controlled by pharmacological treatment. Neurological examination also showed a mild hypertonia, delayed age of closure of anterior fontanelle, high pain threshold and abnormal deep tendon reflexes.

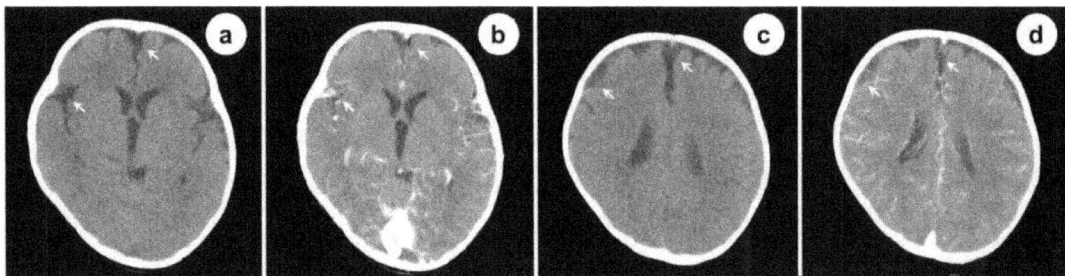

Figure 2: CT image of the brain at the age of 8 months. Note a slight focal cerebral atrophy (arrows) and disproportionate atrophy of frontal lobes. CT scan slices without contrast (a-c) and with contrast (b-d).

She is being treated by Psychiatry due to several behaviour issues: emotional instability, short attention span, autistic-like features, perseveration, anxiety, immaturity, and stereotype movements. In addition, episodes of aggression or self-injurious behaviour were reported. Autistic behaviour was assessed with CARS (Childhood Autism Rating Score) test and the total score obtained was 43, which rated as severe autism. Behaviour was evaluated with Vineland Adaptive Behaviour Scales (VABS), score obtained was 16, which rated as profoundly deficient adaptive behaviour.

Developmental milestones were extremely delayed. The patient was assessed using the Brunet-Lezine Psychomotor Development Scale; score of 9 was obtained, which rated as markedly psychomotor delay. The age when the patient reached the milestones of each developmental area tested (Gross motor skills, Fine motor tasks, Personal-social and Speech) are detailed in Table 2. When the proband was 1 month old, she was enrolled in early intervention programs. She was just able to sit unsupported, but not to walk and to run at the age of 5 years and 3 months. Speech was absent but she could spell simple sounds. She was able to communicate through a few gestures and to follow simple orders due to the application of alternative communication intervention since she was 1 year and 6 months old.

Developmental Area	Milestone	CdLS-TS proband	CdLS*	Standard parameters
Gross motor	Rolls over	12 m	7 m	3 m
	Sits alone	26 m	12 m	5 ½ m
	Crawls	18 m	15 m	-
	Pulls to stand	4 y 6 m	16 m	-
	Cruises	> 5 y 3 m	17 m	9 ½ m
	Walks alone	> 5 y 3 m	24 m	12 m
	Run	> 5 y 3 m	3 y	-
Fine motor	Reaches	~ 10 m	6 m	-
	Grasps	~ 8 m	6 m	-
	Transfers	24 m	12 m	-
Personal/Social	Smiles	1 ½ m	3 m	1 ½ m
	Laughs	3 m	5 m	2 m
	Feeds self: Bottle	18 m	11 m	-
	Feeds self: Fingers	3 y	18 m	5 ½ m
	Feeds self: Cup	> 5 y 3 m	24 m	11 ½ m
	Feeds self: Spoon	> 5 y 3 m	3 y	-
	Clothes: take off	> 5 y 3 m	4 y	3 y 6 m
	Clothes: puts on	> 5 y 3 m	5 y	3 y 6 m
	Toiled trained	> 5 y 3 m	3 y	24 m
Speech	Babbles	18 m	10 m	7 m
	First word	> 5 y 3 m	18 m	10 m
	Understand commands simple	2 y 6 m	2 y 6 m	10 m
	Communicates other gestures	3 y	3 y	12 m
	Puts word together	> 5 y 3 m	4 y 6 m	20 m

Table 2: Psychomotor development. Milestones and ages of acquisition in CdLS-TS proband compared to CdLS* and unaffected individuals (*Age on acquisition of each skill for 50% of CdLS individuals, based on the Kline et al., (Kline *et al.*, 1993)).

3 Approach to Clinical Features of CdLS *vs.* TS

Clinical diagnosis of CdLS was based primarily on the clinical findings like craniofacial features, pre- and post-natal growth delay (weight, length and head circumference at birth below the 3rd centile), intellectual disability, poor psychomotor development, learning disabilities, specific behavioural impairments, congenital cardiovascular abnormalities and hirsutism (Table 1). Interestingly, this patient also showed some keys findings of TS diagnosis in the newborn like the peripheral lymphedema and webbed neck as result of the residua of the fetal lymphedema and cystic hygromas (Bondy, 2007; Gravholt, 2005). Other findings consistent with TS included: *cubitus valgus*, nail hypoplasia, short sternum, broad chest with widely spaced nipples and inefficient sucking and swallowing reflexes in the neonatal period (Table 1). She also had characteristic overlap features of both syndromes, including short stature, low set ears, high arched palate, congenital hip dysplasia, sensorineural hearing loss and speech delay (Bondy, 2007; Kline *et al.*, 2007b; Saenger *et al.*, 2001) (Table 1). In summary, the model patient showed predominant CdLS features, although she could have new TS symptoms like puberty delay in the adolescence.

Following the criteria proposed by Kline *et al.* [2007] (Kline *et al.*, 2007b), the patient had a severe CdLS phenotype, although with mild upper limb anomalies. Interestingly, she showed multiple abnormalities and minor musculoskeletal defects consist with CdLS as small hands and feet, 5th finger clinodactyly, proximally placed thumb, single palmar crease and limited elbow extension (Kline *et al.*, 2007b) (Table 1). By contrast only the bilateral *cubitus valgus* is typical in TS (Bondy, 2007) (Table 1).

The high palate is a feature common in both syndromes, however it is just considered as a secondary diagnostic criteria for CdLS (Kline *et al.*, 2007b), while as a clinical timely marker for the TS (Savendahl & Davenport, 2000). Moreover a high incidence of palate defects was noted more often in CdLS patients, who carried mutations in *SMC1A* gene rather than in *NIPBL* gene (Pie *et al.*, 2010).

Ophthalmologic findings have been reported in a high percentage of CdLS and TS patients (Kline *et al.*, 2007b; Levin *et al.*, 1990; Lloyd *et al.*, 1997). Two large studies in CdLS individuals have revealed the presence of hypertrichosis (96%), synophrys (99%), long eyelashes (99%), myopia (57-58%) and ptosis (44-46%) (Wygnanski *et al.*, 2005; Nallasamy *et al.*, 2006) Nevertheless a remarkable feature in this disorder is the finding of peripapillary pigment rings, which are found in 83% of patients (Barakat *et al.*, 2009). Regarding TS, clinically significant strabismus and hyperopia ocurred in 25-35% of the patients with this condition. Cataracts and nystagmus also occur more commonly in patients with TS. Red-green colour deficiency is present in approximately 8% of the population with TS, a percentage similar to that found in males (Sybert & McCauley, 2004). However, the congenital bilateral glaucoma diagnosed in this proband has been uncommonly described in both disorders, only in three CdLS cases (Lee *et al.*, 2003; Nallasamy *et al.*, 2006) and in three other patients with TS (Lloyd *et al.*, 1997). Hence, it is not certain if there is a true association between glaucoma with CdLS or TS, or if this are just coincidental finding.

The prevalence of congenital heart defects (CHDs) have been reported among 17 to 45% of patients with TS and 13 to 70% of CdLS cases. Clinically, the residual postnatal webbed neck found in the proband, could be able to predict defects common in TS such as bicuspid aortic valve and aortic coarctation (Bondy, 2007, 2008; Pinsker, 2012). However, these cardiovascular anomalies were discarded in our case by echocardiography. But she still had ASD, VSD and PS; typical CHDs in CdLS and rarely seen in TS (<0,5%) (Chatfield *et al.*, 2012; Gravholt, 2004; Kline *et al.*, 2007b; Selicorni *et al.*, 2009; Sybert & McCauley, 2004). Besides, ASD, VSD and PS as isolated defects appear to be the most common in CdLS (Chatfield *et al.*, 2012; Selicorni *et al.*, 2007) (Table 1), though their combination has been just reported in 2 additional cases (Selicorni *et al.*, 2009; Tsukahara *et al.*, 1998).

Traditionally gonadal dysgenesis, with delayed or absent pubertal development and subsequent infertility, has been considered an almost universal feature of TS (Bondy, 2007; Saenger *et al.*, 2001) (Table 1). Besides, it is usually accompanied by an increase in gonadotropins, especially FSH. However, the study reported by Fechner *et al.*, demonstrated that young girls with 45,X/46,XX mosaicism have FSH values close to normal (Fechner *et al.*, 2006), just like it has been detected in the proband. Hence, it could be an important prognostic sign of ovarian structure and function. In fact, it has been previously described that two fifths of girls with 45,X/46,XX mosaicism have spontaneous menarche and even fertility (Sybert & McCauley, 2004).

Individuals with TS clearly have increased risk of autoimmune diseases like celiac disease and thyroiditis, generally associated with antithyroid antibodies (Gravholt, 2004) (Table 1). Autoimmune thyroid disease is common during childhood in TS and has been reported as early as 4 years age. There are some studies that have reported a prevalence of 24% of hypothyroidism in their cohorts (Bondy, 2007). Recently the immunologic features of CdLS, have been described. Interestingly, it has been demonstrated that these individuals have a high risk of developing idiopathic thrombocytopenic purpura or autoimmune hemolytic anemia due to a dysfunction in the Tfh cells (Jyonouchi *et al.*, 2013). Because there are not always overt clinical symptoms, these diseases have to be looked for on a regular basis (Bondy, 2007; Saenger *et al.*, 2001). Overall, endocrine and autoimmune studies were normal in the patient. Only the lipid profile was abnormal due to elevated TG plasma levels. This finding was previously seen only in women with TS, suggesting that the X chromosome deletion could be associated with dyslipidemia (Bondy, 2007).

Neurological involvement in CdLS, primarily includes seizures in 23% of the classic and/or severe cases, with no specific pattern on EEG and most of them respond satisfactorily to pharmacological treatment (Kline *et al.*, 2007b) (Table 1). However, there is little information about seizure semiology, EEG findings and the natural course of epilepsy in CdLS patients. Recently a more detailed description of epilepsy in CdLS individuals has been published, which has disclosed that the most common type of epilepsy in CdLS patients is partial epilepsy, it has a favourable course and responds well to monotherapy with anti-epileptic medication (Verrotti *et al.*, 2013). Nevertheless in TS, seizures or epilepsy are rarely found (Chacko *et al.*, 2012). It is remarkable, that our case shares many of the newly described characteristics of epilepsy reported in CdLS like the age of onset (4 years), type of epilepsy (focal seizures compatible with partial epilepsy) and the favorable outcome with anti-epileptic drug therapy (Depakene ™). Taken into account that the brain is the organ most sensitive to cohesin disruption (Baquero-Montoya *et al.*, 2013; Mannini *et al.*, 2010), the neurological manifestations in this individual could be mainly explained due to the mutation in *NIPBL*.

Radiologic brain findings in CdLS may include enlarged ventricles, enlargement of basal cisterns, thinning or atrophy of white matter (Kline *et al.*, 2007b). In contrast, in TS brain abnormalities are infrequent (Chacko *et al.*, 2012). The focal cerebral atrophy is a non-specific brain anomaly, but perhaps in our case suggests a predominance of the CdLS phenotype. Additional clinical findings that support this hypothesis are the presence of hypertonia in the newborn period as well as the delayed age of closure of anterior fontanelle, high pain threshold and abnormal deep tendon reflexes (Table 1).

Typically development is delayed in CdLS individuals (Kline *et al.*, 1993) (Table 2), with a range from borderline IQ with learning disabilities to profound intellectual disability (ID) (Kline *et al.*, 2007b). The primarily affected developmental milestones are the speech and language (Kline *et al.*, 2007b) (Table 2). On the contrary most individuals with TS have normal intelligence, but some of them might experience cognitive impairments in areas of mathematics, visual-spatial function, executive function and specific aspects of language (Bondy, 2007; Chacko *et al.*, 2012). Our proband had global developmental delay with a predominance of speech impairment (Table 2), being difficult to fit these clinical findings in any of the two syndromes, though there is a slight trend towards CdLS.

The patient's behaviour impairments such as emotional instability, short attention span, perseveration, anxiety, immaturity, self-injurious behaviour and autistic spectrum disorder are striking (Table 1). These findings are classically described in CdLS, where the spectrum of behavioral issues goes from hyperactivity with or without attention deficit disorder, short attention span, aggression to autistic spectrum disorder. These features also correlate with the degree of intellectual disability (Kline *et al.*, 2007b) (Table 1). In turn in TS, specific behaviour problems with severe degree of impairment are not frequent (Bondy, 2007; Chacko *et al.*, 2012).

4   Molecular Analyses

In order to identify disease-causing mutations, the molecular genetic analysis of *NIPBL* was performed, which is the first and main demonstrated cause of CdLS (CDLS1, OMIM 122470) and account for ~70% of cases with classical faces (Krantz *et al.*, 2004; Tonkin *et al.*, 2004). This screening identified a *de novo* heterozygous frameshift mutation in exon 9 of the *NIPBL* gene (c.1445_1448delGAGA; p.(Arg482Asnfs*20)) (Figure 3), which had also been reported in a female CdLS patient from Portugal (Oliveira *et al.*, 2010).

To explore the possibility that the proband could carry the *NIPBL* mutation in mosaic state, the molecular analysis by Sanger sequencing was performed on DNA samples from different embryonic origins: peripheral blood lymphocytes (mesoderm) and oral mucosa epithelial cells (ectoderm). The mutation-related peaks were similar to those of the wild type allele, discarding somatic mosaicism. This suggests that *NIPBL* mutation may have appeared during meiotic division in either spermatogenesis or oogenesis or in early embryonic mitotic cell divisions.

Similar to other frameshift mutations, this one (c.1445_1448delGAGA) results in a predicted stop codon and consecutive truncation of the translational product (p.(Arg482Asnfs*20)). The comparison between sequences of NIPBL and homologous proteins from different species suggests the presence of two phylogenetically differentiated regions: the N-terminal 1150 amino acids which are apparently only conserved in vertebrates; and the C-terminal sequence, found in representative species of all eukaryotes, from yeast to human (Pie *et al.*, 2010; Strachan, 2005; Wierzba *et al.*, 2012). The big exon 9 codifies 209 amino acids located within the N-terminal half of the protein, where it has been found just seven additional mutations but all of them frameshift. Among more than 250 mutations previously reported in *NIPBL*, the fact that most of frameshift mutations are located in this N-terminal half of the protein (~ 48,5% *vs* 24% C-terminal half), suggests that this domain is important although it has not been associated with any function yet (Pie *et al.*, 2010; Strachan, 2005; Wierzba *et al.*, 2012).

5   Genotype-phenotype Correlations

Molecular genetic analysis finally validated the clinical diagnosis of CdLS caused by a heterozygous frameshift *NIPBL* mutation (c.1445_1448delGAGA; p.(Arg482Asnfs*20)) (Figure 3). As mentioned before, this mutation has been previously identified in a female CdLS patient from Portugal (Oliveira *et al.*,

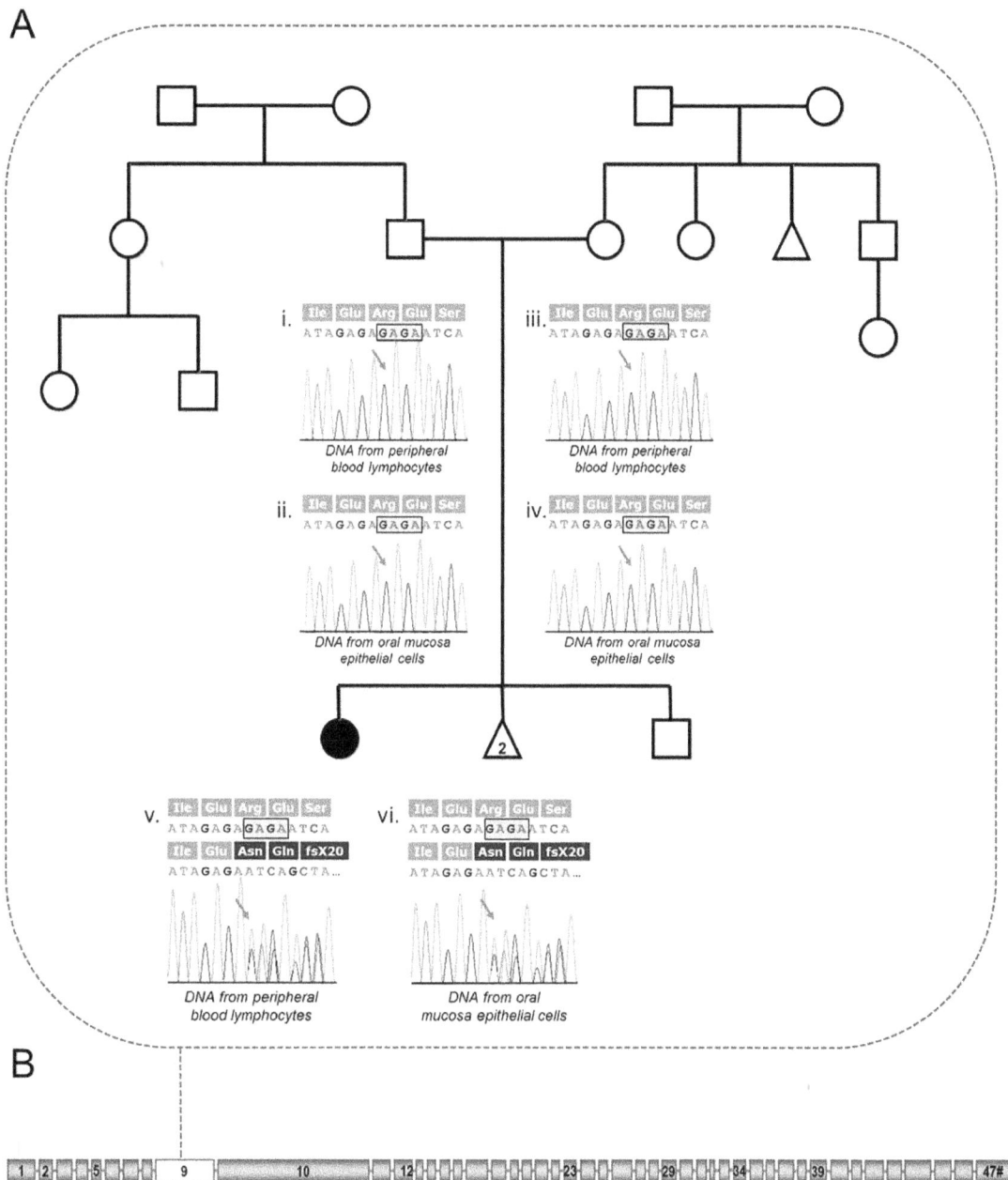

Figure 3: (A) Pedigree of the affected family and partial electropherograms of exon 9 of the *NIPBL* gene. White symbols indicate unaffected individuals, whereas a black symbol indicates the affected individual. The sequencing analysis performed on genomic DNA from the patient peripheral blood lymphocytes (v) and oral mucosa epithelial cells (vi) shows similar heights of the peaks of the allele carrying the c.1445_1448delGAGA mutation in both tissues. Wild-type electropherograms identified in the normal parents are also indicated (i-iv). (B) Schematic model of the *NIPBL* gene. The exon 9 of the *NIPBL* gene is highlighted in white.

2010). This female patient also showed facial dysmorphic features, severe growth retardation, small hands and feet, and no major malformations. Unfortunately, we cannot compare the phenotype of both patients due to the lack of a detailed clinical information of the reported CdLS patient (Oliveira *et al.*, 2010). However, we should emphasize that both patients showed a severe phenotype without limb reduction defects.

According to medical literature, the proband shared the typical phenotypic parameters of *NIPBL* mutation carriers, which are significantly different from those without detectable mutation. Among these features are included: the classic facial features (anteverted nostrils, depressed nasal bridge, short neck and narrowing of the bitemporal diameter), pre-natal and post-natal growth retardation, developmental delay, and even a speech impairment and hearing loss (Bhuiyan *et al.*, 2006; Gillis *et al.*, 2004; Oliveira *et al.*, 2010; Pié *et al.*, 2010; Rohatgi *et al.*, 2010; Selicorni *et al.*, 2007; Yan *et al.*, 2006). Besides, she did not present limb reduction defects, which is consistent with Oliveira's former report, which described that 65% of individuals with *NIPBL* mutations had small hands only or no abnormality of the upper limbs (Oliveira *et al.*, 2010).

In addition, it should be noticed that truncating mutations usually result in haploinsufficiency and led to more severe phenotypes, which seems to be shown by the proband described in this chapter. In fact, this trend has been previously demonstrated in patients with *NIPBL* mutations who carry this kind of mutation (Bhuiyan *et al.*, 2006; Gillis *et al.*, 2004; Oliveira *et al.*, 2010; Pié *et al.*, 2010; Rohatgi *et al.*, 2010; Selicorni *et al.*, 2007; Yan *et al.*, 2006).

6   Cytogenetic and FISH Analyses

To confirm the clinical diagnosis of TS, conventional cytogenetic investigation was performed on metaphase chromosomes prepared from cultured peripheral blood lymphocytes. GTG banding confirmed female gender and showed that her karyotype was 45,X/46,XX, with 24% cells containing only one chromosome X. Parent's karyotypes had to be also examined and were confirmed to be normal.

Most of patients with mosaic form of Turner syndrome (92%) have considerable tissue specific differences in levels of X aneuploidy (Nazarenko et al., 1999), due to that, we decided to perform additional FISH analysis of interphase nuclei of tissues from different germ layers (lymphocytes from mesoderm and buccal epithelial cells from ectoderm) that allowed more precise definition of the cytogenetic diagnosis. This analysis confirmed the presence of 45,X/46,XX mosaicism in both tissues, 28 % of monosomy X in peripheral blood lymphocytes ((nuc ish (DXZ1X1, DYZ1X0)[140], (DXZ1X2 DYZ1X0)[360]) and only 7% of cells in buccal smears ((nuc ish (DXZ1X1, DYZ1X0)[7], (DXZ1X2 DYZ1X0)[83]).

7   Karyotype-phenotype Correlations

The phenotype of one patient with TS would depend upon the temporal and anatomical distribution of 45,X cell populations during developing embryo (Sybert & McCauley, 2004). Therefore, even knowing the degree of 45,X/46,XX mosaicism of leukocytes or buccal epithelial cells from the patient, these tissues may not accurately represent the degree of mosaicism and clinical involvement in other organs more frequently affected such as the gonad and heart (Bondy, 2008; Fechner *et al.*, 2006; Nazarenko *et al.*, 1999).

Due to previously mentioned data, the phenotypic predictions in Turner syndrome that are based on karyotype are unreliable (Davenport, 2010). Even so, some correlations between 45,X/46,XX karyotype and phenotype have been reported. These patients are taller than regular women with TS; who are also the most likely to have spontaneous menarche and fertility. Besides the intellectual and learning disabilities seem to be less common among them (Sybert & McCauley, 2004). However, these positive predictions about the height parameter and cognitive profile are masked by the predominant CdLS features that showed the proband.

8   Molecular Mechanisms Underlying Co-existence of Both Rare Disorders

The coexistence in several patients of these two rare disorders raises the issue of whether there is indeed a cause-effect association. Recently, truncating mutations in *NIPBL* gene have been found in some colorectal cancers related with chromosomal instability and aneuploidy (Barber *et al.*, 2008; Barbero, 2011; Liu & Krantz, 2009). The authors suggested that these mutations could disrupt the chromosome segregation (Barber *et al.*, 2008; Barbero, 2011), carried through cohesion complex, during mitosis and meiosis. Therefore, *NIPBL* mutation might be the cause of the loss of an X chromosome in our proband (Barber *et al.*, 2008; Mannini *et al.*, 2010). Indeed, it must have happened during embryonic mitotic cell divisions, since she also carried a normal cell line. Moreover, this hypothesis could account for numerous chromosomal rearrangements in individuals with CdLS that have been reported over the years (DeScipio *et al.*, 2005; Hoppman-Chaney *et al.*, 2011; Wierzba *et al.*, 2012; Wierzba *et al.*, 2011).

9   Differential Diagnosis

In this case, there is a predominance of CdLS manifestations; therefore the differential diagnosis should be focused in this disorder. Currently there are several conditions demonstrated to overlap with the clinical features of CdLS.

- **Fryns syndrome** is characterized by coarse facies, diaphragmatic hernia (85%), cleft palate (30%) and distal limb hypoplasia (75%). Hypertrichosis, narrow palpebral fissures, flat nasal bridge, upturned nose, micrognathia and cardiac, renal, and genital abnormalities are common in both CdLS and Fryns Syndrome. Individuals with Fryns syndrome have a short upper lip, macrostomia, prenatal polyhydramnios, premature birth and normal birth weight. Inheritance of Fryns syndrome is autosomal recessive (Yucesoy *et al.*, 2008).

- **Fetal alcohol syndrome** is characterized by intrauterine growth retardation, failure to thrive, developmental abdnormalities, microcephaly, facial hirsutism, short palpebral fissures, short upturned nose, smooth underdeveloped philtrum, thin upper lip and cardiac defects. Nevertheless, the hands and feet in this disorder are not small and speech is less affected than in CdLS. Usually the history of alcohol use in the pregnancy is helpful in discriminating this disorder from CdLS (Douzgou *et al.*, 2012).

- **Coffin-Siris Syndrome** is characterized by aplasia or hypoplasia of the distal phalanx or nail of the fifth digit, distinctive facial features (wide mouth with thick, everted upper and lower lips, broad nasal bridge with broad nasal tip, thick eyebrows and long eyelashes, thin vermillion border of the upper lip), moderate to severe developmental/cognitive delay, failure to thrive, feeding difficulties, short stature, ophthalmologic abnormalities, microcephaly, brain malformations and hearing loss. Currently the diagnosis is based on the clinical findings and in the detection of mutations in *ARID1A, ARID1B, SMARCA4, SMARCB1* or *SMCARE1* (Coulibaly *et al.*, 2010).

10   Conclusions

In this chapter, we presented a clinical real case of a female with CdLS due to a mutation in the *NIPBL* gene, and TS with a mosaic 45,X/46,XX karyotype tissue-specific. Recently it has been hypothesized that *NIPBL* could play a role in these rearrangements, mainly because there is a high percentage of CdLS patients, who also carry genomic imbalances. So in the presence of a possible CdLS patient, who also has atypical clinical findings or a severe neurological involvement, it is reasonable to rule out simultaneously chromosomal or genomic rearrangements.

Acknowledgement

We sincerely thank the patient's family for participating in this study. This study was funded by grants from: The Spanish Ministry of Health - Fondo de Investigación Sanitaria (FIS) (Ref.#PI12/01318), the Diputación General de Aragón (Grupo Consolidado B20), European Social Fund (Construyendo Europa desde Aragón), University of Zaragoza (Ref.# PIF-UZ_2009-BIO-02).

References

Baquero-Montoya, C., Gil-Rodriguez, M., Teresa-Rodrigo, M., Hernandez-Marcos, M., Bueno-Lozano, G., Bueno-Martinez, I., Remeseiro, S., Fernandez-Hernandez, R., Bassecourt-Serra, M., Rodriguez de Alba, M., Queralt, E., Losada, A., Puisac, B., Ramos, F., & Pie, J. (2013). Could a patient with SMC1A duplication be classified as a human cohesinopathy? Clinical genetics. doi: 10.1111/cge.12194.

Barakat, M. R., Traboulsi, E. I., & Sears, J. E. (2009). Coat's Disease, Megalopapilla and Cornelia de Lange Syndrome. Ophtalmic Genetics, 30, 106-108.

Barber, T. D., McManus, K., Yuen, K. W., Reis, M., Parmigiani, G., Shen, D., Barrett, I., Nouhi, Y., Spencer, F., Markowitz, S., Velculescu, V. E., Kinzler, K. W., Vogelstein, B., Lengauer, C., & Hieter, P. (2008). Chromatid cohesion defects may underlie chromosome instability in human colorectal cancers. Proceedings of the National Academy of Sciences of the United States of America, 105, 3443-3448.

Barbero, J. L. (2011). Sister chromatid cohesion control and aneuploidy. Cytogenetic and Genome Research, 133, 223-233.

Barisic, I., Tokic, V., Loane, M., Bianchi, F., Calzolari, E., Garne, E., Wellesley, D., & Dolk, H. (2008). Descriptive epidemiology of Cornelia de Lange syndrome in Europe. American Journal of Medical Genetics Part A, 146A, 51-59.

Beck, B. & Mikkelsen, M. (1981). Chromosomes in the Cornelia de Lange syndrome. Human Genetics, 59, 271-276.

Bhuiyan, Z. A., Klein, M., Hammond, P., van Haeringen, A., Mannens, M. M., Van Berckelaer-Onnes, I., & Hennekam, R. C. (2006). Genotype-phenotype correlations of 39 patients with Cornelia De Lange syndrome: the Dutch experience. *Journal Medical Genetics, 43, 568-575.*

Bondy, C. A. (2007). Care of girls and women with Turner syndrome: a guideline of the Turner Syndrome Study Group. *The Journal of Clinical Endocrinology and Metabolism, 92, 10-25.*

Bondy, C. A. (2008). Congenital cardiovascular disease in Turner syndrome. *Congenital Heart Disease, 3, 2-15.*

Braunholz, D., Hullings, M., Gil-Rodriguez, M. C., Fincher, C. T., Mallozzi, M. B., Loy, E., Albrecht, M., Kaur, M., Limon, J., Rampuria, A., Clark, D., Kline, A., Dalski, A., Eckhold, J., Tzschach, A., Hennekam, R., Gillessen-Kaesbach, G., Wierzba, J., Krantz, I. D., Deardorff, M. A., & Kaiser, F. J. (2012). Isolated NIPBL missense mutations that cause Cornelia de Lange syndrome alter MAU2 interaction. *European Journal of Human Genetics, 20, 271-276.*

Calo, S., Gualandri, W., & Radice, C. (1968). [XY-XO mosaicism in a case of Cornelia De Lange syndrome]. *Minerva pediatrica, 20, 2600-2604.*

Chacko, E., Graber, E., Regelmann, M. O., Wallach, E., Costin, G., & Rapaport, R. (2012). Update on Turner and Noonan syndromes. *Endocrinology and Metabolism Clinics of North America, 41, 713-734.*

Chatfield, K. C., Schrier, S. A., Li, J., Clark, D., Kaur, M., Kline, A. D., Deardorff, M. A., Jackson, L. S., Goldmuntz, E., & Krantz, I. D. (2012). Congenital heart disease in Cornelia de Lange syndrome: phenotype and genotype analysis. *American Journal of Medical Genetics Part A, 158A, 2499-2505.*

Coulibaly, B., Sigaudy, S., Girard, N., Popovici, C., Missirian, H.H., Tasei, A.M., & Fernandez, C. (2010). Coffin-Siris syndrome with multiple congenital malformations and intrauterine death: Towards a better delineation of the severe end of the spectrum. *European Journal of Medical Genetics, 53, 318-321.*

Davenport, M. L. (2010). Approach to the patient with Turner syndrome. *The Journal of Clinical Endocrinology and Metabolism, 95, 1487-1495.*

Deardorff, M. A., Bando, M., Nakato, R., Watrin, E., Itoh, T., Minamino, M., Saitoh, K., Komata, M., Katou, Y., Clark, D., Cole, K. E., De Baere, E., Decroos, C., Di Donato, N., Ernst, S., Francey, L. J., Gyftodimou, Y., Hirashima, K., Hullings, M., Ishikawa, Y., Jaulin, C., Kaur, M., Kiyono, T., Lombardi, P. M., Magnaghi-Jaulin, L., Mortier, G. R., Nozaki, N., Petersen, M. B., Seimiya, H., Siu, V. M., Suzuki, Y., Takagaki, K., Wilde, J. J., Willems, P. J., Prigent, C., Gillessen-Kaesbach, G., Christianson, D. W., Kaiser, F. J., Jackson, L. G., Hirota, T., Krantz, I. D., & Shirahige, K.(2012a). HDAC8 mutations in Cornelia de Lange syndrome affect the cohesin acetylation cycle. *Nature, 489, 313-317.*

Deardorff, M. A., Kaur, M., Yaeger, D., Rampuria, A., Korolev, S., Pie, J., Gil-Rodriguez, C., Arnedo, M., Loeys, B., Kline, A. D., Wilson, M., Lillquist, K., Siu, V., Ramos, F. J., Musio, A., Jackson, L. S., Dorsett, D., & Krantz, I. D. (2007). Mutations in cohesin complex members SMC3 and SMC1A cause a mild variant of cornelia de Lange syndrome with predominant mental retardation. *American Journal of Human Genetics, 80, 485-494.*

Deardorff, M. A., Wilde, J. J., Albrecht, M., Dickinson, E., Tennstedt, S., Braunholz, D., Mönnich, M., Yan, Y., Xu, W., Gil-Rodríguez, M. C., Clark, D., Hakonarson, H., Halbach, S., Michelis, L.D., Rampuria, A., Rossier, E., Spranger, S., Van Maldergem, L., Lynch, S.A., Gillessen-Kaesbach, G., Lüdecke, H.J., Ramsay, R.G., McKay, M.J., Krantz, I.D., Xu, H., Horsfield, J. A., & Kaiser, F. J. (2012b). RAD21 mutations cause a human cohesinopathy. *American Journal of Human Genetics, 90, 1014-1027.*

DeScipio, C., Kaur, M., Yaeger, D., Innis, J. W., Spinner, N. B., Jackson, L. G., & Krantz, I. D. (2005). Chromosome rearrangements in cornelia de Lange syndrome (CdLS): report of a der(3)t(3;12)(p25.3;p13.3) in two half sibs with features of CdLS and review of reported CdLS cases with chromosome rearrangements. *American Journal of Medical Genetics Part A, 137A, 276-282.*

Douzgou, S., Breen, C., Crow, Y.J., Chandler, K., Metcalfe, K., Jones, E., Kerr, B., & Clayton-Smith, J. (2012). Diagnosing fetal alcohol syndrome: new insights from newer genetic technologies. *Archives of Disease in Childhood, 97, 812-817.*

Fechner, P. Y., Davenport, M. L., Qualy, R. L., Ross, J. L., Gunther, D. F., Eugster, E. A., Huseman, C., Zagar, A. J., & Quigley, C. A. (2006). Differences in follicle-stimulating hormone secretion between 45,X monosomy Turner syndrome and 45,X/46,XX mosaicism are evident at an early age. The Journal of Clinical Endocrinology and Metabolism, 91, 4896-4902.

Gillis, L. A., McCallum, J., Kaur, M., DeScipio, C., Yaeger, D., Mariani, A., Kline, A. D., Li, H. H., Devoto, M., Jackson, L. G., & Krantz, I. D. (2004). NIPBL mutational analysis in 120 individuals with Cornelia de Lange syndrome and evaluation of genotype-phenotype correlations. American Journal of Human Genetics, 75, 610-623.

Gravholt, C. H. (2004). Epidemiological, endocrine and metabolic features in Turner syndrome. European Journal of Endocrinology / European Federation of Endocrine Societies, 151, 657-687.

Gravholt, C. H. (2005). Clinical practice in Turner syndrome. Nature Clinical Practice Endocrinology & Metabolism, 1, 41-52.

Hjerrild, B. E., Mortensen, K. H., & Gravholt, C. H. (2008). Turner syndrome and clinical treatment. British Medical Bulletin, 86, 77-93.

Hoppman-Chaney, N., Jang, J. S., Jen, J., Babovic-Vuksanovic, D., & Hodge, J. C. (2011). In-frame multi-exon deletion of SMC1A in a severely affected female with Cornelia de Lange Syndrome. American Journal of Medical Genetics Part A, 158A, 193-198.

Jyonouchi, S., Orange, J., Sullivan, K.E., Krantz, I., & Deardorff, M. (2013). Immunologic Features of Cornelia de Lange Syndrome. Pediatrics, doi:10.1542/peds.2012-3815.

Kline, A. D., Grados, M., Sponseller, P., Levy, H. P., Blagowidow, N., Schoedel, C., Rampolla, J., Clemens, D. K., Krantz, I., Kimball, A., Pichard, C., & Tuchman, D. (2007a). Natural history of aging in Cornelia de Lange syndrome. American Journal of Medical Genetics Part C, 145C, 248-260.

Kline, A. D., Krantz, I. D., Sommer, A., Kliewer, M., Jackson, L. G., FitzPatrick, D. R., Levin, A. V., & Selicorni, A. (2007b). Cornelia de Lange syndrome: clinical review, diagnostic and scoring systems, and anticipatory guidance. American Journal of Medical Genetics Part A, 143A, 1287-1296.

Kline, A. D., Stanley, C., Belevich, J., Brodsky, K., Barr, M., & Jackson, L. G. (1993). Developmental data on individuals with the Brachmann-de Lange syndrome. American Journal of Medical Genetics, 47, 1053-1058.

Klosovskii, B. N., Iankova, M. F., Fateeva, E. M., & Damanskaia, L. (1968). [On the problem of the De Lange's syndrome]. Pediatriia, 47, 33-39.

Krantz, I. D., McCallum, J., DeScipio, C., Kaur, M., Gillis, L. A., Yaeger, D., Jukofsky, L., Wasserman, N., Bottani, A., Morris, C. A., Nowaczyk, M. J., Toriello, H., Bamshad, M. J., Carey, J. C., Rappaport, E., Kawauchi, S., Lander, A. D., Calof, A. L., Li, H. H., Devoto, M., & Jackson, L. G. (2004). Cornelia de Lange syndrome is caused by mutations in NIPBL, the human homolog of Drosophila melanogaster Nipped-B. Nature Genetics, 36, 631-635.

Lee, W. B., Brandt, J. D., Mannis, M. J., Huang, C. Q., & Rabin, G. J. (2003). Aniridia and Brachmann-de Lange syndrome: a review of ocular surface and anterior segment findings. Cornea, 22, 178-180.

Levin, A. V., Seidman, D. J., Nelson, L. B., & Jackson, L. G. (1990). Ophthalmologic findings in the Cornelia de Lange syndrome. Journal of Pediatric Ophthalmology and Strabismus, 27, 94-102.

Liu, J. & Krantz, I. D. (2008). Cohesin and human disease. Annual Review of Genomics and Human Genetics, 9, 303-320.

Liu, J. & Krantz, I. D. (2009). Cornelia de Lange syndrome, cohesin, and beyond. Clinical genetics, 76, 303-314.

Liu, J., Z Zhang, Z., Bando, M., Itoh, T., Deardorff, M. A., Clark, D., Kaur, M., Tandy, S., Kondoh, T., Rappaport, E., Spinner, N. B., Vega, H., Jackson, L. G., Shirahige, K., & Krantz, I. D. (2009). Transcriptional dysregulation in NIPBL and cohesin mutant human cells. PLoS biology, 7, e1000119.

Lloyd, I. C., Haigh, P. M., Clayton-Smith, J., Clayton, P., Price, D. A., Ridgway, A. E., & Donnai, D. (1997). Anterior segment dysgenesis in mosaic Turner syndrome. British Journal of Ophthalmology, 81, 639-643.

Mannini, L., Liu, J., Krantz, I. D., & Musio, A. (2010). Spectrum and consequences of SMC1A mutations: the unexpected involvement of a core component of cohesin in human disease. Human Mutation, 31, 5-10.

Musio, A., Selicorni, A., Focarelli, M.L., Gervasini, C., Milani, D., Russo, S., Vezzoni, P., & Larizza, L. (2006). X-linked Cornelia de Lange syndrome owing to SMC1L1 mutations. Nature Genetics, 38, 528-530.

Nallasamy, S., Kherani, F., Yaeger, D., McCallum, J., Kaur, M., Devoto, M., Jackson, L. G., Krantz, I. D., & Young, T. L. (2006). Ophthalmologic findings in Cornelia de Lange syndrome: a genotype-phenotype correlation study. Archives of Ophthalmology, 124, 552-557.

Nasmyth, K. (2011). Cohesin: a catenase with separate entry and exit gates? Nature Cell Biology, 13, 1170-1177.

Nazarenko, S. A., Timoshevsky, V. A., & Sukhanova, N. N. (1999). High frequency of tissue-specific mosaicism in Turner syndrome patients. Clinical genetics, 56, 59-65.

Oliveira, J., Dias, C., Redeker, E., Costa, E., Silva, J., Reis Lima, M., den Dunnen, J. T., & Santos, R. (2010). Development of NIPBL locus-specific database using LOVD: from novel mutations to further genotype-phenotype correlations in Cornelia de Lange Syndrome. Human Mutation, 31, 1216-1222.

Pie, J., Gil-Rodriguez, M. C., Ciero, M., Lopez-Vinas, E., Ribate, M. P., Arnedo, M., Deardorff, M. A., Puisac, B., Legarreta, J., de Karam, J.,C., Rubio, E., Bueno, I., Baldellou, A., Calvo, M. T., Casals, N., Olivares, J. L., Losada, A., Hegardt, F. G., Krantz, I. D., Gomez-Puertas, P., & Ramos, F. J. (2010). Mutations and variants in the cohesion factor genes NIPBL, SMC1A, and SMC3 in a cohort of 30 unrelated patients with Cornelia de Lange syndrome. American Journal of Medical Genetics Part A, 152A, 924-929.

Pinsker, J. E. (2012). Clinical review: Turner syndrome: updating the paradigm of clinical care. The Journal of Clinical Endocrinology & Metabolism, 97, E994-1003.

Ranke, M. B. & Saenger, P. (2001). Turner's syndrome. Lancet, 358, 309-314.

Remeseiro, S. & Losada, A. (2013). Cohesin, a chromatin engagement ring. Current Opinion in Cell Biology, 25, 63-71.

Rohatgi, S., Clark, D., Kline, A. D., Jackson, L. G., Pie, J., Siu, V., Ramos, F. J., Krantz, I. D., & Deardorff, M. A. (2010). Facial diagnosis of mild and variant CdLS: Insights from a dysmorphologist survey. American Journal of Medical Genetics Part A, 152A, 1641-1653.

Saenger, P. (1996). Turner's syndrome. The New England Journal of Medicine, 335, 1749-1754.

Saenger, P., Wikland, K. A., Conway, G. S., Davenport, M., Gravholt, C. H., Hintz, R., Hovatta, O., Hultcrantz, M., Landin-Wilhelmsen, K., Lin, A., Lippe, B., Pasquino, A. M., Ranke, M. B., Rosenfeld, R., & Silberbach, M. (2001). Recommendations for the diagnosis and management of Turner syndrome. The Journal of Clinical Endocrinology & Metabolism, 86, 3061-3069.

Savendahl, L., & Davenport, M. L. (2000). Delayed diagnoses of Turner's syndrome: proposed guidelines for change. Journal of Pediatrics, 137, 455-459.

Seitan, V. C., Banks, P., Laval, S., Majid, N. A., Dorsett, D., Rana, A., Smith, J., Bateman, A., Krpic, S., Hostert, A., Rollins, R. A., Erdjument-Bromage, H., Tempst, P., Benard, C. Y., Hekimi, S., Newbury, S. F., & Strachan, T. (2006). Metazoan Scc4 homologs link sister chromatid cohesion to cell and axon migration guidance. PLOS Biology, 4, e242.

Selicorni, A., Colli, A.M., Passarini, A., Milani, D., Cereda, A., Cerutti, M., Maitz, S., Alloni, V., Salvini, L., Galli, M.A., Ghiglia, S., Salice, P., & Danzi, G. B. (2009). Analysis of congenital heart defects in 87 consecutive patients with Brachmann-de Lange syndrome. American Journal of Medical Genetics Part A, 149A, 1268-1272.

Selicorni, A., Russo, S., Gervasini, C., Castronovo, P., Milani, D., Cavalleri, F., Bentivegna, A., Masciadri, M., Domi, A., Divizia, M. T., Sforzini, C., Tarantino, E., Memo, L., Scarano, G., & Larizza, L. (2007). Clinical score of 62 Italian patients with Cornelia de Lange syndrome and correlations with the presence and type of NIPBL mutation. Clinical genetics, 72, 98-108.

Strachan, T. (2005). Cornelia de Lange Syndrome and the link between chromosomal function, DNA repair and developmental gene regulation. Current Opinion in Genetics & Development, 15, 258-264.

Sybert, V. P. & McCauley, E. (2004). Turner's syndrome. The New England Journal of Medicine, 351, 1227-1238.

Tonkin, E. T., Wang, T. J., Lisgo, S., Bamshad, M. J., & Strachan, T. (2004). NIPBL, encoding a homolog of fungal Scc2-type sister chromatid cohesion proteins and fly Nipped-B, is mutated in Cornelia de Lange syndrome. Nature Genetics, 36, 636-641.

Tsukahara, M., Okamoto, N., Ohashi, H., Kuwajima, K., Kondo, I., Sugie, H., Nagai, T., Naritomi, K., Hasegawa, T., Fukushima, Y., Masuno, M., & Kuroki, Y. (1998). Brachmann-de Lange syndrome and congenital heart disease. American Journal of Medical Genetics, 75, 441-442.

Verrotti, A., Agostinelli, S., Prezioso, G., Coppola, G., Capovilla, G., Romeo, A., Striano, P., Parisi, P., Grosso, S., Spalice, A., Foiadelli, T., Curatolo, P., Chiarelli, F., & Savasta, S. (2013). Epilepsy in patients with Cornelia de Lange syndrome: A clinical series. Seizure, 22, 356-359.

Watrin, E., Schleiffer, A., Tanaka, K., Eisenhaber, F., Nasmyth, K., & Peters, J. M. (2006). Human Scc4 is required for cohesin binding to chromatin, sister-chromatid cohesion, and mitotic progression. Current Biology, 16, 863-874.

Wygnanski-Jaffe, T., Shin, J., Abdolell, M., Jackson, L.G., & Levin, A.V. (2005). Ophthalmologic findings in the Cornelia de Lange syndrome. J AAPOS, 9 (5), 407-15.

Wierzba, J., Gil-Rodriguez, M. C., Polucha, A., Puisac, B., Arnedo, M., Teresa-Rodrigo, M. E., Winnicka, D., Hegardt, F. G., Ramos, F. J., Limon, J., & Pie, J. (2012). Cornelia de Lange syndrome with NIPBL mutation and mosaic Turner syndrome in the same individual. BMC Medical Genetics, 13, 43.

Wierzba, J., Kuzniacka, A., Ratajska, M., Lipska, B. S., Kardas, I., Iliszko, M., & Limon, J. (2011). Cornelia de Lange syndrome associated with a de-novo novel NIPBL splice-site mutation and a coincidental inherited translocation t(3;5)(p13;q11). Clinical Dysmorphology, 20, 222-224.

Yan, J., Saifi, G. M., Wierzba, T. H., Withers, M., Bien-Willner, G. A., Limon, J., Stankiewicz, P., Lupski, J. R., & Wierzba, J. (2006). Mutational and genotype-phenotype correlation analyses in 28 Polish patients with Cornelia de Lange syndrome. American Journal of Medical Genetics Part A, 140, 1531-1541.

Yucesoy, G., Cakiroglu, Y., & Caliskan, E. (2008). Fryns syndrome: case report and review of the literature. Journal of Clinical Ultrasound, 36, 315-317.

Impact of Late-Onset Sepsis on Neurodevelopmental Outcome in Premature Infants: Strategies to Prevent It

Pasqua Betta, Chiara Grasso, Angela D'Ambra, Pietro Sciacca
Department of Paediatrics
University of Catania, Italy

Domenico Maurizio Romeo
Division of Child Neurology
Catholic University, Rome, Italy

1   Introduction

The increased survival of Extremely Low Birth Weight (ELBW) infants has heightened awareness of the importance of assessing and improving long-term outcomes associated with prematurity. It is estimated that almost 15 % of the most immature infants develop cerebral palsy (CP) and approximately half of them develop cognitive and behavioral deficits (Vohr *et al.*, 2000).

Infections are frequent complications among ELBW preterm infants. They are associated with significant morbidity rates, including neurological outcome besides to short-term sequelae and increased risk of death (Stoll & Hansen, 2003). Few studies only reported data on neurodevelopmental follow-up, confirming that preterm infants with a history of sepsis show worse neurodevelopmental outcome compared to control group in early infancy, involving mental and psychomotor retardation, vision and hearing impairment and cerebral palsy (Stoll *et al.*, 2004). Furthermore, differences in the outcome according to sepsis pathogens were reported and infants with Gram-positive sepsis had the poorest neurodevelopmental outcomes (Stoll *et al,* 2002). Sepsis may lead to poor neurodevelopmental outcomes by several mechanisms as: cytokine effects on cerebral hemodynamics with white matter injury, cerebral ischemia reperfusion injury after arterial hypotension, biological immaturity of preterm infants and vulnerability to brain injury during sepsis (Schlapbach *et al.*, 2011). Prompt diagnosis and effective treatment do not protects septic neonates from the risk of late neurodevelopmental impairment. Thus prevention of bacterial and fungal infections is crucial in these settings of unique patients and it is related to the promotion of breast-feeding and hygiene measures, to the adoption of a cautious central venous catheter policy, to the enhancement of the enteric microbiota composition with the supplementation of probiotics and to the medical stewardship concerning H2 blockers. Additional measures may include the use of lactoferrin, fluconazole, nystatin and specific measures to prevent ventilator associated pneumonia (Manzoni *et al.*, 2013).

The oral administration of probiotics reduces the incidence of necrotizing enterocolitis (NEC) in preterm infants, by inhibition or reduction of inflammatory signaling in the intestinal epithelia. But the limited number of clinical trials results in lack of definition of optimal strains, timing, dosage and duration of probiotics administered to VLBW (very low birth weight) preterm infants (Lin *et al.*, 2013). Few studies report on the role of probiotics, used for the prevention of NEC, in neurodevelopmental outcome of preterm infants with sepsis. Sari (Sari *et al.*, 2012) concludes that, although oral probiotics given to preterm infants reduce the incidence of NEC, they do not affect growth, neurodevelopmental and sensory outcomes between 2 and 3 years corrected age. One study (Romeo *et al.*, 2011) reported a different neurodevelopmental outcome in a population of preterm infants between those treated with probiotics and those having no supplementation. The same affirmation is showed in Hunter's study (Hunter *et al.*, 2012). However these studies showed differences in term of based population, timing, dosage and duration of probiotics treatment and a clear comparison is difficult to make.

In the present chapter we wish to determine correlation between neonatal infections and adverse neurodevelopmental and growth results in early childhood, to suggest that a close neurological follow-up, especially during the first 12 months of life, is necessary for infants with a diagnosis of sepsis. We would also specifically explore the role of probiotics in the prevention of late-onset sepsis, of gastrointestinal colonization by *Candida* spp. and in the protection against fungal infections and their ability in reducing the risk of adverse neurological and growth sequelae in early infancy (12 months).

2   Intestinal Microbiota in Newborn

The normal human microflora is a complex ecosystem that somehow for establishing colonization depends on enteric nutrients, but also on the mode of delivery and on a possible administration of antibiotics. At birth, the digestive tract is sterile.. Diet and environmental conditions can influence this ecosystem (Hammerman *et al.*, 2004).

At birth intestinal colonization is derived from organisms in the birth canal and maternal faecal microflora. The microbial imprinting depends on the mode and location of delivery. Literature data shows that infants born in a hospital environment, by caesarean section, have a high component of anaerobic microbial flora (*Clostridia*) and high post of Gram-negative enterobacteria. Those born prematurely by vaginal delivery and breast-fed have a rather rich in *Lactobacilli* and *Bifidobacteria* microflora (Grönlund *et al*, 1999; Hall *et al*, 1990). Diet can influence the microbiota, while the breast-feeding promotes an intestine microbiota in which *Bifidobacteria* predominates, indeed in formula bottle-fed baby coliform, enterococci and bacteroides predominate. *Escherichia coli* and *Streptococcus* are among the first bacteria to colonize the digestive tract. Subsequently, strict anaerobes (*Bacteroides, Bifidobacteri, Clostridium*) are established during the first week of life, when the diet plays a fundamental role (Mackie *et al*, 1999). The pattern of bacterial colonization in the premature neonatal gut is different from the one of the healthy, full term infant gut. Aberrant preterm infants admitted to NICU, born by caesarean section, are more often separated from their mother and kept in an aseptic intensive care setting and treated with broad-spectrum antibiotics. This is the reason why they show a highly modified bacterial flora, consisting of less than 20 species of bacteria, with a predominance of *Staphylococcus* (*Aureus* and *Coagulase negative*) among aerobic micro-organisms, and *Enterobacteriaceae* (*Klebsiella*), among enterococci and anaerobic *Clostridia* (Dai *et al*, 1999; Gothefors, 1989). It is believed that microbial diversity is an important factor in determining the stability of the ecosystem and that it is the fecal loss of diversity that predisposes the preterm gastrointestinal colonization of antibiotic-resistant bacteria and fungi with a consequent potential risk of infection and contribute to the development of necrotizing enterocolitis (Fanaro *et al*, 2003).

2.1   Necrotizing Enterocolitis (NEC)

NEC is a serious anoxic and ischemic disease affecting almost the ileo-colic area of premature newborns. It is characterized by bacteria proliferation and production of gas inside gastric walls (cystic pneumatosis) associated with edema and inflammation. Its incidence rate is 1-3 cases per 1000 newborns, with a mortality rate ranging between 10-50 %. The prematurity is the most important risk factor, as well as the low birth weight (<1500 g). This risk increases after the colonization or the infection of pathogens such as *Clostridium, Escherichia, Klebsiella, Salmonella, Shigella, Campylobacter, Pseudomonas, Streptococcus, Enterococcus, Staphylococcus Aureus* and coagulase negative *Staphylococcus*. Other factors that can increase its incidence are the intestinal immaturity, the decrease of the intestinal motility, the increase of permeability to macromolecules and an excessive volume of milk. Certainly breast feeding represents a protective factor, as it is shown by the decreased incidence of NEC in breast-fed infants. Moreover literature data supporting the benefits of probiotics are increasing in the last decades. The role of intestinal micro-organisms has been largely described, even if it is still not clear. Advances in molecular biology and intestinal microbiology allow a better characterization of the intestinal microbiota in children affected by NEC. Nowadays, literature data describes different methods of characterization of the microbial genotype and of identification of its genes, expression of the specific proteins and production of metabolites

(Deshpande *et al.* 2007). The application of these techniques on bioptic samples of infected and non-infected subjects could improve the comprehension of the persistence of NEC in premature newborns. Deshpande in 2010 published a meta analysis of 11 trials (N= 2176) which confirms the benefit of probiotic supplements in reducing NEC, death and disease in preterm newborns. Furthermore in this study the dramatic effect sizes, the tight confidence intervals, extremely low P values and overall evidence suggest that additional placebo-controlled trials are unnecessary if a suitable probiotic product is available (Desphande *et al.*, 2010).

There is a correlation between NEC and neurodevelopmental impairment in newborns. A recent study of Shah (Shah *et al.*, 2012) proves that the mental developmental index (MDI) and the psychomotor developmental index (PDI) values of the Bayley's scale were significantly greater among infants without NEC than those with NEC. Even after adjustment for use of antenatal glucocorticoids, birth weight, gender, race, surfactant therapy, intraventricular hemorrhage (IVH), bronchopulmonary dysplasia (BPD), sepsis and postnatal steroid treatment, MDI and PDI values remained significantly different between no NEC and NEC groups. NEC provokes neurodevelopmental impairment by several mechanisms. Some of them are mediated by inflammatory cytokines and bacterial products, others by vasodilatation and arterial hypotension that may cause cerebral ischemia and reperfusion injury in an immature brain (Figure 1 g-h). As literature actually says we can conclude that the diagnosis of stage II or greater NEC is associated with an increased risk of adverse long-term neurodevelopmental outcome in preterm ELBW infants.

3   Neonatal Sepsis

Sepsis is the response of the organism at the invasion of tissues, fluids or body cavity by pathogens or potentially pathogens microorganisms. Clinical signs associated with sepsis are temperature instability, irritability, apathia, feeding difficulties, prolonged capillary refill, apnea, tachycardia and tachypnea; laboratory signs of sepsis are elevated C-reactive protein, left shift or leucopenia. Proven sepsis is defined as a positive result on one or more bacterial or fungal cultures in an infant with clinical and/or laboratoristic signs of infection. Suspected sepsis is defined by the presence of clinical and/or laboratoristic signs of infection without any positive bacterial or fungal culture. A sepsis is defined early-onset (EOS) if it occurs at ≤72 hours of life; while it is late-onset (LOS) when it occurs at >72 hours.

3.1   Bacterial Infections

Bacterial infections continue to cause a high burden on neonatal morbidity and mortality (Stoll *et al.*, 2003). Approximately 1.5 % of VLBW infants suffer from early-onset sepsis and about 36 % from late-onset sepsis, with mortality rates ranging from 10 % to 30 %. Mortality is higher in African-American preterm infants (24,4 %) (Shane & Stoll 2013).

Group B streptococci cause 38 % of early-onset sepsis and they are followed by *Escherichia coli* (24%). In VLBW infants Gram-negative pathogens are isolated most frequently than in full-term newborns and they are correlated with an increased risk of death (Hornik *et al*, 2012).

Gram-positive organisms cause 70 % of late-onset infections. Of these, coagulase-negative *Staphylococcus* is the most common pathogen (48 % of all infections) and it is followed by *Staphylococcus aureus* (10 %). *Enterococcus* spp. causes the 3 % of late onset sepsis, group B *Streptococcus* the 2 % and Gram-negative organisms the 18 %. The most frequent are *Escherichia Coli* (5 %), *Klebsiella* (4 %),

Pseudomonas (3 %), *Enterobacter* (2,5 %) and *Serratia* (2 %). Sometimes more than one organism can be found (Stoll *et al*, 2002).

Neonatal risk factors of early onset sepsis are prematurity, low birth weight, male gender and the presence of other neonatal disease such as respiratory distress, asphyxia, congenital immunodeficiency disorders or congenital metabolic disorders. Maternal risk factors of early onset sepsis are rupture of membrane greater than 18 hours, maternal fever during labor or intra-amniotic infections, maternal drug addiction, group B streptococcal (GBS) vaginal colonization (Shane & Stoll 2013). The universal screen for GBS colonization during pregnancy and the recommendation for intra-partum antibiotic prophylaxis (IAP) in colonized women reduced significantly the rates of early-onset GBS sepsis (Boyer & Gotoff, 1986).

Late-onset sepsis complicate the extreme prematurity, they usually have slower onset and course, lower mortality but they more often involve the nervous central system (NCS). The risk of late-onset infections increases with decreasing birth weight and gestational age, with prolonged hospitalization and with the protracted use of central venous catheters (Stoll *et al* 2002).

Initial clinical manifestations of sepsis are nonspecific and they can be associated with complications such as respiratory distress, disseminated intravascular coagulation (DIC), necrotizing enterocolitis (NEC), persistent pulmonary hypertension of the newborn (PPHN) or septic shock. Group B streptococcal is often responsible of fulminant sepsis, Gram-negative organisms instead are often associated with an early endotoxin-associated septic shock while coagulase-negative *Staphylococcus* is the most common pathogen associated with a more insidious course of the sepsis. Symptomatic newborns, with or without risk factors, without any non-infectious cause that can explain the set of clinical signs, should undergo a careful physical examination, blood tests and cultures and should initiate empirical antibiotic therapy (Stolfi & Pedicino, 2009). The studying of the epidemiology of pathogens responsible of sepsis can be useful to identify infants with possible infection and to select appropriate empiric antimicrobial therapy while waiting a targeted therapy (Shane & Stoll, 2013).

3.2   Fungal Infections

Fungal infections (primarily *Candida* spp.) have become increasingly important as causal agents of infection in preterm infants. They currently are the third most common cause of late-onset sepsis in VLBW preterm infants at the NICU, with an estimated incidence of 1.6 – 9 % in VLBW infants, but up to 15% in ELBW, and with a crude mortality rate around 30 – 75 %. *Candida Albicans* has been and still is the species most frequently isolated, although *Candida parapsilosis* and other species of Candida are more often reported as a cause of invasive candidiasis. Clinical manifestations of systemic candidiasis may not be specific, especially in an infant already in critical condition, moreover blood cultures were positive just in 50% of the patients with invasive fungal disease (IFI) (Silva *et al.*, 2009).

Among the known risk factors, colonization by *Candida* spp. is the most important predictor of IFI. This association between colonization and infection has been proven for all sites that can be monitored with serial cultures. In particular, previous colonization can often be found before any IFI, if properly investigated. It is estimated that about 60 % of VLBW infants can be colonized during the first month of life in the NICU, and many of these can be infected after being colonized. In this regard, in 1986 Baley calculated that out of 100 VLBW infants in NICU, 33 developed fungal colonization, and 7 of them proceeded to IFI (Baley *et al.*, 1986).

Of all the sites of colonization, the gastrointestinal tract (investigated with cultures from throat swabs, gastric aspirates, fecal or rectal swabs) seems to be the one with the highest predictive value for subsequent dissemination in case of colonization. The fungal colonization at different levels of the intestinal tube is a well-known risk factor for subsequent dissemination and systemic fungal disease in preterm infants. The positivity of the rectal swab was taken by some authors as an expression of fungal colonization in toto (Pappu-Katikaneni *et al.* 1990). Moreover, the preterm baby in NICU is highly at risk for intestinal microecology disorders with proliferation of pathogenic microflora (including fungi). This is due to the fact that the infant undergoes to long-term treatments with broad-spectrum antibiotics, and often has difficulties in establishing and maintaining the oral feeding. In these special patients, the enteric tube is considered the most important reservoir and site of colonization for all types of pathogens and it is also considered as the site from which most frequently a low systemic fungal dissemination can start.

It has been shown that you can sometimes prevent the incidence of IFI by reduction of intestinal fungal colonization. Therefore research has focused its efforts towards the identification of the optimal prophylactic strategy especially in premature infants. However, at date, there is still no clear indication: prophylaxis with antifungal agents in fact still raises concerns about the tolerability and about the potential selection of resistant strains (Manzoni *et al.* 2013).

4   Pathogenesis

The body's response to infections is the pathophysiological basis of sepsis (Hotchkiss & Karl, 2003). Severe sepsis is the syndrome due to the complication of the organ failure in sepsis (Skrupky *et al.* 2011). The theory of an uncontrolled immunitary response is not enough to explane the pathophysiology of sepsis. Many animals studies where guinea-pigs died from "cytokine storm" and where the administration of drugs that block these mediators improved survival, do not reflect the clinical pictures in humans (Flink & Heard, 1990; Deitch, 1998). This is due to a revaluation of the fundamental meaning of the pathophysiology of sepsis. Cytokines, such as TNFα and IL1, have damaging effects in sepsis but also beneficial ones (Hotchkiss & Karl, 2003): the use of TNF or IL1 antagonists in fact is often associated with a higher mortality except for specific subgroups of patients (Fisher *et al,* 1996). Other news about pathophysiology of sepsis gather from recent discovered about toll like receptors (TLRs). These receptors exist to serve as an early warning of infection and to help mount an expeditious response. It is possible that in selected individuals down modulation of this pathway may be advisable but it must be done in a graded fashion and perhaps only after the initial immune response has been activated (Skrupky *et al.* 2011).

Although there is still considerable debate, a growing consensus is that sepsis initiates both a pro- and anti-inflammatory response that begin rapidly after life threatening infection. Although both, pro- and anti-inflammatory processes, begin promptly after sepsis onset, in general there is predominance of an initial hyperinflammatory phase whose magnitude is determined by a number of factors including pathogen virulence, bacterial load, host genetic factors, and host comorbidities. Sepsis can be considered a race to the death between invading pathogens and the host immune response where pathogens seek an advantage by disabling selected aspects of host defenses including inducing apoptotic death of immune cells, decreasing monocyte major histocompatibility complex class-2 expression, increasing expression of negative co-stimulatory molecules, inducing anti-inflammatory cytokines production, and increasing suppressor cells (Skrupky *et al.* 2011). This could explain the results of the Hotchkiss's autopsy study that shows a discordance between histologic findings and the degree of organ dysfunction in patients who died from sepsis (Hotchkiss *et al.* 1999). Skrupky *et al.* in their work of 2011 affirm that much organ dysfunction in patients with sepsis can be explained by "cell hibernation" which results from defence mechanisms reducing cellular processes to basic roles. To date, although occasionally a patient with sepsis may die of refractory shock, more frequently the exact cause of death remains elusive even after the autopsy (Hotchkiss & Karl, 2003).

4.1   Sepsis May Lead to Poor Neurodevelopmental Outcome by Several Mechanisms

Preterm infants are at risk for infection throughout their hospitalization with various long-term complications, including adverse neurodevelopmental (ND) outcome (Adams-Chapman, 2012). A study on extremely premature infants born earlier than 28 weeks of gestational age, shows that proven sepsis independently increases the risk for poor neurodevelopmental outcomes at 2 years of age. The presence of sepsis, BPD, brain injury, and retinopathy of prematurity (ROP) is highly predictive of adverse outcomes. Sepsis is among the 4th main risk factor influencing long-term outcomes in this population, together with BPD, brain injury, and ROP. All of these have a greater impact on the outcome than the gestational age, the birth weight and the gender (Schlapbach et al., 2011). Mechanisms by which sepsis can lead to poor neurodevelopmental outcome are:

1. *Bacterial products and the cytokine storm.* Pathogens stimulate the dendritic cells which induce TCD4+ cells to produce pro-inflammatory cytockines, including TNFα and IFNγ, and to activate B lymphocytes to produce specific antibodies. Pathogens also activate the NFkB gene in macrophage with the production of TNFα, IL1 and IL10. In the course of the systemic inflammatory response syndrome, this cytokine storm can directly damage the highly vulnerable premature brain (Wu & Colford, 2000) and other organs, such as the lung and retina. Additional support for this hypothesis comes from magnetic resonance imaging studies demonstrating white-matter injury associated with bacterial infections and NEC in premature infants (Shah et al., 2008). In accordance, the recent study by Martin, reports a higher risk of neurodevelopmental dysfunction and microcephaly in NEC infants with late bacteremia (Martin et al., 2010). Of note, postnatal infections result in increased white-matter injury in premature infants (Chau et al., 2009).

2. *Arterial hypotension during sepsis may cause cerebral ischemia-reperfusion injury.* Because of varying institutional practices in the definition and treatment of hypotension (Barrington, 2007). Arterial hypotension is mediated by pro-inflammatory cytokines and by the activation of neutrophils that increased vascular permeability and by the induction of nitric oxide synthase (iNOS) with the subsequent increase of the nitric oxide (NO).

Moreover sepsis may be an indicator of disease severity in extremely preterm infants. For example, prolonged mechanical ventilation is associated with a higher sepsis risk (Stoll et al., 2002).
Susceptibility to sepsis may also reflect the biological immaturity. These developing brain of these infants may be more vulnerable to injury (Figure 1 g-h).

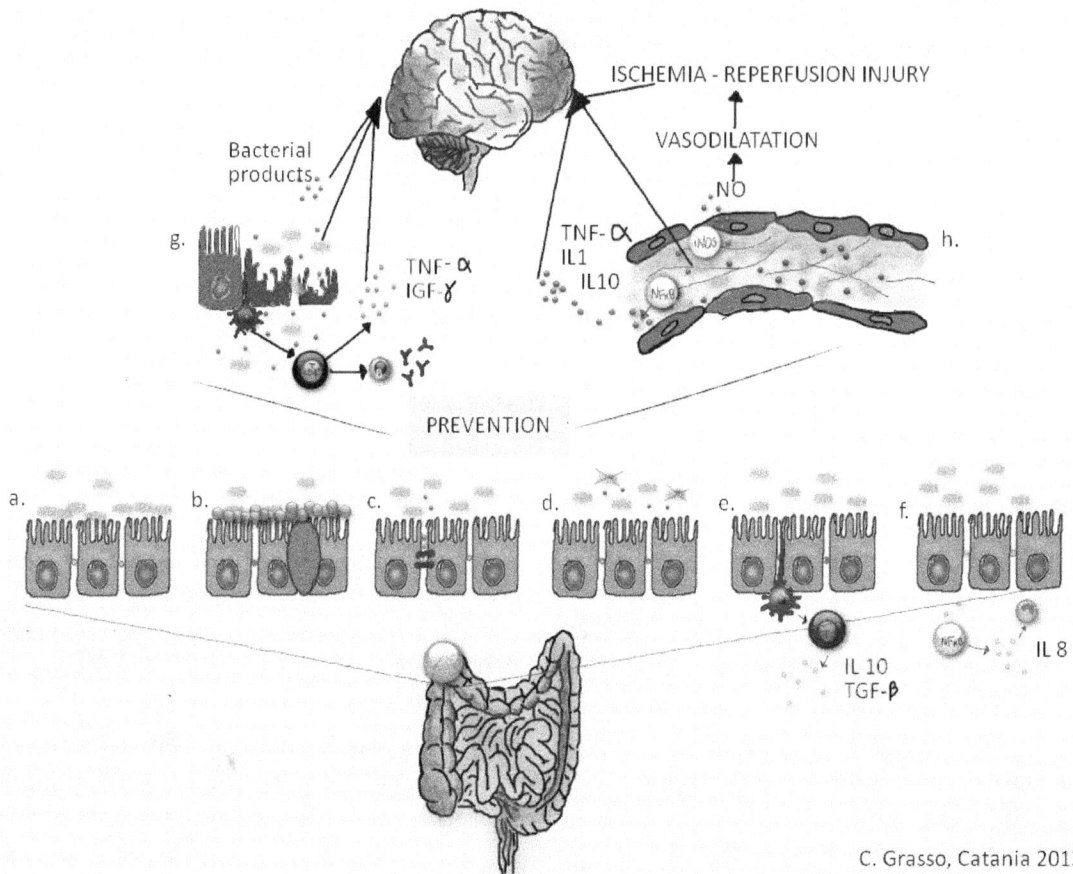

Figure 1: Role of probiotics in decreasing the incidence of necrotizing enterocolitis (NEC) (g.), sepsis (h.) and neurological impairment in preterm newborns. Probiotics (green sticks) can prevent NEC or sepsis by several mechanisms: a. Forming a physical barrier against the pathogens (brown sticks). b. Stimulating the Goblet Cells to produce a barrier of mucus (blue rounds). c. Reinforcing the apical tight-junctions of the enterocytes. d. Producing antimicrobial factors which kill pathogenic microorganisms e.Stimulating the innate immune system by signaling dendritic cells. f. Preventing or triggering an innate immune response by initiating TNF production by epithelial cells and inhibiting (or activitating) NFκB in macrophage and dampening (or priming) the host immune response. 1 g-h During NEC (g.) or sepsis (h.) neurological damage can be caused by the direct action of pathogens and their products; by the cytokine storm.

5   Neonatal Sepsis and Neurodevelopmental Outcome

Pre and postnatal infections in preterm infants represent a risk for inflammatory-mediated white matter injury (WMI) to the immature brain, with possible neurobehavioral impairments (Shah *et al.*, 2012). These brain abnormalities are seen even when the infection is only clinical without positive cultures. But in these cases only serial quantitative brain imaging could detect the impact of postnatal infection at term-equivalent age, suggesting an impairment of the brain in developing (Chau *et al.*, 2009).

Shah *et al.* demonstrated that sepsis/NEC in preterm infants is associated with a higher prevalence and severity of WMI on MRI at term-equivalent age and a delayed cognitive and motor development at 2 years of age (Shah *et al.*, 2008).

So far, the largest study to date to evaluate the impact of neonatal infection on adverse outcomes in early childhood was conducted on more than 6.000 preterm newborns with infection and followed at 18-22 months of corrected age, in which 41% of infected infants (any clinical sepsis, bloodstream infection, or meningitis) and 57% of infants with fungal sepsis had at least one adverse neurodevelopmental outcome. The prevalence of adverse neurodevelopmental outcome in infants with fungal sepsis (Stoll *et al.*, 2004) were as follows:

- Mental developmental index of less than 70   - 34%

- Psychomotor developmental index of less than 70 - 24%

- Cerebral Palsy   - 18%

- Visual impairment   - 14%

- Hearing impairment   - 5%

On the other hand, in a recent analysis, the Swiss Neonatal Network evaluated neurodevelopmental outcomes of preterm infants with a GA of 24-27 weeks at 2 years of age. 25% percent of these infants had culture-proven sepsis, which was independently associated with an increased risk of cerebral palsy. (Schlapbach *et al.*, 2011)

Thus, rigorous neurodevelopmental follow-up of these high-risk newborns is needed, to early identify those infants at risk of ND outcome and possibly reduce the risk of neurological impairment (Romeo *et al.*, 2013). The identification of differences and variations in development of preterm infants should be interpreted cautiously, as it could identify infants as having problems when their developmental course is simply different (Rosenbaum *et al.*, 2006). Therefore finding appropriate instruments for the assessments of these infants is crucial not only for individual patient but also for families and society; furthermore the possibility for an early identification of neurodevelopmental delay implies an early intervention with beneficial effects on development.body's response to infections is the pathophysiological basis of sepsis (Hotchkiss & Karl, 2003). Severe sepsis is the syndrome due to the complication of the organ failure in sepsis (Skrupky *et al.* 2011). The theory of an uncontrolled immunitary response is not enough to explane the pathophysiology of sepsis. Many animals' studies where guinea-pigs died from "cytokine storm" and where the administration of drugs that block these mediators improved survival, do not reflect the clinical pictures in humans (Flink & Heard, 1990; Deitch, 1998). This is due to a revaluation of the fundamental meaning of the pathophysiology of sepsis. Cytokines, such as TNFα and IL1, have damaging effects in sepsis but also beneficial ones (Hotchkiss & Karl, 2003): the use of TNF or IL1 antagonists in fact is often associated with a higher mortality except for specific subgroups of patients (Fisher *et al*, 1996). Other news about pathophysiology of sepsis gather from recent discovered about toll like receptors (TLRs). These receptors exist to serve as an early warning of infection and to help mount an expeditious response. It is possible that in selected individuals down modulation of this pathway may be advisable but it must be done in a graded fashion and perhaps only after the initial immune response has been activated (Skrupky *et al.* 2011).

Although there is still considerable debate, a growing consensus is that sepsis initiates both a pro- and anti-inflammatory response that begins rapidly after life threatening infection. Although both, pro- and anti-inflammatory processes, begin promptly after sepsis onset, in general there is predominance of an initial hyperinflammatory phase whose magnitude is determined by a number of factors including pathogen virulence, bacterial load, host genetic factors, and host comorbidities. Sepsis can be considered a race to the death between invading pathogens and the host immune response where pathogens seek an advantage by disabling selected aspects of host defenses including inducing apoptotic death of immune cells, decreasing monocyte major histocompatibility complex class-2 expression, increasing expression of negative co-stimulatory molecules, inducing anti-inflammatory cytokines production, and increasing suppressor cells (Skrupky *et al.* 2011). This could explain the results of the Hotchkiss's autopsy study that shows a discordance between histologic findings and the degree of organ dysfunction in patients who died from sepsis (Hotchkiss *et al.* 1999). Skrupky et al. in their work of 2011 affirm that much organ dysfunction in patients with sepsis can be explained by "cell hibernation" which results from defence mechanisms reducing cellular processes to basic roles. To date, although occasionally a patient with sepsis may die of refractory shock, more frequently the exact cause of death remains elusive even after the autopsy (Hotchkiss & Karl, 2003).

6   Prevention is Possible

Prompt diagnosis and effective treatment do not protect septic neonates from the risk of late neurodevelopmental impairment. Thus prevention of bacterial and fungal infection is crucial in these patients. Prevention strategies are based on the promotion of breast-feeding and of hygiene measures, the adoption of a cautious central venous catheter policy, the restriction of the use of H2 blockers or of proton pump inhibitors and the enhancement of the enteric microbiota composition with the supplementation of probiotics. Additional measures may include the use of lactoferrin, fluconazole, and nystatin and specific measures to prevent ventilator associated pneumonia (Manzoni *et al.* 2013).

6.1   Prophylaxis of Bacterial Mediated Sepsis

Preterm newborns at risk for sepsis, either because of clinical signs and symptoms or pregnancy-related risk factors, must be submitted to empirical antibiotic therapy. Before the 72nd hours of age the combination between ampicillin and aminoglycoside is recommended (Polin RA, 2012). Cephalosporins should be never used as empiric therapy except if gram-negative meningitis is suspected. They in fact can due the development of multi-resistant gram negative bacterial strains and of candidiasis (Manzoni *et al.* 2011). Among third-generation cephalosporins, ceftriaxone interferes with the bilirubin-albumin binding so the use of cefotaxime is preferred (Shane & Stoll 2013). Antimicrobial therapy must be reassessed as soon as culture results became known. Duration of therapy recommended is of 10 days in case of bacteriemia without a focus, while it is prolonged to 21 days in case of meningitis. In suspected sepsis with negative cultures, optimal therapeutic strategy is unknown. Some studies recommend to prolong antimicrobial therapy until clinical normalization (Stolfi *et al.* 2009) but several others describe the association between antimicrobial treatment for greater than 5 days in newborns with culture-negative clinical sepsis with increased risk of death or NEC (Shane & Stoll, 2013; Kuppala *et al*, 2011). If there is no clinical evidence of infection and if any organism is not isolated, the antibiotic therapy can be discontinued after 48-72 hours (Stolfi *et al.* 2009). Intra-partum antibiotic prophylaxis (IAP) with ampicillin in women, who are colonized by GBS, reduced significantly the rates of EO GBS sepsis but it does not prevent LOS (Boyer & Gotoff, 1986).

6.2   Prophylaxis of Fungal Mediated Sepsis

Because of the high mortality rate and the neurodevelopmental impairment associated with fungal sepsis in VLBW infants, prevention with nystatin, miconazole, and fluconazole has been studied in the highest-risk patients. Manzoni and colleagues in Italy published the results of their multicenter, randomized, placebo-controlled trial investigating two different fluconazole doses (3 mg/kg and 6 mg/kg) compared with a placebo group. In 322 infants who weighed less than 1500 g, investigators reported a significant difference in the incidence of fungal infections between the fluconazole prophylaxis groups compared to the placebo patients. There were no significant differences between the 3 mg/kg and the 6 mg/kg group (Manzoni et al., 2007).

Fluconazole is an excellent drug for prophylaxis because of its long half-life, high tissue concentration, low lipophilicity, and low protein binding. The one concern with fluconazole prophylaxis is the potential for the emergence of resistance over time, and this issue is under further study. Dosing with 3 mg/kg twice weekly is effective and limits exposure, cost, and potential adverse effects. When initiated around birth, prophylaxis should be administered for 6 weeks or less in patients with a birth weight of less than 1000 g or less than 6 weeks if intravenous access is no longer needed. For patients with a birth weight of more than 1000 g, prophylaxis must be continued until intravenous access is no longer needed and until adequate enteral feedings are achieved (Manzoni et al., 2007).

6.3   Probiotics: a Viable Weapon

Neonatal infections are frequent complications of ELBW infants receiving intensive care. The most valid indication of the probiotic remains the decrease of intestinal infections. In fact, the literature shows that the probiotic can reduce the severity and number of episodes of diarrhea.

6.3.1   Mechanism of Action

Probiotics can prevent sepsis by several mechanisms:

- forming a physical barrier against the pathogens (Figure 1 a).

- stimulating the Goblet Cells to produce mucus that forms a mechanical barrier (Figure 1 b).

- reinforcing the apical tight-junctions of the enterocytes and thus preventing the penetration of the pathogens (Figure 1 c).

- producing antimicrobial factors which kill pathogenic microorganisms (Figure 1 d).

- stimulating the innate immune system by signaling dendritic cells which then lead to the induction of TREG cells and to the production of anti-inflammatory cytokines including IL-10 and TGF-β

- preventing or triggering an innate immune response by initiating TNF production by epithelial cells and inhibiting (or activating) NFκB in macrophage dampening (or priming) the host immune response by influencing the production of IL-8 and subsequent recruitment of neutrophils to sites of intestinal injury (Figure 1 f).

6.3.2   Probiotics and Necrotizing Enterocolitis

Weizman made a double-blind placebo-controlled study using a formula supplemented with *Lactobacillus* (L.) *reuteri or B. bifidium* for 12 weeks. In the group of infants in therapy with probiotics less gastrointestinal infectious episodes have been demonstrated, fewer episodes of fever compared to placebo, with consequent reduction of antibiotic therapy. The improvement of perinatal care has led to increased survival of high-risk infants (ELBW, respiratory distress, surgery). For this reason one of the neonatal research priorities is the prevention and the treatment of sepsis in NEC and bronchopulmonary dysplasia (Weizman & Alsheikh, 2006). In view of the role of mediators of inflammation in BPD and in sepsis is therefore important to modulate the immune response in these young patients. Some studies have shown that probiotics can alter the intestinal microflora and reduce the growth of pathogenic microorganisms in the intestines of preterm infants, decreasing the incidence of necrotizing enterocolitis and sepsis (Figure 1). Deshpande in 2010 found a significant difference in developing definite NEC between neonates in the control group (no probiotics) compared with neonates in the probiotics group. Moreover he affirmed that the numbers needed to treat (NNT) with probiotics to prevent 1 case of NEC was 25 and confirmed the benefits of probiotic supplements in reducing death and disease in preterm neonates (Deshpande *et al*, 2010).

6.3.3   Probiotics and Fungal Infections

A study performed in rats with immune deficiency has been shown that the administration of *Lactobacillus rhamnosus* GG (LGG) reduced the risk of colonization and sepsis by *Candida*. One of our retrospective study, performed in 2002 at the University of Catania, showed that supplementation from birth for at least 4-6 weeks of a symbiotic (*Lactogermine plus* 3.5 x109 ucf/day) decreased the incidence and the intensity of gastrointestinal colonization of *Candida*, and subsequently its related infections in a group of preterm infants. Another randomized study on 80 preterm infants has confirmed that the administration of LGG (at a dose of 6 billion ufc/day) from the first day of life for a period of 6 weeks reduced the fungal enteric colonization with no side effects (Romeo *et al,* 2011). Newborns submitted to greater surgical interventions (esophageal atresia, diaphragmatic hernia, intestinal malformations) have an increased risk of bacterial and/or fungal infections due to the use of drains, central venous catheter, tatal parenteral nutrition (TNP), persistent nose-gastric probe that can be the cause of serious sepsis or pneumonias. In a recent study we presented at ESPHGAN, we demonstrated that surgical infants admitted to our NICU and supplemented with probiotics have a reduced risk of bacterial and *Candida* infections and an improved in clinical outcome (Betta *et al*, 2007). Furthermore in our study newborns treated with probiotics healed in 19±9.3 days of anti-mycotic treatment while newborns who didn't received probiotics healed in 40.7±16.2 days (p<0.05). In our experience the administration of probiotics has allowed a more rapid eradication of the infection with a lower number of total days of anti-mycotic therapy (Romeo *et al.*2006) (Figure 2). In another recently published study on preterm infants, the use of probiotics appeared to be effective in the prevention of both bacterial and fungal infections, in the attenuation of gastrointestinal symptoms and in a more rapid weaning from TPN with a reduction in the central venous catheter time and the number of days in hospital. These results were evident both in a group of preterm baby and in a group of surgical newborn treated with a supplementation of probiotics. A new prospecter, multicenter, double-blind, randomized placebo-controlled trial in 11 tertiary care NICUs evaluated the capacity of bovine lactoferrin (BLF) supplementation in VLBW newborns with birth weights of <1000 grams. Infants treated with BLF or with BLF and *Lactobacillus rhamnosus* GG (LGG) compared with placebo had

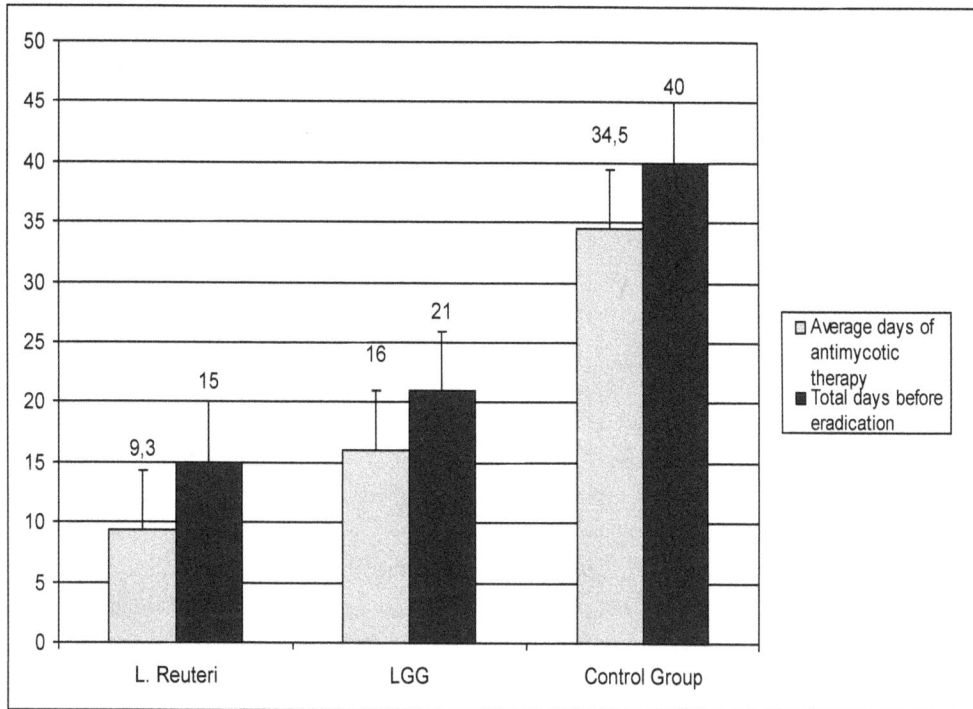

Figure 2: Role of probiotics (Lactobacillus reuteri and Lactobacillus rhamnosus GG) in decreasing the duration of antimycotic therapy and in achieving more quickly the healing by invasive fungal infections (IFI) (Romeo MG et al., 2006).

lower incidence of the first LOS episode (P< 0.001 for BLF plus LGG vs control) (Manzoni *et al.* 2009). The secondary analysis of data from this study show that in newborns treated with BLF or with BLF and LGG compared with placebo, invasive fungal infections (IFI) (P< 0.002 for BLF plus LGG vs control) and the progression rate colonization-infection (P< 0.02 for BLF plus LGG vs control) was significant lower (Manzoni *et al.* 2012). However in Desphande meta-analysis no significant difference in the risk for sepsis between the probiotics and control group neonates was found (Deshpande *et al.*, 2010). Only one of the 11 trial included in his study reported significantly lower risk for sepsis in the probiotic group (Stratiki *et al.*, 2007).

6.3.4   Probiotics and Neurodevelopmental Outcome

Although oral administration of probiotics has proven to be effective in reducing the incidence of sepsis and NEC in preterm infants, the role on neurodevelopmental outcome in this population of infants is controversial and studied only by a few authors.

Both the studies of Sari (Sari *et al.*, 2012) and of Chou (Chou *et al.*, 2010) reported that oral probiotic administered to VLBW infants reduce the incidence and severity of NEC but did not affect growth, neuromotor, neurosensory, and cognitive outcomes at 18 to 22 months corrected age using the Bayley Scale of Infant Development Second Edition (BSID-II). On the other hand, in a recent work (Romeo *et al.* 2011) reported a study on 249 preterm infants with sepsis with supplementation of two types of probiotics (*Lactobacillus* (L.) *reuteri, and L. rhamnosus*), they performed a structured neurological assessment using the Hammersmith Infant Neurologic Examination (HINE) at 12 months. A statistically significant higher incidence of suboptimal scores in the control group was found rather than in both the probiotic ones, concluding that probiotic supplementation may improve the neurological status of these preterm infants. However these studies present significant differences on based population, timing, dosage, and duration of probiotics treatment and to make a clear comparison is quite difficult. In the study of Romeo et al the supplementation of probiotics was given within 72 hours after hospitalization, whereas in the others studies probiotics were given later, on the 7th day after birth when most complications like IVH and periventricular leukomalacia (PVL), and even the inflammatory processes, had already occurred. Furthermore, the based population was clearly different with higher incidence of high risk infants in the studies of Chou (Chou *et al.*, 2010) and Sari (Sari *et al.*, 2012). Romeo in his work shows the potential beneficial effects of *L. reuteri* supplementation on clinical and physiological variables related to gut function, consistently higher than *L. rhamnosus* and control groups. *L. reuteri* improves feeding tolerance, bowel habits and gastric motility by increasing the gastric emptying rate and reducing the fasting antral area, and then reducing episodes of regurgitation. The first and foremost factor is the bacterial tolerance to both acid and alkaline environments. *L. reuteri* is reported to be highly resistant to the acid pH and to the antibiotic treatment (Romeo *et al.* 2011). *L. reuteri* has also the ability to successfully inhibit the growth of pathogens by a combination of different mechanisms including excretion of lactic and acetic acids or other short chain fatty acids, hydrogen peroxide, antimicrobial substances and bacteriocins. Furthermore *L. reuteri*, when comes in contact with other bacteria found in the human gut, converts glycerol into a potent, broad-spectrum antimicrobial that was termed 'reuterin'. It is a low molecular weight, neutral, water-soluble compound (3-hydroxy propionaldehyde) capable of inhibiting growth of species representing several bacterial genera as well as yeasts, fungi, protozoa and viruses. Reuterin action is local and it is not systemically absorbed. (Connolly E, 2004). Finally in the study of Romeo, the follow-up was based on a structured neurological assessment at 12 months corrected age, possibly underlining the role of probiotics at early ages. Longitudinal follow-up is therefore needed to explore the effect of probiotics from the first months to pre-school age using structured psychomotor scales, as BSID-II (Romeo *et al.*, 2011).

7   Conclusions

Sepsis is still a serious problem for the neonatal intensive care units. Today improvements in neonatal care allow survival of lower birth weight and lower gestational age infants who have a major duration of hospitalization and more need of parenteral nutrition and of others invasive maneuvers. This is related with a major risk of late onset-sepsis. Despite their usefulness in preventing bacterial sepsis is still under discussion, probiotics in addition to other strategies of prevention, are useful to prevent fungal infection. They in this way decrease morbidity and mortality in ELBW and especially reduce long-lasting neurological sequelae. Certainly more randomized and controlled studies about longitudinal follow-up from the first months to pre-school age of newborns who were admitted at the NICU, are therefore needed to explore long-lasting effects of probiotics.

Abbreviations

BLF—bovine lactoferrin

BPD—bronchopulmonary dysplasia
BSID-II—Bayley Scale of Infant Development Second Edition
CONS—coagulase-negative Staphylococcus
CP—cerebral palsy
DIC—disseminated intravascular coagulation
ELBW—extremely low birth weight
EOS—early-onset sepsis
GA—gestational age
GBS—group B streptococcal
HINE—Hammersmith Infant Neurologic Examination
IFI—invasive fungal infection
IFNγ—gamma-interferon
IL—interleukin
iNOS—inducible nitric oxide sinthase
IVH—intraventricular hemorrhage
LGG—*Lactobacillus rhamnosus* GG
LOS—late-onset sepsis
MDI—mental developmental index
MRI—magnetic resonance imaging
N—number
NCS—nervous central system
ND—neurodevelopmental
NFkB—nuclear factor kappa-light-chain-enhancer of activated B cells
NICU—neonatal intensive care unit
NEC—necrotizing enterocolitis
NNT—numbers needed to treat
NO—nitric oxide
PDI—psychomotor developmental index
PPHN—persistent pulmonary hypertension of the newborn
PVL—periventricular leukomalacia
ROP—retinopathy of prematurity
TLRs—toll like receptors
TNFα—tumor necrosis factor α
TPN—total parenteral nutrition
VLBW—very low birth weight
WMI—white matter injury

References

Adams-Chapman I. (2012) Long-term impact of infection on the preterm neonate. Semin Perinatol. 36(6):462-470.

Baley J.E., Kliegman R.M., Boxerbaum B., Fanaroff A.A. (1986) Fungal colonization in the very low birth weight infant. Pediatrics, 78(2):225-232

Barrington K. (2007) Time for pressure tactics. Pediatrics, 119(2):396–397.

Betta P.; Sciacca P.; Trovato L. et al. (2007) Probiotics in the prevention of Bacterial and Candida infections in newborns submitted to greater surgical interventions and admitted in NICU. Retrospective Group Controlled Study. ESPGHAN, Barcelona, May 9-12, 2007

Boyer K.M., Gotoff S.P. (1986) Prevention of early-omset neonatal group B streptococcal disease with selective intrapartum chemoprophylaxis. N Engl J Med, 314:1665-1669.

Chou I.C., Kuo H.T., Chang J.S., Wu S.F., Chiu H.Y., Su B.H. et al.(2010) Lack of effects of oral probiotics on growth and neurodevelopmental outcomes in preterm very low birth weight infants. J Pediatr., 156(3):393-396.

Chau V., Poskitt, K.J., McFadden, D.E., Bowen-Roberts, T., Synnes, A., Brant, R., Sargent, M.A., Soulikias, W. & Miller S.P. (2009). Effect of chorioamnionitis on brain development and injury in premature newborns. Ann Neurol. , 66(2):155–164

Connolly E. (2004) Lactobacillus reuteri ATCC 55730 A clinically proven probiotic. Nutrafoods; 3(1):15–22.

Dai D. & Walker W.A. (1999) Protective nutrients and bacterial colonization in the immature human gut. Adv Pediatr,46:353-382

Deitch E.A. (1998) Animal models of sepsis and shock: a review and lessons learned. Shock;12:411-420.

Deshpande G., Rao S. & Patole S. (2007) Probiotics for prevention of necrotising entercolitis in preterm neonates with very low birth weight: a systematic reiew of randomised controlled trials. Lancet, 369:1614-20.

Deshpande G., Rao S., Patole S. & Bulsara M. Updated Meta-analysis of Probiotics for Preventing Necrotizing Enterocolitis in Preterm Neonates. (2010) Pediatrics, 5:921-930.

Fanaro S., Chierici R., Guerrini P. & Vigi V. (2003) Intestinal microflora in early infancy: composition and development Acta Paediatr Suppl, 91:48-55.

Fisher C.J. Jr, Agosti J.M., Opal S.M., Lowry S.F., Balk R.A., Sadoff J.C., Abraham E., Schein R.M. & Benjamin E. (1996) Treatment of septic shock with the tumor necrosis factor receptor:Fc fusion protein. The soluble TNF receptor sepsis study group. N Engl J Med;334:1697-1702.

Flink M.P. & Heard S.O. (1990) Laboratory models of sepsis and septic shock. J Surg Res. 49:186-196.

Gareau M.G., Sherman P.M. & Walker W.A. (2010) Probiotics and the gut microbiota in intestinal health and disease. Nat Rev Gastroenterol Hepatol., 7:503-514.

Gothefors L. (1989) Effects of diet on intestinal flora. Acta Paediatr Scand Suppl, 351:118-21.

Grönlund M.M., Lehtonen O.P., Eerola E. & Kero P. (1999) Fecal microflora in healthy infants born by different methods of delivery: permanent changes in intestinal flora after cesarean delivery. J Pediatr Gastroenterol Nutr, 28:19-25

Hall M.A., Cole C.B., Smith S.L., Fuller R. & Rolles C.J. (1990) Factors influencingthe presence of faecal Lactobacilli in early infancy. Arch Dis Child, 65:185-8.

Hammerman C., Bin-Nun A. & Kaplan M. (2004). Germ warfare: probiotics in defence of premature gut. Clin Perinat,31: 489-500.

Hornik C.P., Fort P., Clark R.H., et al. (2012) Early and late onset sepsis in very-low-birth-weight infants from a large group of neonatl intensive care units. Early Hum Dev, 88(Suppl 2):S69-S74.

Hotchkiss R.S. & Karl I.E. (2003). The pathophysiology and Treatment od sepsis. N Engl J Med. 348(2):138-150.

Hotchkiss R.S., Swanson P.E., Freeman B.D., Tinsley K.W., Cobb J.P., Matuschak G.M., Buchman T.G. & Karl I.E. (1999) Apoptotic cell death in patients with sepsis, shock, and multiple organ dysfunction. Crit Care Med;27:1230-1251.

Hunter C., Dimaguila M.A., Gal P., Wimmer J.E. Jr, Ransom J.L., Carlos R.Q., Smith M., Davanzo C.C. (2012) Effect of routine probiotic, Lactobacillus reuteri DSM 17938, use on rates of necrotizing enterocolitis in neonates with birthweight < 1000 grams: a sequential analysis. BMC Pediatr. 4; 12:142.

Kuppala V.S., Meinzen-Derr J., Morrow A.L. & Schibler K.R. (2011) Prolonged initial empiric antibiotic treatment is associated with adverse outcomes in premature infants. J Pediatr,159:720-725.

Lin H.Y., Chang J.H., Chung M.Y. & Lin H.C. (2013) Prevention of necrotizing enterocolitis in preterm very low birth weight infants: Is it feasible? J Formos Med Assoc, 20:1-8.

Mackie R.I., Sghir A. & Gaskins H.R. (1999) Developmental microbial ecology of the neonatal gastrointestinal tract. Am J Clin Nutr, 69:1035S-1045S.

Manzoni P., De Luca D., Stronati M., Jacqz-Aigrain E., Ruffinazzi G., Luparia M., Tavella E., Boano E., Castagnola E., Mostert M. & Farina D. (2013). Prevention of nosocomial infections in neonatal intensive care units. Am J Perinatol, 30(2):81-88.

Manzoni P., Rinaldi M., Cattani S., Pugni L., Romeo M.G., Messner H., Stolfi I., Decembrino L., Laforgia N., Vagnarelli F., Memo L., Bordignon L., Saia O.S., Maule M., Gallo E., Mostert M., Magnani C., Quercia M., Bollani L., Pedicino R., Renzullo L., Betta P., Mosca F., Ferrari F., Magaldi R., Stronati M., Farina D.; Italian Task Force for the Study and Prevention of Neonatal Fungal Infections, Italian Society of Neonatology. (2009) Bovine lactoferrin supplementation for prevention of late-onset sepsis in very low-birth-weight neonates: a randomized trial. JAMA 7;302(13):1421-1428.

Manzoni P., Rizzollo S., Decembrino L., Ruffinazzi G., Rossi Ricci A., Gallo E., Stolfi I., Mostert M., Stronati M. & Farina D. (2011) Recent avances in prevention of sepsis in the premature neonates in NICU. Early Hum Dev;87(Suppl 1):S31:S33.

Manzoni P., Stolfi I., Messner H., Cattani S., Laforgia N., Romeo M.G., Bollani L., Rinaldi M., Gallo E., Quercia M., Maule M., Mostert M., Decembrino L., Magaldi R., Mosca F., Vagnarelli F., Memo L., Betta P.M., Stronati M., Farina D.; Italian Task Force for the Study and Prevention of Neonatal Fungal Infections–the Italian Society of Neonatology. (2012). Bovine lactoferrin prevents invasive fungal infections in very low birth weight infants: a randomized controlled trial. Pediatrics;129(1):116-123.

Manzoni P., Stolfi I., Pugni L., Decembrino L., Magnani C., Vetrano G., Tridapalli E., Corona G., Giovannozzi C., Farina D., Arisio R., Merletti F., Maule M., Mosca F., Pedicino R., Stronati M., Mostert M. & Gomirato G.; Italian Task Force for the Study and Prevention of Neonatal Fungal Infections; Italian Society of Neonatology. (2007) A multicenter, randomized trial of prophylactic fluconazole in preterm neonates. N Engl J MedJun 14, 356(24):2483-2495.

Martin C.R., Dammann O., Allred E.N., Patel S., O'Shea T.M., Kuban K.C. & Leviton A. (2010). Neurodevelopment of extremely preterm infants who had necrotizing enterocolitis with or without late bacteremia. J Pediatr., 157(5):751–756.

Pappu-Katikaneni L.D., Rao K.P. & Banister E. (1990). Gastrointestinal colonization with yeast species and Candida septicemia in very low birth weight infants. Mycoses, 33:20–23.

Polin R.A. & Committee on Fetus and Newborn. (2012). Management of neonates with suspected or proven early-onset bacterial sepsis. Pediatrics 2012; 129:1006-1015.

Romeo M.G., Betta P., Trovato L. & Oliveri S. (2006) Ruolo del probiotico nella prevenzione delle infezioni in una Unità di Terapia Intensiva Neonatale 12° Congresso Nazionale di Neonatologia Acta Neonatologica & Pediatrica 206:208 Montecatini SIN.

Romeo D.M., Cioni M., Palermo F., Cilauro S. & Romeo M.G. (2013) Neurological assessment in infants discharged from a neonatal intensive care unit. Eur J Paediatr Neurol.17(2):192-198.

Romeo M.G., Romeo D.M., Trovato L, Oliveri S., Palermo F., Cota F. & Betta P. (2011). Role of probiotics in the prevention of the enteric colonization by Candida in preterm newborns: incidence of late-onset sepsis and neurological outcome. J Perinatol, 31(1):63-69.

Rosenbaum P. (2006) Classification of abnormal neurological outcome. Early Hum Dev. 82: 167-171.

Sari F.N., Eras Z., Dizdar E.A., Erdeve O., Oguz S.S., Uras N. & Dilmen U. (2012). Do oral probiotics affect growth and neurodevelopmental outcomes in very low-birth-weight preterm infants? Am J Perinatol., 29(8):579-586.

Schlapbach L. J., Aebischera M., Mark Adams M., Natalucci G., Bonhoeffer J., Latzin P., Nelle M., Bucher A.U., Latal B. & the Swiss Neonatal Network and Follow-Up Group. (2011). Impact of Sepsis on Neurodevelopmental Outcome in a Swiss National Cohort of Extremely Premature Infants. Pediatrics, 128(2), e348 -e357.

Shah D.K., Doyle L.W., Anderson P.J., Bear M., Daley A.J., Hunt R.W. & Inder T.E. (2008). Adverse neurodevelopment in preterm infants with postnatal sepsis or necrotizing enterocolitis is mediated by white matter abnormalities on magnetic resonance imaging at term. J Pediatr, 153(2):170–175.

Shah T.A., Meinzen-Derr J., Gratton T., Steichen J., Donovan E.F., Yolton K., Alexander B., Narendran V. & Schibler K.R. (2012) Hospital and neurodevelopmental outcomes of extremely low-birth-weight infants with necrotizing enterocolitis and spontaneous intestinal perforation. J Perinatol.,32(7):552-558.

Shane A.L. & Stoll B.J. (2013) Recent Developments and Current Issues in the Epidemiology, Diagnosis, and Management of Bacterial and Fungal Neonatal Sepsis. Am J of Perinatol., 30:131-142.

Silva A.P., Miranda I.M., Lisboa C., Pina-Vaz C., & Rodrigues A.G. (2009). Prevalence, Distribution, and Antifungal Susceptibility Profiles of Candida parapsilosis, C. orthopsilosis, and C. metapsilosis in a Tertiary Care Hospital. J. Clin. Microbiol., 47(8):2392–2397.

Skrupky L.P., Kerby P.W. & Hotchkiss R.S. (2011) Advances in the management of sepsis and the understanding of key immunologic defects. Anesthesiology, 115(6):1349-62.

Stratiki Z., Costalos C., Sevastiadou S. et al. (2007) The effect of a Bifidobacter supplemented bovine milk on intestinal permeability of preterm infants. Early Hum Dev,83(9):575–579

Stolfi I., Pedicino R. & Gruppo di Studio Infettivologia Neonatale. (2009) Manuale fdi Infettivologia Neonatale. Biomedia 279-308.

Stoll B.J. & Hansen N. (2003). Infections in VLBW infants: studies from the NICHD Neonatal Research Network. Semin Perinatol, 27(4):293–301.

Stoll B.J., Hansen N.I., Adams-Chapman I., Fanaroff A.A., Hintz S.R., Vohr B., Higgins R.D. et National Institute of Child Health and Human Development Neonatal Research Network. (2004). Neurodevelopmental and growth impairment among extremely low-birth-weight infants with neonatal infection. JAMA, 292(19), 2357–2365.

Stoll B.J., Hansen N., Fanaroff A.A., Wright L.L., Carlo W.A., Ehrenkranz R.A., Lemons J.A., Donovan E.F., Stark A.R., Tyson J.E., Oh W., Bauer C.R., Korones S.B., Shankaran S., Laptook A.R., Stevenson D.K., Papile L.A. & Poole W.K. (2002) Late-onset sepsis in very low birth weight neonates: the experience of the NICHD Neonatal Research Network. Pediatrics, 110(2 pt 1):285–291.

Vohr B.R., Wright L.L., Dusick A.M.., Mele L., Verter J., Steichen J.J., Simon N.P., Wilson D.C., Broyles S., Bauer C.R., Delaney-Black V., Yolton K.A., Fleisher B.E., Papile L.A. & Kaplan M.D. (2000). Neurodevelopmental and functional outcomes of extremely low birth weight infants in the National Institute of Child Health and Human Development Neonatal Research Network, 1993-1994. Pediatrics, 105(6):1216-26.

Weizman Z. & Alsheikh A. (2006) Safety and tolerance of a probiotic formula in early infancy comparing two probiotic agents: a pilot study. J Am Coll Nutr, 25(5):415-419.

Wu Y.W. & Colford J.M. Jr. (2000). Chorioamnionitis as a risk factor for cerebral palsy: a meta-analysis. JAMA, 284(11):1417–1424.

Brain Network Reorganization in Neurodevelopmental Disorders Revealed by Dynamic Autoregressive Neuromagnetic Causal Imaging

Richard Eugene Frye
Department of Pediatrics
University of Arkansas for Medical Science, Little Rock, USA

Jacqueline Liederman
Department of Psychology
Boston University, Boston, USA

1   Introduction

Functional and structural neuroimaging have provided great insight into brain function in typical individuals and about brain reorganization in neurological disease. However, in some brain based diseases, particularly neurodevelopmental disorders such as dyslexia and autism, neuroimaging studies have provided somewhat contradictory findings. In some cases this is due to the fact that brain activation studies only provide part of the information needed to understand these disorders. In such cases, connectivity needs to be considered. New connectivity techniques, particularly those that measure effective connectivity, consider not only connectivity between brain regions but also how different brain regions influence one another. In this manuscript we discuss a method that uses Granger causality to measure effective connectivity in magnetoencephalography (MEG) recordings. This technique, called Dynamic Autoregressive Neuromagnetic Causal Imaging (DANCI), has been applied to MEG recording of children and adults with dyslexia and autism. We demonstrate how DANCI can be used to understand how the top-down and bottom-up influences of various brain regions are fundamentally altered to reorganize the brain's neural network in neurodevelopmental disorders. In our previous studies we have used this technique to demonstrate that different patterns of connectivity correlate with functional abilities in cognitive abilities such as language in individuals with neurodevelopmental disorders. In this chapter we describe the fundamental theory behind DANCI as well as the methods for applying DANCI to MEG data. We then show how to design analyses and experiments to use DANCI to answer questions regarding fundamental changes in brain organization.

2   Reorganization of Neural Networks in Neurodevelopmental Disorders

The exact neuropathological abnormalities that define neurodevelopmental disorders such dyslexia and autism are still being uncovered. Although it is clear that there are abnormalities in functional brain activity, the results of functional neuroimaging studies for neurodevelopmental disorders, such as dyslexia, are inconsistent. In functional neuroimaging studies on dyslexic individuals, atypical brain activation has been noted in three cortical areas, including the inferior frontal areas (IFAs), the temporoparietal areas (TPAs), and the ventral occipital-temporal areas (VOTAs; (Pugh *et al.*, 2000). The TPAs are most consistently reported to demonstrate atypical functional activation in studies of individuals with dyslexia. Relative under-activation of the left TPA and over-activation of the right TPA has been reported in dyslexic readers during early childhood (Simos *et al.*, 2002), later childhood (Temple *et al.*, 2003), adolescence (Simos *et al.*, 2002), and adulthood (Shaywitz *et al.*, 2003). Several studies have indicated that atypical TPA functional activation can change with remediation. However, the exact changes in right and left TPA functional activation have been inconsistent across studies. Some studies report an increase in left TPA activation in children with dyslexia who respond to intensive intervention (Simos *et al.*, 2007). However, other studies report that functional activation of both the right and left TPAs increase following interventions in children with dyslexia (Temple *et al.*, 2003). The reason for these contradictory findings is not clear. One of the complications of these experiments is that the level of task difficulty can have a major effect on activation of the various brain regions. Indeed, dyslexic readers may finding certain reading tasks more difficult than typical readers and the difficulty of the task changes for the dyslexic reader after a successful intervention (Fisher *et al.*, 2012).

Rather than simply considering these findings as contrary, these findings might suggest that there is another way to look at functional neuroimaging data. For example, instead of considering the brain of individuals with neurodevelopmental disorders as being less or more activated than the typically developing brain, these mixed results suggest that the neural networks in the brain of individuals with neurodevelopmental disorders might be organized differently than the neural networks in the brain of typically developing individuals. A clear example of this can be seen in dyslexia. In individuals with a childhood history of dyslexia (i.e., specific reading disability), brain organization as a young adult appears to be critically important in the eventual development of reading ability (Frye *et al.*, 2010; 2012; Shaywitz *et al.*, 2003). In a landmark study using functional magnetic resonance imaging (fMRI), Shaywitz *et al.* (2003) demonstrated that young adults with a history of dyslexia in childhood who develop accurate but non-fluent reading skills show marked reorganization of the brain's neural network as compared to typically developing individuals. This reorganization was not seen in those with a history of dyslexia in childhood who failed to develop adequate reading skills as young adults. In fact, individuals with persistently poor reading skills into adulthood demonstrated brain activation that looked more like the typically developing control group than the young adults with a history of dyslexia in childhood who developed adequate reading skills in young adulthood.

This reorganization implies that the neural networks in the brain of individuals with neurodevelopmental disorders are connected differently than those with typical development. Many studies support the notion for abnormalities in neuroconnectivity underlying dyslexia (Frye *et al.*, 2008; 2011) and autism (Ellmore *et al.*, 2013; Li *et al.*, 2012). However, the findings from neuroconnectivity studies have been contrary and, sometimes, inconsistent, leaving in question the exact significance of neuroconnectivity abnormalities in these neurodevelopmental disorders (Frye *et al.*, 2011; Vissers *et al.*, 2012). In fact, some studies have reported both increases and decreases in connectivity in the same subject populations. For example, in individuals with autism, resting-state connectivity between the posterior cingulate gyrus and other cortical area regions, as compared to controls, is increased to some regions and decreased to others (Monk *et al.*, 2009). Furthermore, the relationship between connectivity and cognitive function is inconsistent. For example, separate studies have demonstrated that poorer social skills are associated with both increased (Anderson *et al.*, 2011) and decreased (Weng *et al.*, 2010) resting-state connectivity in the default mode network.

Newer connectivity techniques allow the study of effective connectivity. Using such techniques it is possible to determine the influence of different cortical areas on each other, not just whether cortical areas are connected to one another. Two model-based effective connectivity techniques are called structural equation modeling and dynamic causal modeling. These techniques require the experimenter to specify a particular set of causal connections between brain areas and then estimate free parameters for these models. These models restrict the number of possible causal connections. These techniques can be especially powerful for experiments in which the detail of brain connectivity is well known or when there is a limited amount of neuroimaging data to fit to the model (model-based techniques require less degrees of freedom). However, when the details of brain connectivity is still poorly identified such techniques can limit discover of unique patterns of connectivity. For example, studies which applied these techniques to the reading networks of the brain have only evaluated a subset of possible connections between cortical areas -- some studies have only examined one direction of influence (Levy *et al.*, 2009) while others have limited the analysis to only the left hemisphere (Bitan *et al.*, 2009; Cao *et al.*, 2008; Quaglino *et al.*, 2008).

In contrast to these *model-driven* techniques for measuring effective connectivity, Granger causality (GC) is a *data-driven* technique that empirically calculates the direction and strength of connectivity with minimal assumptions about the structure of the neural network (Frye *et al.*, 2010; 2011; 2012; Wu *et al.*, 2011). GC is based on the assumption that causes precede effects. To determine the temporal relationship between neurophysiological signals, the GC technique uses autoregressive (AR) models to analyze the temporal relation within and between signals. Essentially, if a particular neurophysiological signal can predicted another neurophysiological signal better than that signal can predict itself, it is considered to be driving the signal. Recently, using Granger causality to analyze magnetoencephalography (MEG) recordings, Frye *et al.* (2010; 2012) have shown that the organization of the brain network just prior to decoding a phonological stimulus is critically important in individuals who suffered from dyslexia during childhood. Specifically, individuals with a history of dyslexia who performed better on the phonological task in the scanner demonstrated greater top-down control from the IFAs to other brain areas and less influence of the right TPA on the left TPA.

3   Advantages of Magnetoencephalography for Measuring Connectivity

Over the last 30 years, neuroimaging has revolutionized our ability to study the nervous system, provided insight into the basic architecture and principles of brain function and increased our understanding of clinical neurological disorders. Over the past two decades, measures of connectivity have been applied to functional neuroimaging data derived from fMRI and positron emission tomography (PET) (Ramnani *et al.*, 2004). Such neuroimaging methods measure changes in brain metabolism due to neural activity. Indeed, connectivity techniques applied to fMRI have identified neural systems that were not obvious on functional activation maps. However, fMRI and PET measure brain activation on a time scale of seconds while brain systems operate on a millisecond time scale. Thus, only very stable and prolonged connections between brain areas can be measured with metabolic techniques. Thus, prolonged brain states, such as those that regulate and represent emotion, may be best represented by such technique, while brain operations which are required to operate on quickly changing stimuli, such as language, may be better studied by other techniques which have greater temporal resolution. More recently, measures of anatomic connectivity derived from diffusion tensor imaging have provided detailed information regarding the organization, integrity and architecture of white matter connectivity in the brain (Sherbondy *et al.*, 2005). Diffusion tensor imaging reveals relatively static or long-term changes in connectivity on the order of months or years. Such techniques can be very useful for examining the consequences of brain reorganization with therapeutic interventions.

Quick dynamic change in neural activation and connectivity that involve the rapid interplay between many cognitive areas cannot be appreciated with metabolic neuroimaging techniques. The importance of this is highlighted when considering sensory and language systems. For example, underlying key building blocks of auditory and visual language are processed rapidly and automatically. For example, auditory syllables are processed in approximately one-fifth of a second, and words are processed in approximately one-third of a second. Indeed, the processing of these language stimuli requires the cooperation and integration of activity in frontal, temporal, parietal and occipital areas within this subsecond processing time frame. Indeed, in a classic example of dramatic reorganization, a congenitally blind person's crossmodal pattern of activation was revealed by MEG. Somatosensory input rapidly activated visual cortex via the posterior parietal cortex toV5 and V3 and eventually to V1. In sighted people this se-ries of activations to visual cortex was not found (Ioannides *et al.*, 2013).

Whole-head MEG measures fluctuations in the local magnetic field results from the simultaneous post-synaptic activation of approximately 10,000 pyramidal cells in the cortical gray matter (Hamalainen, 1992). By combining the strengths of several other neuroimaging methods, MEG represents a significant advance in neuroimaging for both clinical and research applications. Like metabolically based neuroimaging tools, such as PET and fMRI, MEG can provide a functional map of the location of brain activity with reasonable spatial resolution[1]. However, by measuring the changes in the brain's magnetic field on a millisecond time scale, MEG recordings provide an approximately three order of magnitude greater temporal resolution than metabolic-based functional neuroimaging tools. This allows MEG to provide visualization of the spatiotemporal dynamics of cortical activation. Indeed, the evolution of brain activity through time, the flow of activation from one cortical area to another and the dynamic interactions between cortical areas can be visualized and qualitatively studied with MEG.

The high temporal resolution of electroencephalography (EEG), another noninvasive neurophysiologic neuroimaging technique, also allows the dynamics of brain connectivity to be examined. EEG has used connectivity techniques for decades and has embraced the measurement of connectivity direction, such as GC, partial directed coherence, and directed transfer function (Astolfi *et al.*, 2005). Until the development of DANCI, the only measures of effective connectivity that have been applied to MEG data used a rough index of directionality (Leuthold *et al.*, 2005). We have investigated the applicability of the GC technique to both signal and source space MEG data. This investigation was fueled by the discovery that language networks responsible for both visual and auditory phonological decoding undergo rapid wide-spread activation with complex spatiotemporal dynamics (Frye *et al.*, 2005; 2006a; 2006b). Such empirical observations were derived from qualitative analysis of sequential dynamic statistical parameter mapping images viewed as movies. In order to provide a quantitative analysis tool, we developed an empirical analysis technique to provide images of neural connectivity based on few assumptions of the neural network structure. We demonstrated that traditional measures of GC could be applied to source space MEG in order to visualize the dynamic changes in brain activation using DANCI (Frye *et al.*, 2007). More recently we demonstrated how DANCI could be used to visualize the widely distributed cortical network structure active while preparing to phonologically decode a non-word stimulus in normal and dyslexic readers (Frye *et al.*, 2010; 2012).

3   Dynamic Autoregressive Neuromagnetic Causality Imaging (DANCI)

3.1   Interconnected Neural Networks

Most connectivity techniques use the pair-wise approach. However, such an approach presents limitation since it only considers the interaction between two signals (Figure 1A). The brain is a highly-connected neural network with more than two sources of activity. Models of interconnectivity become increasingly complex as the number of simultaneously active interconnected sources increase (i.e., three signals, Figure 1B, and five signals, Figure 1C). In fact, for S sources, there are S * (S-1) causal connections. Thus, if the connectivity between two sources is considered (i.e., the pair-wise approach), potentially important

---

[1]   It should be noted that an exact comparison of the spatial resolution between fMRI and MEG cannot be made since localization of MEG signal is performed using a model-based approach and are therefore estimated. In comparison fMRI signals are measured with a predefined spatial resolution.

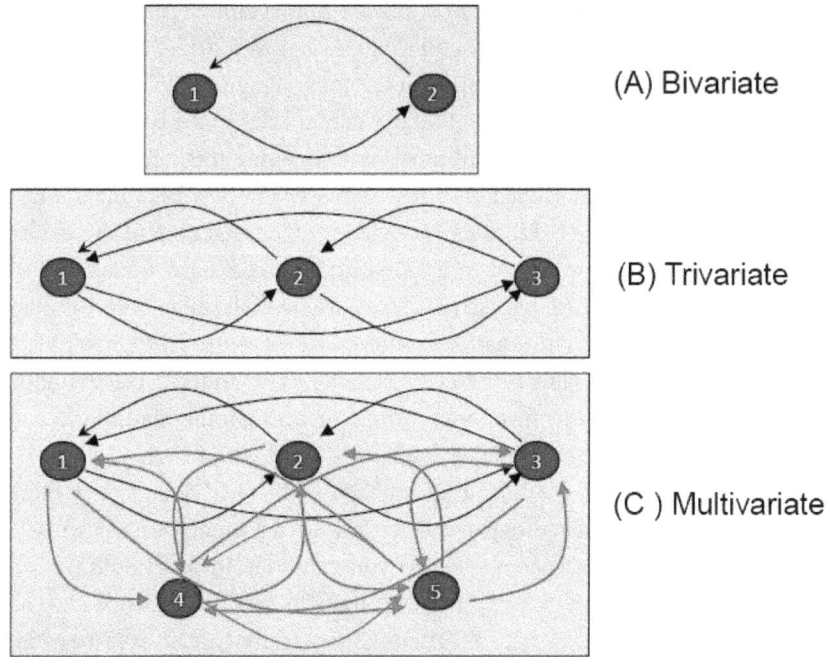

Figure 1: Interaction between signals. Signal sources are represented by circles and causal interactions between sources are represented by arcs with arrows. (A) Pair-wise causality models represent the directed interaction between only two signals (bivariate). (B) More complicated models represent the directed interactions of three signals (trivariate). (C) The number of directed interactions starts to grow geometrically when addition signals (in this case five) are considered.

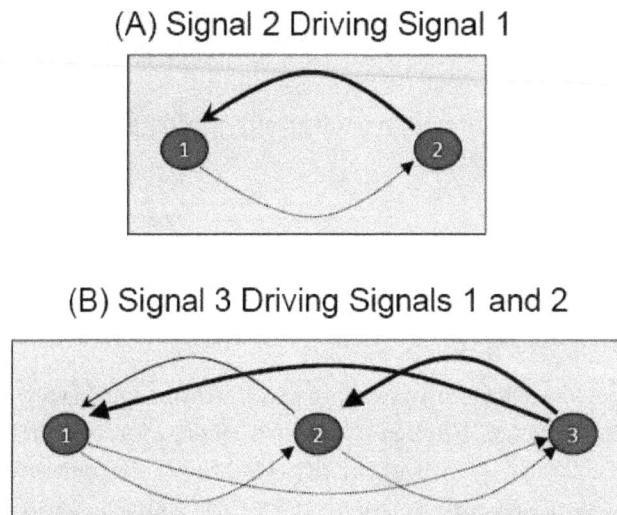

Figure 2: Multiple source analysis. Increasing the number of signals simultaneous considered ensures that the model represents the proper network architecture. For example, in (A) signal 2 appears to be driving signal 1 but really a latent, unconsidered signal (signal 3) in (B) is driving both signals 1 and 2.

interactions will be ignored. For example, source 2 would appear to be the primary driver of source 1, if the pair-wise approach was used (Figure 2A). However, it becomes obvious that source 3 is driving both sources 1 and 2 if all sources are considered simultaneously (Figure 2B). Once the latent source (i.e., source 3) is unconcealed and taken into account, the true causal influence of source 2 on source 1 can be measured.

The possibility of such latent sources in larger interconnected networks like the brain is one justification for considering multiple sources simultaneously. Such complex interactions are the rule rather than the exception in biological neural networks, making them important to consider in models of the nervous system. Inferring an incorrect relationship between two sources due to the use a pair-wise analysis was called 'prima facie cause' by Granger (C.W.J. Granger, 1980). In fact this limitation of connectivity analysis motivated the development of more sophisticated connectivity techniques. Indeed, complex, multichannel models allow the influence of any particular source to be determined given the influence of all other sources.

3.2   Computational Methods for Calculating Granger Causality

The complex interaction between multiple brain regions can be considered using an implementation of GC we recently described called DANCI[2] (Frye & Wu, 2011). DANCI uses least-squares linear regression (LSLR) to model the interactions between a large number of MEG sensors (Frye *et al*, 2007) or sources (Frye *et al.*, 2007), or EEG electrodes (Pollonini *et al.*, 2010). Originally Granger (1969) described the LSLR approach for calculating autoregressive (AR) model coefficients and GC. However, over the last two decades researchers, particularly those in the signal analysis field, have adopted the Levinson, Wiggins, Robinson (LWR) algorithm, a maximum entropy method, to solve the system of equations associated the GC analysis. Recently, we demonstrated that the LSLR method was far superior to the LWR method in terms of accuracy and speed for calculating and solving the coefficients of the complex AR models (Frye & Wu, 2011). In addition, we also demonstrated the superiority of the DANCI approach for the calculations of effective connectivity as compared to other potential measures of effective connectivity, including directed transfer function, partial directed coherence, squared partial directed coherence, full frequency directed transfer function and direct directed transfer function (Wu *et al.*, 2011). In fact, recently we have demonstrated that DANCI can provide an excellent measure of connectivity with a very low theoretical error rate (Frye, 2013).

3.3   Pairwise Autoregressive Models

Linear AR models are traditionally used to calculate GC since they have considerable flexibility and can model interactions within and between multiple signals simultaneously, thereby provide a powerful technique for studying the connections between signals in the nervous system. An AR process can be defined for a time series $A = [a(t): 1...T]$. The AR process is assumed to have a periodic component so that any time t it can be predicted by the signal at some past time. The signal $a(t)$ given by

$$a(t) = c_1 * a(t-1) + c_2 * a(t-2) + c_3 * a(t-3) \tag{1}$$

where $a(t)$ is a signal that is dependent on the past three values at times $t-1$, $t-2$ and $t-3$. The influence of the previous values of the signal is given by the coefficients c_1, c_2 and c_3 for times $t-1$, $t-2$ and

---

[2] DANCI MATLAB software functions are freely available at: http://openwetware.org/wiki/Frye:_Function_Reference_(Granger_Causality_Project).

$t - 3$, respectively. The number of previous time values considered defines the order of the model. The model order is three in Equation (1). Since real signals are not completely deterministic, we must consider that the predicted value of signal $a(t)$ is associated with some error $e_{a|a}(t)$. This error represents the portion of the signal $a(t)$ at time t which is not accounted for by the given previous values of $a(t - 1)$, $a(t - 2)$ and $a(t - 3)$. This stochastic definition is given by

$$a(t) = c_{a,1} * a(t-1) + c_{a,2} * a(t-2) + c_{a,3} * a(t-3) + e_{a|a}(t) \qquad (2)$$

A generalization of the model for any order P is given by

$$a(t) = \sum_{j=1}^{p} c_{a,j} * a(t-j) + e_{a|a}(t) \qquad (3)$$

Where error $e_{a|a}(t)$ represents the portion of the signal a(t) at time t that is not accounted for given the previous values of $a(t - 1)...a(t - P)$. In a manner similar to the AR case, a periodic signal can also be predicted by another periodic signal rather than itself. The case where the time series $B = [b(t): 1...T]$ predicts the time series A is given by

$$a(t) = \sum_{j=1}^{p} c_{b,j} * b(t-j) + e_{a|b}(t) \qquad (4)$$

Where the model order is P and $e_{a|b}(t)$ represents the error in predicting $a(t)$ given the previous time point of $b(t - 1)...b(t - P)$. The signal $a(t)$ can also be predicted by its own past activity as well as activity of another signal. In order to formulate such a model, we combine Equations (3) and (4) to produce Equation (5).

$$a(t) = \sum_{j=1}^{p} c_{a,j} * a(t-j) + \sum_{k=1}^{p} c_{b,j} * b(t-k) + e_{a|ab}(t) \qquad (5)$$

Equation (5) demonstrates that signal $a(t)$ at time t is being predicted by the previous activity of both $a(t - 1)...a(t - P)$ and $b(t - 1)...b(t - P)$. $e_{a|ab}(t)$ represents the error in predicting $a(t)$ given the previous time point of $a(t - 1)...a(t - P)$ and $b(t - 1)...b(t - P)$.

3.4   Calculating Granger Causality in Pairwise Models

Granger causality measures the influence of one signal on another. This measure is based on the relative change in the model error when time series are added to improve the prediction of the dependent signal. For example, we can measure the error accounted for by adding the time series B to Equation (5) by comparing the error terms of Equations (3) and (5). The traditional causality measure is given by a ratio of the variance of the model before and after the addition of the new time-series. This value is calculated using Equation (6):

$$F_a = \ln \frac{Var(e_{a|a})}{Var(e_{a|ab})} \qquad (6)$$

3.5   Solving the Pairwise Models

The LSLR approach for solving the AR equations require a model to be specified as

$$Y = X\beta + e \qquad (7)$$

where Y is the matrix of dependent values, X is the design matrix containing the independent variables, β is the model coefficients and e is the model error. Once the data are specified in this form, β is calculated by solving,

$$\beta = \left(X'X\right)^{-1}\left(X'Y\right) \tag{8}$$

In order to solve the AR Equation outlined in Equation (7) we specify one row of the vector Y and matrix X for one data observation o as:

$$Y^o = \left[a^o(t)\right] \tag{9}$$

$$X^o = \left[a^o(t-1) \ldots a^o(t-P) \quad b^o(t-1)\ldots b^o(t-P)\right] \tag{10}$$

This can then be generalized for multiple observations by specifying vector Y and matrix X for observations $o = 1\ldots O$ as:

$$Y = \left[Y^1\ldots Y^O\right]' \tag{11}$$

$$X = \left[X^1\ldots X^O\right]' \tag{12}$$

3.6   Implementing Multichannel Models

AR models can be generalized to model the mutual influence of S signals with T time points in time series $A = [a_s(t) : s = 1..S, t = 1..T]$. A system of AR models of order P is given as:

$$a_1(t) = \sum_{j=1}^{p} C_{1,1,j} a_1(t-j) + \sum_{j=1}^{p} C_{1,2,j} a_2(t-j) + \cdots + \sum_{j=1}^{p} C_{1,S,j} a_S(t-j) + e_{1|1\ldots S}(t)$$

$$a_2(t) = \sum_{j=1}^{p} C_{2,1,j} a_1(t-j) + \sum_{j=1}^{p} C_{2,2,j} a_2(t-j) + \cdots + \sum_{j=1}^{p} C_{2,S,j} a_S(t-j) + e_{2|1\ldots S}(t) \tag{13}$$

$$\ldots\ldots$$

$$a_S(t) = \sum_{j=1}^{p} C_{S,1,j} a_1(t-j) + \sum_{j=1}^{p} C_{S,2,j} a_2(t-j) + \cdots + \sum_{j=1}^{p} C_{S,S,j} a_S(t-j) + e_{S|1\ldots S}(t)$$

In this set, each equation represents a signal $a_s(t)$ at time t that is being predicted by previous values of itself and all other signals. For example, in Equation (13), coefficients $c_{1,1,j}$ ($j = 1..P$) quantitatively describe the influence of the activity of $a_1(t)$ on itself, coefficients $c_{1,2,j}$ ($j = 1..P$) quantitatively describe the influence of the activity of $a_2(t)$ on $a_1(t)$, and coefficients $c_{1,s,j}$ ($j = 1\ldots P$) quantitatively describe the influence of signal $a_s(t)$ on $a_1(t)$, etc. Likewise coefficients $c_{s,1,j}$ ($j = 1\ldots P$) describe the quantitative influence of signal $a_1(t)$ on signal $a_s(t)$. This set of equations allows the influence of all signals of interest to be considered simultaneously. In order to formulate this problem for LSLR we modify our definition of matrix X for one data observation o (previously Equation 10) to Equation 14:

$$X^o = \left[a_1^o(t-1)\ldots a_1^o(t-P) \; a_2^o(t-1)\ldots a_2^o(t-P)\ldots \; a_S^o(t-1)\ldots a_S^o(t-P)\right] \tag{14}$$

In addition, Y (previously defined as Equation 11) can be redefined as Equation 15:

$$Y_s = \left[a_s^1(t) \dots a_s^o(t) \right] \tag{15}$$

The coefficients for Equation 13 can be calculated using Equation 16:

$$c_s = \left(X'X \right)^{-1} \left(X'Y_s \right) \tag{16}$$

Each signal can be solved by redefining vector Y with the values for each specific signal or source. The error vector for the system of equations is defined by Equation 17 and then the mean squared error must be calculated using Equation 18.

$$e_{s|1\dots S} = Xc_s - Y_s \tag{17}$$

$$mse_{s|1\dots S} = \frac{\sum_{i=1}^{O} e_{s|1\dots S}^2}{O} \tag{18}$$

In order to determine the influence of one signal on another and calculate GC, the independent signal (i.e., the one influencing the signal of interest) needs to be eliminated from the systems of equations and the error of the equation system needs to be recalculated. The AR models for a signal s in Equation (13) already accounts for the influence of all of signals. We can eliminate the signal of interest by reconstructing the matrix X^o leaving out the signal of interest. For example, if we were interested in the influence of signal 2 on any other signal s, we would reformulate X^o as demonstrated in Equation (19), recalculate the LSLR and derive the error vector $e_{s|1,3\dots S}$.

$$X^o = \left[a_1^o(t-1) \dots a_1^o(t-P) \; a_3^o(t-1) \dots a_3^o(t-P) \dots a_S^o(t-1) \dots a_S^o(t-P) \right] \tag{19}$$

The GC measure representing the influence of signal 2 on signal s given all of the other signals 1 to S (expect for 2) would be calculated with Equation (20):

$$F_{2 \to s} = \ln \frac{mse_{s|1,3\dots S}}{mse_{s|1\dots S}} \tag{20}$$

Using the approach above, we constructed a matrix of GC values to represent the influence of each MEG sensor on every other MEG sensor. We then evaluated the significance of each GC value in order to consider only the connections which represented significant connectivity. The same measure of error that is used to calculate GC can also be used in a partial F-test in order to calculate the significance of the GC value. Equation (21) outlines the calculation of this F-distributed value which has P and $O \times T - S \times P - 1$ degrees-of-freedom in the numerator and denominator, respectively. Granger used the same symptom 'F' to signify GC, making the notation confusing.

$$F_{P,O*T-S*P-1}^{2 \to s} = \frac{\dfrac{O \cdot (mse_{s|1,3\dots S} - mse_{s|1\dots S})}{P}}{\dfrac{O \cdot mse_{s|1\dots S}}{O \cdot T - S \cdot P - 1}} \tag{21}$$

To empirically derive the structure of the network we can use Equation (21) to determine the connections truly exist within the network. The F-value in Equation (21) provides an indication of statistical significant of the GC value.

4   Interpreting Granger Causality in Neuroimaging Experiments

In order to quantitatively analyze GC values, in our recent studies we constructed a linear mixed-model (Frye *et al.*, 2010; 2012). In order to ensure we only examine true network connections, we use a very conservative alpha ($p \leq 10^{-4}$), as calculated from the F-value derived with Equation (21), in order to eliminate non-significant connection from the analysis. We then use a statistical analysis to determine whether GC values were different between different conditions and whether the GC values depend on the individual's behavioral performance during the task. We felt that it was important to look at both factors because our previous studies on dyslexia found that the relation between behavioral performance and connectivity was not necessarily the same for different reading groups and that individual behavioral performance as well as history of dyslexia both independently predicted the pattern of connectivity in the brain (Frye *et al.*, 2011). Thus, our previous models contained the fixed-effects of both reading groups and a covariate for performance with an additional interaction between these effects. When applying statistical models to experiments with effective connectivity, we must also examine the direction of effective connectivity (i.e., to or from a cortical area). Thus, since there are two directions of connectivity for each connection (in vs. out) an additional fixed-effect of connectivity direction was included in the statistical model models. Lastly, when we apply a model to examine the changes in connectivity in a certain area of the brain, we also need a factor to account for the area of the brain to/from which the connectivity is coming from or going to. For example, if we are examining how a TPA is connected to the other brain areas that we believe are important for language (i.e., 5 other areas, specifically right and left IFA, right and left VOTA and the contralateral TPA) an additional fixed-effect, which represented brain area, needs to be included in the model. Thus, a final model is created with fixed-effects of area (5 levels), reading group, and connectivity direction (in v. out) with a covariate representing performance. In our previous studies we used the 'mixed' procedure of SAS 9.1 (SAS Institute Inc., Cary, NC) to evaluate the model. For mixed-models, variables are also designated to represent the repeated measurements so the individual variance can be taken into accounted. In our previous studies, the participants' cortical areas and connectivity direction were entered as random effects in the mixed-model as well as a variable to account for the individual participant (Frye *et al.*, 2010; 2012).

The general mixed-model in the matrix form is given by Equation (22) where y is the dependent variable, which in this case is connectivity between two cortical regions, X is the design matrix for the fixed effects and covariate, β is a vector containing the parameters of the fixed effects and covariate, Z is the design matrix for the random effects, γ contains the parameters of the random effects and ε is the variance-covariance matrix of the model error.

$$y = X\beta + Z\gamma + \varepsilon \qquad (22)$$

The key assumption of the mixed model are that both γ and ε have the expected value of zero (i.e., $E(\gamma) = 0$ and $E(\varepsilon) = 0$) and known covariance structure given by the matrixes Var (γ) and Var(ε). The values for each row of the design matrix X are given by Equation (23) where c is the constant with value 1, *area* is the cortical *area* represented by the five dummy variables $area_1 \ldots area_5$ (i.e., for analysis of the left

TPA, dummy variables would be set up to represent the other cortical regions that the left TPA is connected to, for example $area_1 = 1$ for left IFA and 0 otherwise, $area_2 = 1$ for left VOTA and 0 otherwise, etc.), inout is connectivity direction represented by a dummy variable (i.e., inward = 0, outward = 1), read is reading group as represented by a dummy variable (i.e., dyslexia = 1, typical = 0) and d_p is the centered d-prime value for the particular participant, p. The behavioral performance measure, d_p, is a measure of the ability of the participant to discriminate between the correct choice (i.e., the signal) and the incorrect choice (i.e., noise) as defined by signal detection theory.

$$
\begin{aligned}
x(t,v,h,a_{p,v}) = \big[& c\ area_1\ area_2\ area_3\ area_4\ area_5\ inout\ read\ d_p(area_1 \times inout).... \\
& (area_5 \times inout)(area_1 \times read)....(area_5 \times read)(area_1 \times d_p).... \\
& (area_5 \times d_p)(inout \times read)(inout \times d_p)(read \times d_p)(area_1 \times inout \times read).... \\
& (area_5 \times inout \times read)(area_1 \times inout \times d_p)....(area_5 \times inout \times d_p) \\
& (area_1 \times read \times d_p)....(area_5 \times read \times d_p)(inout \times read \times d_p) \\
& (area_1 \times inout \times read \times d_p)....(area_5 \times inout \times read \times d_p) \big]
\end{aligned}
\tag{23}
$$

The values for each row of the random-effects design matrix Z are given by Equation (24) where p is the participant where p_i is 1 for participant i and 0 otherwise. The mixed-model was calculated using the restricted maximum likelihood method.

$$
z(p,\ area,\ inout) = \big[p_1....p_{17}\ area_1\ area_2\ area_3\ area_4\ area_5\ inout \big]
\tag{24}
$$

5   An Application of DANCI for Understanding Reorganization of Brain Connectivity in Neurodevelopmental Disorders

In our previous studies we have examined connectivity between important language regions of the brain, specifically, the right and left IFAs, TPAs and VOTAs. The results described below are based on a sample of 10 typical readers and 7 dyslexic readers, all native English speakers between the ages of 18 and 45 years, with normal or corrected vision, normal hearing, and no history of severe psychiatric or neurological illnesses or attention defects. Poor reading performance was confirmed for the dyslexic readers using standard reading tests and all participants were screened for attention problems. While in the MEG scanner, the participants were asked to decide whether two non-words rhymed. This task specifically taps into phonological function. Preliminary studies developed the task to be equated for difficulty across the two reading groups to ensure performance was equal across dyslexic and typical readers as reported in our other studies (Fisher *et al.*, 2012). Below we provide some interesting results from our experiment as an example of an application of DANCI but do not provide a comprehensive analysis of the results as this is beyond the scope of this chapter.

First, in our experiments, several frequency bands of brain activity were analyzed separately since different frequency bands have been linked to different cognitive processes. For example, gamma band activity has been linked to binding features of a visual object, local feature integration and polysensory integration (Fries, 2007) and the transient coupling and uncoupling of local neural networks (Lachaux *et al.*, 2008), while beta band activity has been linked to large-scale integration of brain activity such as top-down frontal control of parietal and occipital areas (Gross *et al.*, 2004; 2006) and multimodal integration between cortical lobes (von Stein *et al.*, 1999). Due to the fact that we are analyzing multiple frequencies with multiple repeated statistical models, the potential effect of inflated alpha need to be mitigated using the Bonferroni method. Since there are 6 frequency bands (low, medium and high beta and low medium and high gamma) examined, the alpha for statistical significance in the models is corrected to account for this fact, so that an alpha of $0.05/6 =\sim 0.008$ is used as the cutoff for significance in the statistical models.

Second, effective connectivity analysis assumes stationarity (i.e., that connectivity is not changing within the time period analyzed). For fMRI data, this assumption is not problematic since the hemodynamic signal changes much slower than the sampling rate of the signal and the entire sampling window. MEG has more than 100 times the temporal resolution of fMRI and thus can resolve much shorter intervals between the cortical areas driving other cortical areas. However, the higher temporal resolution does not easily meet the requirement of stationarity since changes in connectivity could occur within a certain temporal window selected for analysis. Using a short window can mitigate this issue, but guidelines for choosing the window size have not been investigated in MEG (Ding *et al.*, 2000; Frye *et al.*, 2007; Pollonini *et al.*, 2010). For this reason, we analyzed effective connectivity before the onset of the experimental trial, just before presentation of the stimulus. During this pre-stimulus period, brain activity reflects a relatively static preparatory state (Liang *et al.*, 2002), allowing the assumption of stationarity with respect to brain connectivity. This also provides a large number of samples to analyze (i.e., one per trial), thereby increasing reliability of the estimates and decreasing both Type I and Type II errors (Frye, 2013). It is also possible (and potentially very interesting) to analyze the MEG signal during stimulus processing. This would require careful investigation of the length of the time windows in which the signal is sufficiently stationary for valid analysis. Interestingly the optimal length of the time window during analysis of a dynamically changing MEG signal can change as brain activity evolves. We have discussed this in our previous publication (Frye *et al.*, 2007).

Recently we reported the differences in connectivity between the IFAs and other brain regions in the typical and dyslexic readers (Frye *et al.*, 2010). Here we describe the overall connectivity between the left and right IFAs and key language regions (irrespective of connectivity direction or individual performance) for the three beta frequency bands and three gamma frequency bands. We find that connectivity between the left and right IFAs is greater to the right TPA as compared to other brain regions for the low beta frequency range (Figure 3A). This is not true for the middle and high beta frequency ranges where the left and right IFAs demonstrated similar connectivity across to the other regions of interest (Figure 3B, C). For the gamma frequency range we see a slightly different pattern of overall connectivity. For low, medium and high gamma bands, there is significantly greater connectivity between the left and right IFAs with both TPAs as compared to other brain areas (Figure 4A, B, C).

In Figures 5 and 6 we depict both the inward and outward connectivity between key language areas and other brain areas for the low beta frequency range. We demonstrate interesting differences in the patterns of inward and outward connectivity between the dyslexic and typical reading groups. Specifically, in the typical reading group, the left IFA demonstrates greater outward as compared to inward connectivity to other brain regions, consistent with the idea that the frontal regions of the brain are providing top-down activation of key language areas in preparation for incoming language information. This significant difference in the balance between inward vs. outward connectivity is not seen in other language region in the typical reader. However, for the dyslexic reader, a very different pattern is seen. There is more inward as compared to outward connectivity from the left IFA to other regions of the brain suggesting

(A) Low Beta

(B) Middle Beta

(C) High Beta

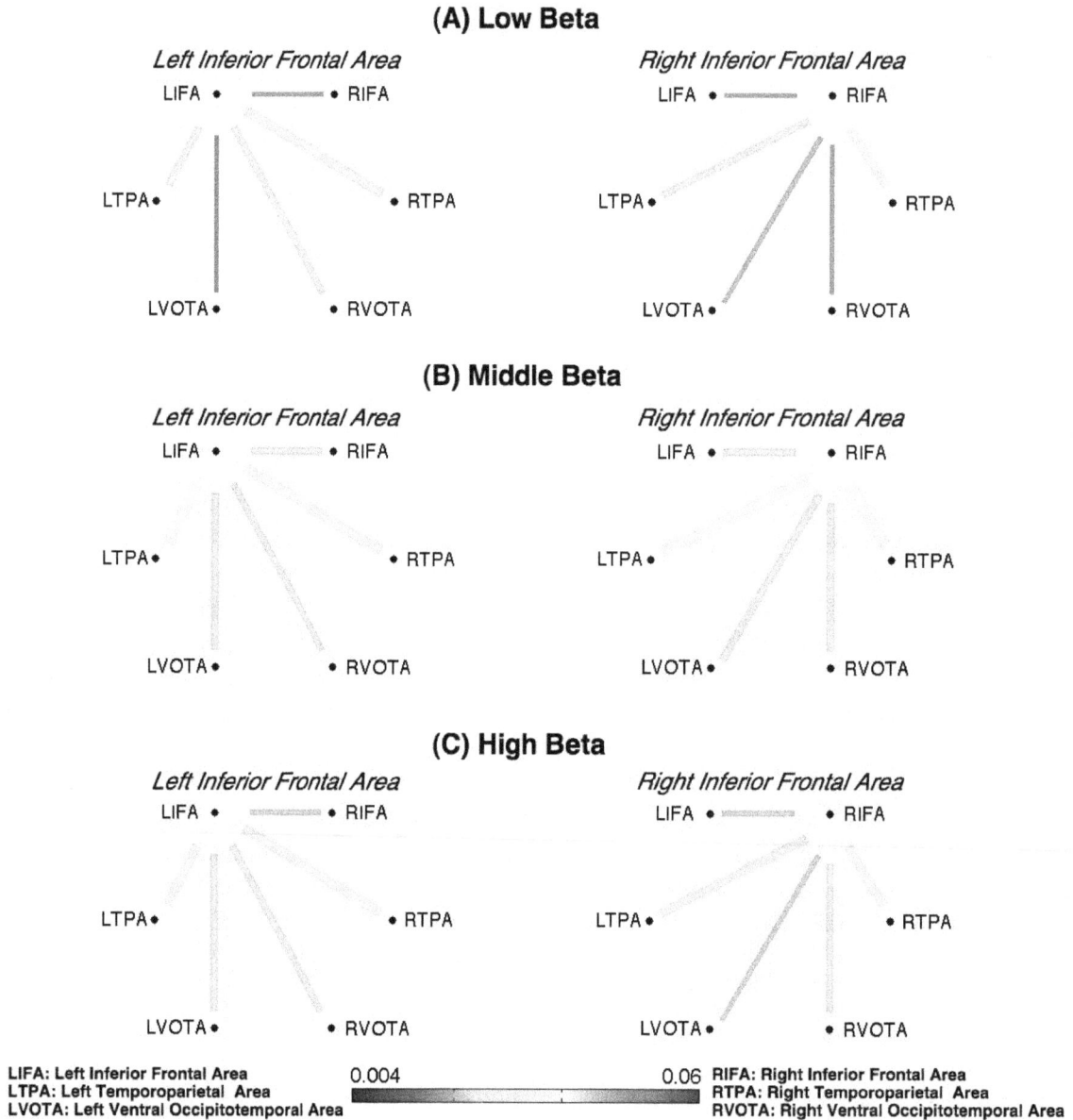

LIFA: Left Inferior Frontal Area
LTPA: Left Temporoparietal Area
LVOTA: Left Ventral Occipitotemporal Area

0.004   0.06

RIFA: Right Inferior Frontal Area
RTPA: Right Temporoparietal Area
RVOTA: Right Ventral Occipitotemporal Area

Figure 3: Overall connectivity from the left (left side of the figure) and right (right side of the figure) IFAs and other key brain regions for word processing (specifically the contralateral IFA and right and left TPAs and VOTAs) for three beta frequency ranges. Connectivity between both the left and right IFA and the right TPA is greater than connectivity with other regions of interest only for the low beta frequency range (A) but not the middle (B) and high (C) beta frequency range.

(A) Low Gamma

Left Inferior Frontal Area

LIFA ●   ● RIFA

LTPA●   ● RTPA

LVOTA●   ● RVOTA

Right Inferior Frontal Area

LIFA ●   ● RIFA

LTPA●   ● RTPA

LVOTA●   ● RVOTA

(B) Middle Gamma

Left Inferior Frontal Area

LIFA ●   ● RIFA

LTPA●   ● RTPA

LVOTA●   ● RVOTA

Right Inferior Frontal Area

LIFA ●   ● RIFA

LTPA●   ● RTPA

LVOTA●   ● RVOTA

(C) High Gamma

Left Inferior Frontal Area

LIFA ●   ● RIFA

LTPA●   ● RTPA

LVOTA●   ● RVOTA

Right Inferior Frontal Area

LIFA ●   ● RIFA

LTPA●   ● RTPA

LVOTA●   ● RVOTA

LIFA: Left Inferior Frontal Area
LTPA: Left Temporoparietal Area
LVOTA: Left Ventral Occipitotemporal Area

0.35   0.65

RIFA: Right Inferior Frontal Area
RTPA: Right Temporoparietal Area
RVOTA: Right Ventral Occipitotemporal Area

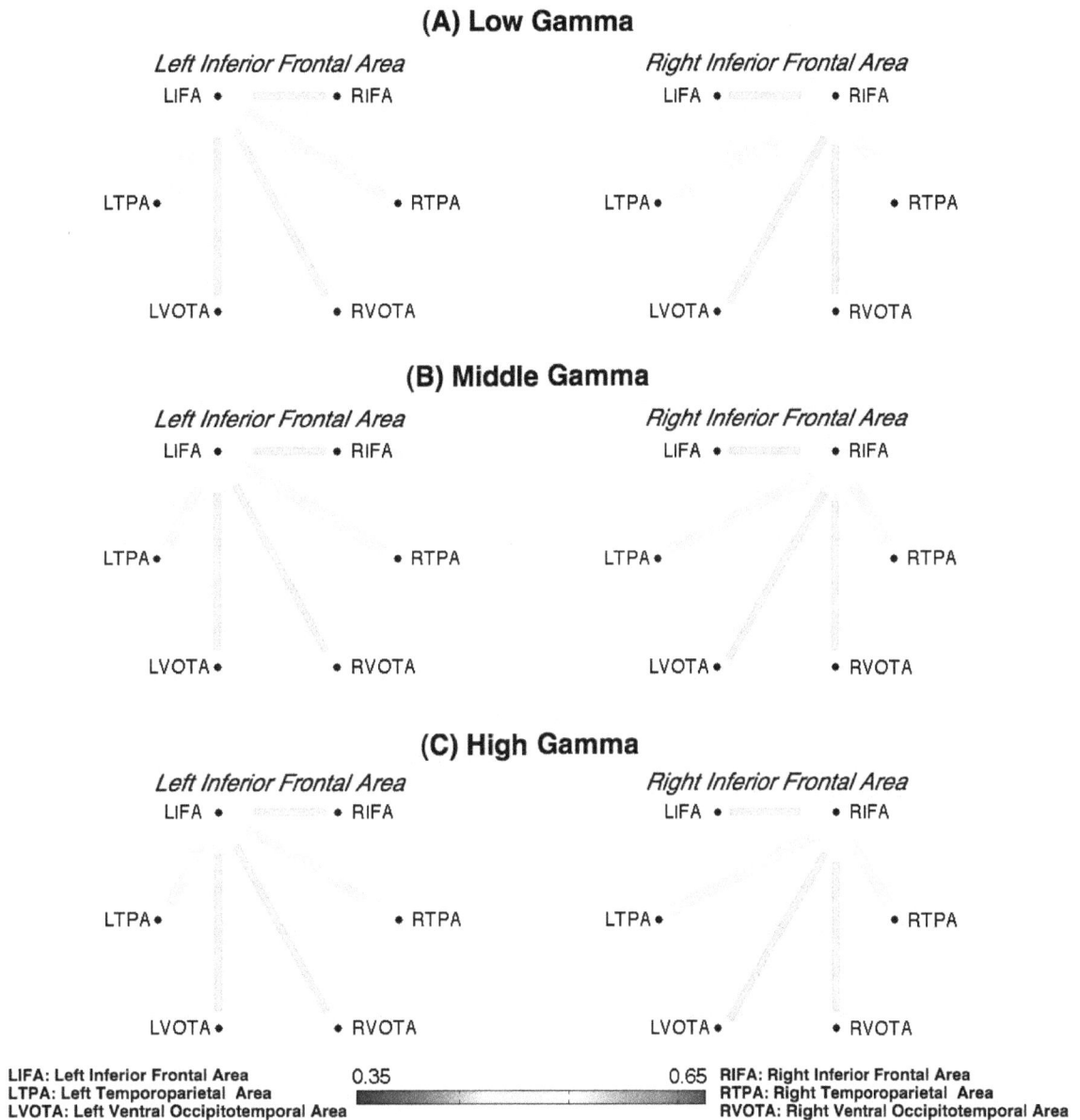

Figure 4: Overall connectivity from the left (left side of the figure) and right (right side of the figure) IFAs and other key brain regions for word processing (specifically the contralateral IFA and right and left TPAs and VOTAs) for three gamma frequency ranges. Connectivity between both the left and right IFA and both the right and left TPAs is greater than connectivity with other regions of interest for all three gamma frequency ranges.

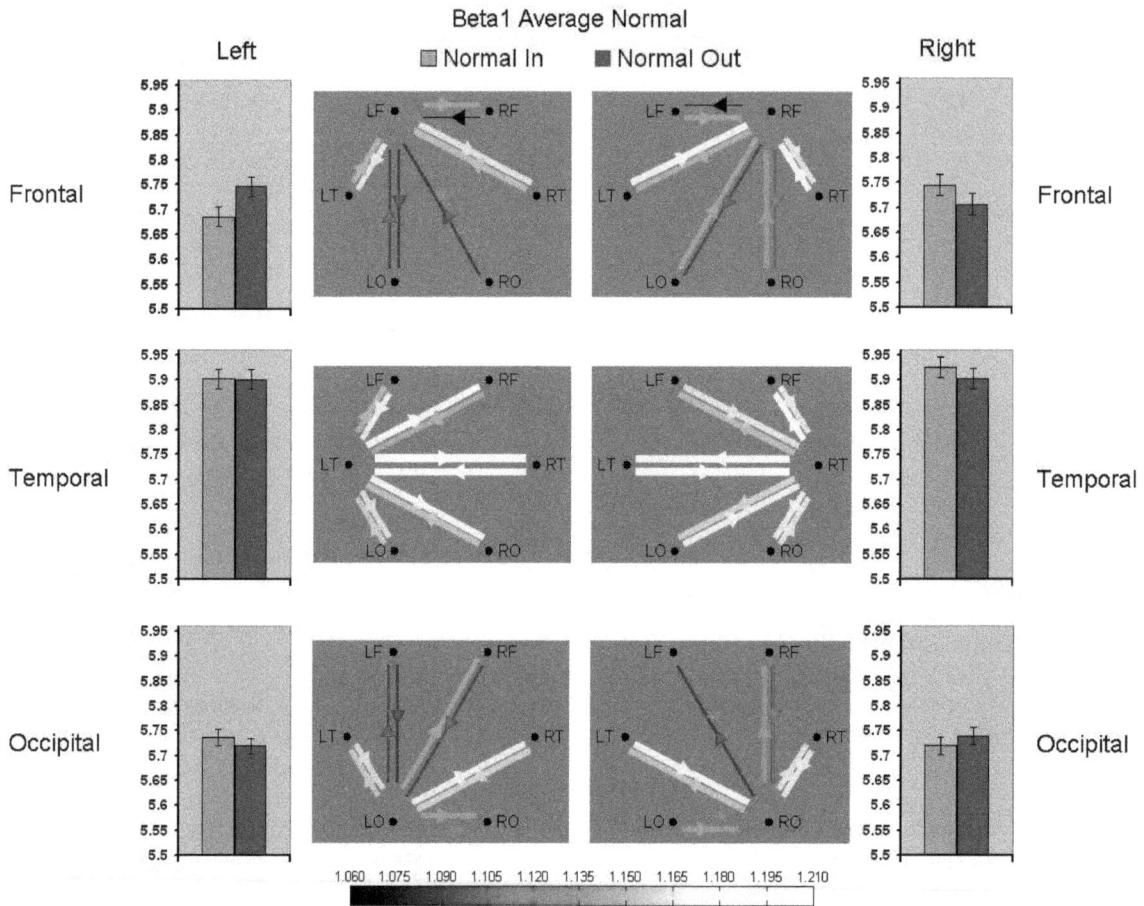

Figure 5: Both inwards and outwards connectivity from key regions important for word processing to and from other key regions in the low beta frequency range for typical readers. The left inferior frontal area (LF) demonstrates greater outward as compared to inward connectivity to other regions indicating top-down control of language networks by the left frontal area in typical readers. Abbreviations: LF= left inferior frontal area, RF = right inferior frontal area; LT = left temporoparietal area; RT = right temporoparietal area; LO = left ventral occipitotemporal area; RO = right occipitotemporal area.

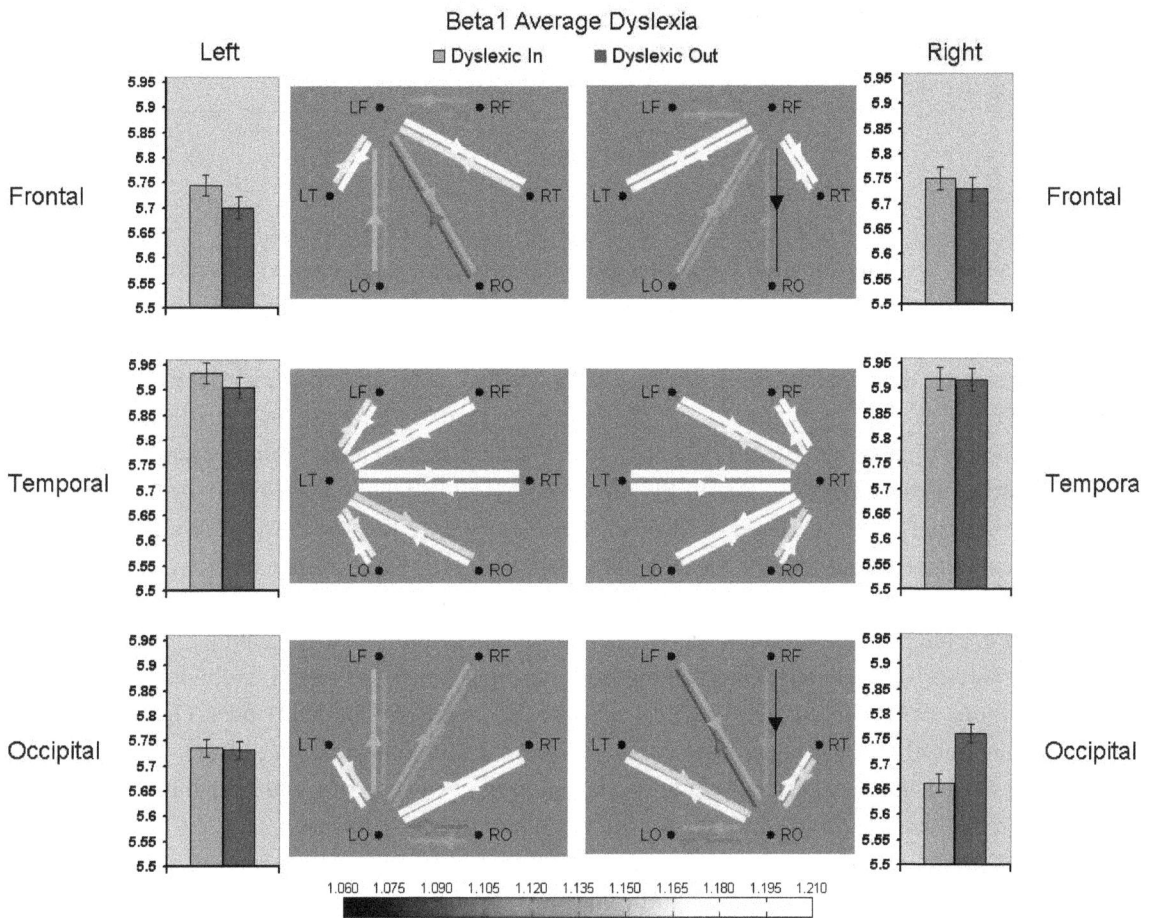

Figure 6: Both inwards and outwards connectivity from key regions important for word processing to and from other key regions in the low beta frequency range for dyslexic readers. The left inferior frontal area (LF) demonstrates greater inward as compared to outward connectivity indicating a failure of top-down control of language networks by the frontal areas in dyslexic readers. The right ventral occipitotemporal area (RO) demonstrates greater outward connectivity suggesting that the overall word processing network is driven by bottom-up processes in dyslexic readers. Abbreviations: LF= left inferior frontal area, RF = right inferior frontal area; LT = left temporoparietal area; RT = right temporoparietal area; LO = left ventral occipitotemporal area; RO = right occipitotemporal area.

that the left IFA is being driven by other brain regions in a bottom-up manner. In fact, for the dyslexic readers there is greater outward as compared to inward connectivity in the right ventral occipitotemporal area to other regions of the brain, suggesting that the network of key language areas in the dyslexic brain is driven in a bottom-up fashion. Interestingly, in our recent study we demonstrated that the balance between inward vs. outward connectivity in the left IFA is related to performance for dyslexic readers, further suggesting that the balance of inward vs. outward connectivity is important.

6   Discussion

The neuroimaging literature supports the notion of neural network reorganization in neurodevelopmental disorders such as dyslexia. We have described the use of a technique for analyzing effective connectivity using Granger Causality called Dynamic Autoregressive Neuromagnetic Causality Imaging (DANCI) which has been recently described in detail (Frye & Wu, 2011), compared to other effective connectivity techniques (Frye & Wu, 2011; Wu *et al.*, 2011) and used in several MEG studies examining neurodevelopmental disorders (Frye *et al.*, 2012; Frye *et al.*, 2010). When used to analyze the preparatory prestimulus period during a cognitive task, this technique can offer an excellent Type I and Type II error rate (Frye, 2013). We have demonstrated how this technique can be used to analyze MEG data from individuals with dyslexia in order to determine the associated changes in the brain's language network.

Future studies can apply this technique to neurodevelopmental disorders besides dyslexia. Autism is a neurodevelopmental disorder that is ripe for the application of this technique. For example, a recent meta-analysis of functional neuroimaging studies suggests that, in general, individuals with autism demonstrate more activity in posterior cortical regions (i.e., temporal, parietal and occipital areas) and less activity in frontal cortical regions, as compared to controls (Samson *et al.*, 2012), suggesting that individuals with autism have enhanced resource allocation to areas involved with visual processing, suggesting preferential use of visual pathways for information processing (Samson *et al.*, 2012). Clearly examining the direction of the connectivity between the occipital areas and other brain regions would provide important information regarding the significance of this pattern of reorganization.

The DANCI technique has the potential to be used in many additional ways. First, it may be possible to analyze the MEG signal during active stimulus processing, although further studies will be needed to determine the potential stationarity of the MEG signal under such condition. Although MEG signals provide high temporal resolution, the continual changing nature of the signal can provide an issue regarding stationarity. There are several metrics to examine this aspect of signal dynamics that can be used. We have discussed an approach to this issues in our previous publication (Frye *et al.*, 2007). Second, it is important to determine which types of brain activity would be optimally measured and analyzed by DANCI. Slowly changing processes, such as emotional states, may better be approached with metabolic neuroimaging techniques while DANCI and MEG may better serve cognitive processes that are rapidly changing such as language. Third, it is important to realize that the AR models used in the example presented above assume linear relationships between cortical sources. Despite being linear models, non-linear terms can be integrated into linear AR models. In our previous work we have demonstrated that our AR models fit very well to the MEG data as demonstrated using diagnostic statistics (Frye & Wu, 2011). Further investigation of non-linear phenomenon in the brain using DANCI would indeed be interesting.

Clearly further studies can benefit from examining causal brain activity using effective connectivity techniques such as DANCI. Such information will provide a greater understanding of brain reorganization in neurodevelopmental and other neurological disorders. Such understand will provide insight into the development of novel treatments for neurodevelopmental and neurological disorders as well as allow the careful examination of changes in brain organization with therapy and development.

References

Anderson, J. S., Druzgal, T. J., Froehlich, A., DuBray, M. B., Lange, N., Alexander, A., L,, . . . Lainhart, J. E. (2011). *Decreased interhemispheric functional connectivity in autism. Cerebral Cortex, 21(5), 1134-1146.*

Astolfi, L., Cincotti, F., Mattia, D., de Vico Fallani, F., Lai, M., Baccala, L., . . . Babiloni, F. (2005). *Comparison of different multivariate methods for the estimation of cortical connectivity: simulations and applications to EEG data. Conf Proc IEEE Eng Med Biol Soc, 5, 4484-4487.*

Bitan, T., Cheon, J., Lu, D., Burman, D. D., & Booth, J. R. (2009). *Developmental increase in top-down and bottom-up processing in a phonological task: an effective connectivity, FMRI study. J Cogn Neurosci, 21(6), 1135-1145.*

Cao, F., Bitan, T., & Booth, J. R. (2008). *Effective brain connectivity in children with reading difficulties during phonological processing. Brain Lang, 107(2), 91-101.*

Ding, M., Bressler, S. L., Yang, W., & Liang, H. (2000). *Short-window spectral analysis of cortical event-related potentials by adaptive multivariate autoregressive modeling: data preprocessing, model validation, and variability assessment. Biol Cybern, 83(1), 35-45.*

Ellmore, T. M., Li, H., Xue, Z., Wong, S. T., & Frye, R. E. (2013). *Tract-Based Spatial Statistics Reveal Altered Relationship Between Non-verbal Reasoning Abilities and White Matter Integrity in Autism Spectrum Disorder. J Int Neuropsychol Soc, 19(6), 723-728. doi: 10.1017/S1355617713000325*

Fries, P. (2007). *A mechanism for cognitive dynamics: neuronal communication through neuronal coherence. . Trends Cognitive Scence, 9, 474-480.*

Frye, R. E. (2013). *A lack of statistical pitfalls in the comparison of multivariate causality measures for effective causality. Comput Biol Med, 43(7), 962-965. doi: 10.1016/j.compbiomed.2013.02.001*

Frye, R. E., Hasan, K., Xue, L., Strickland, D., Malmberg, B., Liederman, J., & Papanicolaou, A. (2008). *Splenium microstructure is related to two dimensions of reading skill. Neuroreport, 19(16), 1627-1631.*

Frye, R. E., Liederman, J., Hasan, K. M., Lincoln, A., Malmberg, B., McLean, J., 3rd, & Papanicolaou, A. (2011). *Diffusion tensor quantification of the relations between microstructural and macrostructural indices of white matter and reading. Hum Brain Mapp, 32(8), 1220-1235. doi: 10.1002/hbm.21103*

Frye, R. E., Liederman, J., McGraw-Fisher, J., Halgren, E., & Dale, A. (2005). *Cortical Dynamics of Phonological Processing in Dyslexic and Normal Readers. Paper presented at the International Dyslexia Association, Denver, CO.*

Frye, R. E., Liederman, J., McGraw Fisher, J., & Wu, M. H. (2012). *Laterality of Temporoparietal Causal Connectivity during the Prestimulus Period Correlates with Phonological Decoding Task Performance in Dyslexic and Typical Readers. Cerebral Cortex, 22(8), 1923-34. doi: 10.1093/cercor/bhr265.*

Frye, R. E., McGraw Fisher, J., Coty, A., Ahlfors, S., Halgren, E., Papanicolaou, A., & Liederman, J. (2006). *Organization of large-scale spatiotemporal networks in young adults with a history of dyslexia. Paper presented at the International Society for Brain Electrotomography, Cheiti, Italy.*

Frye, R. E., McGraw Fisher, J., Coty, A., Liederman, J., & Halgren, E. (2006). *Dyslexic Readers Fail to Use Large Scale Neural Network During Phonological Decoding. Paper presented at the International Neuropsychological Society, Boston, MA.*

Frye, R. E., Wu, M.-H., Liederman, J., & McGraw Fisher, J. (2010). *Greater pre-stimulus effective connectivity from the left inferior frontal area to other areas is associated with better phonological decoding in dyslexic readers. Frontiers in Systems Neuroscience, 4. doi: 10.3389/fnsys.2010.00156*

Frye, R. E., Wu, M., & Zouridakis, G. (2007). *Dynamic Autoregressive Neuromagnetic Causality Imaging (DANCI). Paper presented at the Proceedings of the WSEAS International Conference on Computers, Crete, Greece.*

Frye, R. E., Wu, M., Zouridakis, G., McGraw Fisher, J., Liederman, J., & Halgren, E. (2007). *Changes in cortical connectivity in young adults with a history of reading disability. Paper presented at the Society of Neuroscience Meeting, San Diego, CA.*

Frye, R. E., & Wu, M. H. (2011). *Multichannel least-squares linear regression provides a fast, accurate, unbiased and robust estimation of Granger causality for neurophysiological data. Comput Biol Med, 41(12), 1118-1131. doi: 10.1016/j.compbiomed.2011.04.012*

Frye, R. E., Wu, M. H., Liederman, J., & Fisher, J. M. (2010). *Greater Pre-Stimulus Effective Connectivity from the Left Inferior Frontal Area to other Areas is Associated with Better Phonological Decoding in Dyslexic Readers. Front Syst Neurosci, 4, 156, doi: 10.3389/fnsys.2010.00156.*

Granger, C. W. J. (1969). *Investigating causal relations by econometric models and cross-spectral methods. Econometrica, 37(3), 424-438.*

Granger, C. W. J. (1980). *Testing for causality: a personal viewpoint. J Econ Dyn Control, 2, 329-352.*

Gross, J., Schmitz, F., Schnitzler, I., Kessler, K., Shapiro, K., Hommel, B., & Schnitzler, A. (2004). *Modulation of long-range neural synchrony reflects temporal limitations of visual attention in humans. Proc Natl Acad Sci U S A, 101(35), 13050-13055.*

Gross, J., Schmitz, F., Schnitzler, I., Kessler, K., Shapiro, K., Hommel, B., & Schnitzler, A. (2006). *Anticipatory control of long-range phase synchronization. Eur J Neurosci, 24(7), 2057-2060.*

Hamalainen, M. S. (1992). *Magnetoencephalography: a tool for functional brain imaging. Brain Topogr, 5(2), 95-102.*

Ioannides, A. A., Liu, L., Poghosyan, V., Saridis, G. A., Gjedde, A., Ptito, M., & Kupers, R. (2013). *MEG reveals a fast pathway from somatosensory cortex to occipital areas via posterior parietal cortex in a blind subject. Front Hum Neurosci, 7, 429. doi: 10.3389/fnhum.2013.00429*

Lachaux, J. P., Jung, J., Mainy, N., Dreher, J. C., Bertrand, O., Baciu, M., . . . Kahane, P. (2008). *Silence is golden: transient neural deactivation in the prefrontal cortex during attentive reading. Cerebral Cortex, 18(2), 443-450.*

Leuthold, A. C., Langheim, F. J., Lewis, S. M., & Georgopoulos, A. P. (2005). *Time series analysis of magnetoencephalographic data during copying. Exp Brain Res, 164(4), 411-422.*

Levy, J., Pernet, C., Treserras, S., Boulanouar, K., Aubry, F., Demonet, J. F., & Celsis, P. (2009). *Testing for the dual-route cascade reading model in the brain: an fMRI effective connectivity account of an efficient reading style. PLoS One, 4(8), e6675.*

Li, H., Xue, Z., Ellmore, T. M., Frye, R. E., & Wong, S. T. (2012). *Network-based analysis reveals stronger local diffusion-based connectivity and different correlations with oral language skills in brains of children with high functioning autism spectrum disorders. Hum Brain Mapp. doi: 10.1002/hbm.22185*

Liang, H., Bressler, S. L., Ding, M., Truccolo, W. A., & Nakamura, R. (2002). *Synchronized activity in prefrontal cortex during anticipation of visuomotor processing. Neuroreport, 13(16), 2011-2015.*

McGraw Fisher, J., Liederman, J., Johnsen, J., Lincoln, A., & Frye, R. E. (2012). *A demonstration that task difficulty can confound the interpretation of lateral differences in brain activation between typical and dyslexic readers. Laterality: Asymmetries of Body, Brain and Cognition, 17(3), 340-360.*

Monk, C. S., Peltier, S. J., Wiggins, J. L., Weng, S. J., Carrasco, M., Risi, S., & Lord, C. (2009). *Abnormalities of intrinsic functional connectivity in autism spectrum disorders. Neuroimage, 47(2), 764-772.*

Pollonini, L., Pophale, S., Situ, N., Wu, M. H., Frye, R. E., Leon-Carrion, J., & Zouridakis, G. (2010). *Information communication networks in severe traumatic brain injury. Brain Topogr, 23(2), 221-226. doi: 10.1007/s10548-010-0139-9.*

Pugh, K. R., Mencl, W. E., Jenner, A. R., Katz, L., Frost, S. J., Lee, J. R., . . . Shaywitz, B. A. (2000). *Functional neuroimaging studies of reading and reading disability (developmental dyslexia). Mental Retardation and Developmental Disabilities Research Reviews, 6(3), 207-213.*

Quaglino, V., Bourdin, B., Czternasty, G., Vrignaud, P., Fall, S., Meyer, M. E., . . . de Marco, G. (2008). *Differences in effective connectivity between dyslexic children and normal readers during a pseudoword reading task: an fMRI study. Neurophysiol Clin, 38(2), 73-82.*

Ramnani, N., Behrens, T. E., Penny, W., & Matthews, P. M. (2004). *New approaches for exploring anatomical and functional connectivity in the human brain. Biol Psychiatry, 56(9), 613-619.*

Samson, F., Mottron, L., Soulières, I., & Zeffiro, T. A. (2012). *Enhanced visual functioning in autism: An ALE meta-analysis. Hum Brain Mapp.*

Shaywitz, S. E., Shaywitz, B. A., Fulbright, R. K., Skudlarski, P., Mencl, W. E., Constable, R. T., . . . Gore, J. C. (2003). *Neural systems for compensation and persistence: young adult outcome of childhood reading disability. Biol Psychiatry, 54(1), 25-33.*

Shaywitz, S. E., Shaywitz, B. A., Fulbright, R. K., Skudlarski, P., Mencl, W. E., Constable, R. T., . . . Gore, J. C. (2003). *Neural systems for compensation and persistence: young adult outcome of childhood reading disability. Biol Psychiatry, 54(1), 25-33.*

Sherbondy, A., Akers, D., Mackenzie, R., Dougherty, R., & Wandell, B. (2005). *Exploring connectivity of the brain's white matter with dynamic queries. IEEE Trans Vis Comput Graph, 11(4), 419-430.*

Simos, P. G., Fletcher, J. M., Bergman, E., Breier, J. I., Foorman, B. R., Castillo, E. M., . . . Papanicolaou, A. C. (2002). *Dyslexia-specific brain activation profile becomes normal following successful remedial training. Neurology, 58(8), 1203-1213.*

Simos, P. G., Fletcher, J. M., Foorman, B. R., Francis, D. J., Castillo, E. M., Davis, R. N., . . . Papanicolaou, A. C. (2002). *Brain activation profiles during the early stages of reading acquisition. J Child Neurol, 17(3), 159-163.*

Simos, P. G., Fletcher, J. M., Sarkari, S., Billingsley, R. L., Denton, C., & Papanicolaou, A. C. (2007). *Altering the brain circuits for reading through intervention: a magnetic source imaging study. Neuropsychology, 21(4), 485-496.*

Temple, E., Deutsch, G. K., Poldrack, R. A., Miller, S. L., Tallal, P., Merzenich, M. M., & Gabrieli, J. D. (2003). *Neural deficits in children with dyslexia ameliorated by behavioral remediation: evidence from functional MRI. Proc Natl Acad Sci U S A, 100(5), 2860-2865.*

Vissers, M. E., X Cohen, M., & Geurts, H. M. (2012). *Brain connectivity and high functioning autism: A promising path of research that needs refined models, methodological convergence, and stronger behavioral links. Neuroscience & Biobehavioral Reviews, 36(1), 604-625. doi: 10.1016/j.neubiorev.2011.09.003*

von Stein, A., Rappelsberger, P., Sarnthein, J., & Petsche, H. (1999). *Synchronization between temporal and parietal cortex during multimodal object processing in man. Cereb Cortex, 9(2), 137-150.*

Weng, S. J., Wiggins, J. L., Peltier, S. J., Carrasco, M., Risi, S., Lord, C., & Monk, C. S. (2010). *Alterations of resting state functional connectivity in the default network in adolescents with autism spectrum disorders. Brain Research, 1313, 202-214.*

Wu, M. H., Frye, R. E., & Zouridakis, G. (2011). *A comparison of multivariate causality based measures of effective connectivity. Comput Biol Med, 41(12), 1132-1141. doi: 10.1016/j.compbiomed.2011.06.007.*

Brain Herniation

Gaurav Jain
Department of Anaesthesia
Institute of Medical Sciences, Banaras Hindu University, Varanasi, India

Ghanshyam Yadav
Department of Anaesthesia
Institute of Medical Sciences, Banaras Hindu University, Varanasi, India

Rohit Varshney
Department of Anaesthesia
Teerthanker Mahaveer Medical College, Moradabad, India

1   Introduction

A wide range of abnormal imaging characteristics are evaluated daily, representing various intracranial pathologies like tumour, oedema, haemorrhage, or brain herniation. Brain herniation represents a shift of brain parenchyma across the various anatomical boundaries formed by intracranial bony ridges and dural folds. This usually occurs when an expanding mass lesion including tumours, hematomas, infarctions, infection, or haemorrhage exhausts the limited capacity of intracranial cavity (Andrews *et al.*, 1986; Cuneo *et al.*, 1979; Cruz *et al.*, 2001; Dagnew *et al.*, 2002; Reich *et al.*, 1993; Ropper, 1986). Any insult to the blood supply or the ventricular system can also result in rise of intracranial pressure (ICP), with consequent mass effect upon adjacent compartments and subsequent herniation. Furthermore, other causes of cerebral herniation such as acute hydrocephalus, hepatic encephalopathy, regional or diffuse cerebral oedema by ischemia or infarction and therapeutic lumber cerebrospinal fluid (CSF) drainage are also common (Cuneo *et al.*, 1979; Lidofsky *et al.*, 1992; Reich *et al.*, 1993; Ropper, 1986; Muhonen & Zunkeler, 1994; Weinberg *et al.*, 2003).

Development of herniation due to mass effect depends upon many factors including patient age, size/location/progression rate of mass lesion, and pressure gradient between mean blood pressure, CSF, and brain tissue (Andrews *et al.*, 1986; Cuneo *et al.*, 1979; Cruz *et al.*, 2001; Dagnew *et al.*, 2002; Reich *et al.*, 1993; Ropper, 1986). Although it may affect any age group, elderly patients are at a higher risk of insult. This is due to more space for mobility of cerebral tissue owing to increased CSF content, large ventricles and cerebral atrophy. However, initial neurological findings are minimal in older individuals, due to less compression of brain tissue. Young patients have small, closely apposed basilar cisterns and ventricles, allowing less compensation for any mass effect. Therefore, neurological manifestations of brain herniation are most severe in younger individuals. Herniation can be a slow process resulting from a gradually expanding mass lesion such as subdural hematoma/tumour, or may develop rapidly after an acute traumatic event like epidural/subdural haemorrhage (Andrews *et al.*, 1986; Cuneo *et al.*, 1979; Cruz *et al.*, 2001; Dagnew *et al.*, 2002; Reich *et al.*, 1993; Ropper, 1986). Chronic lesions usually present as severe anatomic herniation with few initial neurological manifestations. In contrast, a rapidly enhancing mass lesion may result in profound and dreaded neurological deficits.

Anatomically, four varieties of cerebral herniation are described. These include: subfalcine, transtentorial (ascending or descending), tonsillar and transphenoidal herniation (Figure 1) (Reich *et al.*, 1993; Meyer, 1920; Scheinker, 1945). A fifth variety, transcalvarial herniation, has also been described. The most common sites are transtentorial, either upward or downward, and subfalcine herniation. The key to gain complete knowledge of brain herniation requires a thorough understanding of anatomic characteristics of brain, intracranial compartments, and dural folds.

2   Anatomical Considerations

The cranium is a rigid bony structure occupying the brain tissue, CSF, blood vessels and meninges. The meninges are protective coverings of the brain that lines the internal cavity to the cranium. Meninges consist of three membranous connective tissue layers: dura mater, arachnoid mater and pia mater. The dura mater is a tough, thick external fibrous membrane consisting of two layers. The outer periosteal layer is intimately adhered to the skull; the inner visceral layer projects inwards to form dural reflections. It divides the cranial cavity into various compartments and protects the brain against excessive movement.

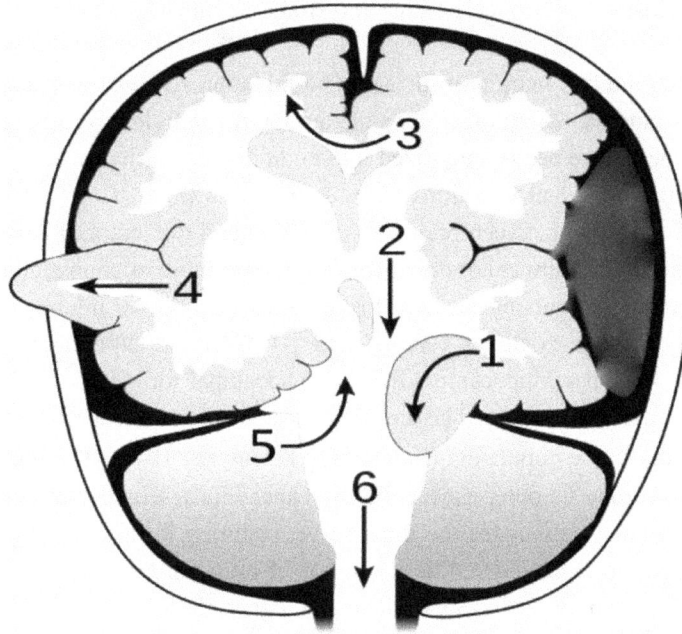

Figure 1: Brain Herniation. 1: Uncal; 2: Descending; 3: Subfalcine; 4: transcalvarial 5: Ascending; 6: Tonsillar.

These dural reflections are known as falx cerebri, tentorium cerebelli, falx cerebelli and the diaphragm sellae.

The falx cerebri is a sickle-shaped inward reflection that separates the cerebral hemispheres. The falx cerebri is adhered in the midline to the inner surface of the calvaria, extending anteriorly from crista galli to the internal occipital protuberance posteriorly (Gray, 1974). Further posteriorly, falx cerebri continuous as the tentorium cerebelli. Falx cerebri is narrow anteriorly but broadens posteriorly, which makes it more resistant to any pressure effect in the posterior portion. For this reason, subfalcine herniations are more common anteriorly. The falx cerebri encloses the superior sagittal sinus along its upper margin and the inferior sagittal sinus along its lower margin. The superior sagittal sinus drains directly into the sinus confluence while inferior sagittal sinus drains into the straight sinus (Gray, 1974).Falx cerebri is in close relationship with anterior cerebral artery (ACA) anteriorly, cingulate gyrus inferiomedially, and internal cerebral veins, vein of Galen and deep subependymal veins posteriorly. Any mass effect in this region can lead of brain ischemia/infarction as a result of arterial compression or brain parenchymal congestion/raised ICP due to compression of venous system (Gray, 1974).

The tentorium cerebelli is a crescent shaped lamina that separates the occipital lobes of cerebral hemispheres from the cerebellum. It resides in the cerebrocerebellar fissure, attached anteriorly to the clinoid processes of the sphenoid bone, anterolaterally to the petrous part of the temporal bone, and posterolaterally to the internal surface of occipital and the parietal bone (Gray, 1974). Superiomedially, tentorium cerebelli continues as falx cerebri; giving it a tent-like appearance. The concave anteriomedial margin of the tentorium between the two clinoid processes is free, leaving a semiovular opening known as tentorial notch or incisura through which the brainstem extends into the infratentorial compartment.

Tentorium cerebelli encloses the transverse sinus, and straight sinus which empties into the sinus conflu-ence (Gray, 1974).

The space between the free margin of incisura and the brain stem varies considerably in size, from virtually no space to as much as 7 mm on either side, among the individuals (Sunderland, 1958). The di-mensions of tentorial notch have been categorized into eight distinct varieties. Alder and Milhorat (2001) have observed wide inter-individual variations in the exposed portions of cerebellar parenchyma within the incisura and poor correlation between brain stem position and the tentorial edge. This pattern poten-tially alters the susceptibility for upward or downward transtentorial herniation among the individuals.

The principal structures coursing through the incisura include the midbrain, occulomotor nerve, posterior communicating artery, posterior cerebral artery (PCA) and superior cerebellar artery (SCA). The medial margin of uncus, parahippocampal gyrus, hippocampal formation and first six cranial nerves are also intimately related to the incisura. The length, course and anatomical relationship of third nerve to the skull base vary widely in the population (Sunderland & Hughes, 1946). The pupillo-constrictor fibres of third nerve are placed along its outer aspect and are exceedingly sensitive to external pressure. Thus, any mass effect in this region pressurizes the third nerve, resulting in loss of pupillary constriction. For this reason pupillary dilation is considered as a symbol of transtentorial herniation (Adler & Milhorat, 2001; Cuneo *et al.,* 1979; Ropper, 1986; Sunderland & Hughes, 1946). The PCA and anterior choroidal artery (ACHA) are vulnerable to occlusion by downward transtentorial herniation. In contrast, SCA is sensitive to upward herniation from the infratentorial compartment. Occlusion of the ACHA results in infarction of vital structures including the optic tract, temporal lobe, basal ganglia, cerebral peduncles, and midbrain (Grossman & Yousem, 1994). Occlusion of the SCA results in cerebellar infarction while PCA occlusion results in occipital lobe infarction (Komaki & Handel, 1974). Histological changes in-clude neuronal swelling with lipid vacuolization and peripherally placed nuclei. Surviving neurons be-come pyknotic and fibrous gliosis ensues. Anatomically, midbrain consists of four components: tectum, tegmentum, ventricular mesocoelia and cerebral peduncles. The mid brain contains many vital structures including third and fourth cranial nerve nuclei, the red nuclei, substantia nigra, periaqeductal gray matter, neurons of reticular activating system, aqueduct of sylvius and numerous interneuronal connections be-tween the cerebral cortex and the lower brain stem or spinal cord. Thus any mass effect in this region leads to profound neurological deficits. The subarachnoid space inside the incisura is divided into various basilar cisterns including quadrigeminal cistern posteriorly, and the interpeduncular and suprasellar cis-terns anteriorly (Sunderland & Hughes, 1946; Nguyen *et al.,* 1989). They act as hydraulic buffers to pre-vent any pressure effect upon the midbrain. Compression of these cisterns is regarded as a hallmark sign of transtentorial herniation. It is also considered as a negative prognostic sign in condition of intracerebral hematoma or contusion (Ross *et al.,* 1989; Toutant *et al.,* 1984).

3   Pathophysiology

3.1   Subfalcine Herniation

The subfalcine herniation is considered as one of the most common variety of brain herniation. It occurs when a supratentorial mass causes a midline shift of brain tissue under the falx cerebri together with lat-eral displacement of the falx cerebri (Osborn, 1996). Though, subfalcine herniation can occur in isolation, the usual presentation is in conjunction with transtentorial herniation (Taveras, 1996). This could be due to generalized effect of clinical pathology, but does not necessarily signify severe clinical presentation.

S. No.	Type	Causes
1.	Developmental	Malformed posterior fossa CSF loss through open spinal defect
2.	Traumatic	Pneumocephalus Epidural/subdural Intracerebral haemorrhage Brain contusion
3.	Infectious	Brain abscess Empyema Meningitis Encephalitis
4.	Metabolic	Hepatic encephalopathy Toxic-metabolic encephalopathy
5.	Vascular	Aneurysm Ischemic stroke Hydrocephalus Hypertensive encephalopathy
6.	Neoplastic	Supratentorial/infratentorial tumours
7.	Therapeutic	Over-drainage of CSF through ventriculo-peritoneal shunting Graft herniation during translabyrinthine craniotomy

Table 1: Aetiology of brain herniation

Due to its inferiomedial location, cingulate gyrus is the most commonly involved portion in sub-falcine herniation. The severity of herniation may vary from mild form with minimal midline shift to complete herniation of the cingulate gyrus and the adjoining parenchyma. Continued mass effect upon the cingulate gyrus can lead to brain parenchymal ischemia or necrosis (Loevner, 1999). Owing to its rigid fibrous assembly, falx cerebri protects the brain against any movement; so even a few millimetres of midline shift is considered significant. Further rise in mass effect compresses the ventricular system including ipsilateral lateral ventricles and foramina of Monro. This results in enlargement of contralateral lateral ventricles with consequent obstructive hydrocephalus (Osborn, 1996). The ACA and its tributaries (the callosomarginal, pericallosal, and frontopolar arteries) course between the falx cerebri and the adjacent frontal and parietal lobes; they are vulnerable to compression by any mass effect in the anterior portion of supratentorial compartment (Osborn, 1996; Loevner, 1999). As the cingulate gyrus extends under the falx, distal ACA gets occluded and consequently ischemia/infarction develops in the supplied portion, leading to contralateral leg weakness (Taveras, 1996; Hassler, 1967; Sohn & Levine, 1967; Barr & Gean, 1994). Complications such as vascular aneurysms have also been reported due to compression of the ACA in subfalcine herniation (Nakstad, 1986). When the lesion is located posteriorly, the internal cerebral veins, vein of Galen, or the deep subependymal veins may get involved, leading to brain congestion and rise in ICP (Sohn & Levine, 1967; Ecker, 1948).

3.2 Transtentorial Herniation

Transtentorial herniation is a dreaded complication, which has an acute presentation, rapid progression and lethal outcome. Transtentorial herniation was first described by Hill in 1896. It is the upward or downward shift of neural parenchyma across the tentorium at the level of incisura (Elguera, 1962). Due to minimal space within the tentorial notch, only a few millimetres midline shift of brain stem is sufficient to cause significant compression (Elguera, 1962; Schwarz & Rosner, 1941; Smyth & Henderson, 1938). Further increase in pressure upon the brainstem, compresses the aqueduct of sylvius and cardiorespiratory centres, which can be fatal (Schwarz & Rosner, 1941; Taveras, 1996). Transtentorial herniation can be further subcategorized into ascending, descending and uncal herniation.Early or unilateral herniation is more accurately called uncal herniation. The terms craniocaudal, rostrocaudal, central or bilateral descending transtentorial herniation, are more appropriately termed as "descending transtentorial herniation".

3.3   Uncal Herniation

Uncal herniation, a subtype of descending transtentorial herniation, was first described by James Collier in 1904. It occurs when innermost portion of temporal lobe, the uncus is pushed inferiomedially across the free edge of the tentorium cerebella. Furthermore, uncus obliterates the supracellar cistern, compresses the occulomotor nerve and cerebral peduncles, and obliterates the aqueduct of sylvius (Meyer, 1920; Jefferson, 1938; Howell, 1959; Kernohan & Woltman, 1929; Marshall et al., 1983). The stalk of pituitary gland may also get stretched across the sellar diaphragm, leading to pituitary infarction (Howell, 1959). Pressure effect upon third nerve causes loss of parasympathetic innervation, resulting in pupillary dilation and loss of light reflex. Pupillary dilation is followed by the motor effects of third nerve compression which precipitates as downward and outward deviation of eye, due to loss of innervation to all ocular muscles except those supplied by fourth and sixth cranial nerve (Barr, 1994; Kernohan & Woltman, 1929). The neurological deficit occurs in this sequence because the parasympathetic fibres are located outer to somatomotor fibres in third nerve, hence compressed first. Further increase in mass effect, compresses the midbrain leading to loss of both parasympathetic and sympathetic innervation bilaterally. This results in mid-positioned (4-5 mm) pupils not reacting to light. Uncal herniation can also compress the PCA resulting in ischemia of ipsilateral primary visual cortex, with consequent contralateral visual field defects in both eyes (Homonymous hemianopia). Pressure effect upon the ipsilateral cerebral peduncle (comprises corticospinal and corticobulbar fibres) results in contralateral hemiparesis. In contrast, uncus may also compress contralateral cerebral peduncle against the tentorium cerebelli, resulting in ipsilateral hemiparesis (false localizing sign), and known as Kernohan's notch (Kernohan & Woltman, 1929; Marshman et al., 2001). Uncal herniation may also precipitate duret haemorrhage in midbrain and pons, which can be fatal.

3.4   Descending Herniation

Descending transtentorial herniation occurs when a midline/bilateral supratentorial mass pushes the diencephalon and/or the parahippocampal gyrus inferiomedially from the supratentorial space, into the incisura (Stovring, 1977; Sheinker, 1945). Jennett and stern (1960) showed that enlargement of supratentorial mass results in a pressure gradient between the supra and infratentorial compartment; maximum over the tentorium, intermediate under the tentorium and minimum in the spinal subarachnoid space. This pressure gradient is responsible for inferiomedial displacement of brain tissue (Hahn & Gurney, 1985). Imaging studies have documented that nearly 50% of patients with transtentorial herniation also develop downward shift of brain stem and concurrent cerebellar tonsillar herniation (Reich, 1993). Typical pathological manifestations include inferiomedial displacement of parahippocampal gyrus and diencephalon, obliteration of basilar cisterns, and compression of occulomotor nerve, midbrain and posterior cerebral/ACHA (Sheinker, 1945; Stovring, 1977, Blinkov et al., 1992). With further increase in herniation, pons and medulla are also compressed (Feldmenn, 1988). In severe cases, occlusion of small perforating branches supplying the upper brain stem results in brain stem haemorrhage (Duret haemorrhage) (Howell,1959; Kernohan & Woltman, 1929; Thompson & Salcman, 1988). Haemorrhage may also occur due to reperfusion injury after initial ischemia. Haemorrhage may further compromise the cardiorespiratory centres, which may be fatal (Sheinker, 1945).

3.5   Ascending herniation

Ascending transtentorial herniation results from upward migration of brain parenchyma through the incisura due to an expanding mass lesion within in the posterior fossa (Ecker, 1948). Common causes are hematoma, infarction, infection or tumour. It may however, rarely be seen after graft herniation into posterior fossa during translabyrinthine craniotomy. Herniated brain tissue includes central lobule, culmen, and cerebellar vermis, which compresses the dorsal mid brain, fourth ventricle, pretectum and the cerebral aqueduct (Sheinker, 1945). Pretectal compression leads to loss of vertical eye movements (Reich *et al.*, 1993; Sunderland, 1958; Osborn, 1996). Increasing pressure effect compresses the pons, leading to loss of sympathetic innervation descending through the pontomedullary region. Thus, the unopposed parasympathetic papillary supply to the eye leads to small minimally reactive pupil, termed as 'pontine pupil' (Cuneo *et al*, 1979; Sunderland, 1958; Alder & Milhorat, 2002; Ross *et al,* 1989). However, coexistent compression of midbrain and third nerve may also cut the parasympathetic supply, leading to mid-positioned or even dilated fixed pupil (Cuneo *et al.*, 1979). With increasing upward herniation obstructive hydrocephalus develops, and the quadrigeminal cistern and superior cerebellar cistern becomes obliterated (Osborn, 1991; Osborn, 1996; Speigelman, 1989). The distal part of SCA and PCA may get compressed, resulting in infarction of cerebellar hemisphere and occipital lobe. Increasing mass effect also compresses the vein of Galen and the basal vein of Rosenthal, which further exacerbates the neuronal congestion, resulting in rise in ICP and secondary haemorrhagic infarction of diencephalon (Reich *et al.*, 1993; Cuneo *et al.*, 1979).

3.6   Tonsillar herniation

In Tonsillar herniation, increased pressure gradient within the posterior fossa pushes the cerebellar tonsils through the foramen magnum, which compresses the lower part of brain stem and upper spinal cord, having life threatening consequences (Reich *et al.*, 1993; Cuneo *et al.*, 1979; Ross *et al.*, 1989; Meyer, 1920; Kernohan & Woltman, 1929). Common causes are again the same, but it has also been observed in condition of malformed posterior fossa. It occurs usually in conjunction with ascending or descending transtentorial herniation in majority of cases (Meyer, 1920). The lumber puncture in presence of supratentorial mass causes sudden decline in CSF pressure below the level of foramen magnum. This augments the cephalocaudal pressure gradient, which results in tonsillar herniation with consequent sudden decline in vital parameters of patient. For this reason, lumber puncture is contraindicated in presence of intracranial tumour (Ramsey, 1994). Acute tonsillar herniation can cause significant compression upon the medulla, posterior inferior cerebellar arteries and fourth ventricle which can be fatal (Cuneo *et al.*, 1979). Ischemia and infarction of cerebellar tonsil, lower cerebellum and entire lower brain stem and upper spinal cord may occur due occlusion of vertebral arteries, their branches and the origin of anterior spinal artery (Reich *et al.*, 1993; Cuneo *et al.*, 1979). Tonsillar herniation of cerebellum is also termed as chairi malformation. Clinical symptomatology may be subtle or patient may exhibit Lhermitte's phenomenon, defined as dyesthesia in arms and legs upon forward bending of head (Reich *et al.*, 1993; Cuneo *et al.*,

1979). It is considered to be due to pressure upon anterior spinal cord tracts. Compression of ventricular system may result in obstructive hydrocephalus (Cuneo *et al.*, 1979).

3.7   Transphenoidal (transalar) herniation

Transphenoidal herniation occurs when mass lesion shifts brain tissue across the sphenoid wing. There are two types of transphenoidal herniation, anterior/ascending and posterior/descending. Posterior herniation occurs when the frontal lobe extends posteriorly and inferiorly over the greater sphenoid ridge, causing posterior displacement of the sylvian fissure and the middle cerebral artery (Taveras, 1996). Anterior herniation occurs when the temporal lobe, sylvian fissure, and middle cerebral artery are shifted anterosuperiorly over the sphenoid wing. Alar herniations are difficult to demonstrate on imaging and clinical symptomatology is also subtle.

3.8   Transcalvarial herniation

It is the herniation of oedematous brain tissue through a bony defect, either due to a congenital bony anomaly, trauma, otitis media or following decompressive craniectomy (Figure 2). For external herniation to occur, three pre-requisites have been described: presence of a bony defect, a dural defect, and increased intracranial pressure (Ramsden *et al.*, 1985). The oedema following decompressive craniectomy is known to result from hyperperfusion of brain parenchyma or increased capillary permeability resulting from decrease in interstitial hydrostatic pressure (Stiver, 2009). This may led to pinching of cerebral vessels, epidural haematoma or injury to the herniating brain parenchyma at the level of defect edge, resulting in ischemia and necrosis of the affected portion. This manifestation is more common in cases where decompression is performed through small sized craniectomy defect (Yang *et al.*, 2008). For this reason, it is always advised to perform sufficient sized craniectomy and optimal decompression, allowing brain to expand outward without constriction.

4   Radiological Aspects

Under the emergent condition, due to easy availability and speed of imaging, cranial computed tomography (CT) should be obtained without any delay to identify the underlying primary pathology that requires immediate medical attention and/or surgical intervention. However, magnetic resonance imaging (MRI) may subsequently be needed for more accurate categorization of mass lesion and associated complications.

4.1   Subfalcine herniation

Imaging signs include unilateral mass effect such as haemorrhage or tumour causing subfalcine shift of brain to the contralateral side, asymmetry of the anterior falx with a widened CSF space on the contralateral anterior falx (Osborn, 1996; Loevner, 1999) (Figure 3). There may be ipsilateral lateral ventricle compression with contralateral lateral ventricle and atria dilation. Other finding includes truncation of anterior aspect of ipsilateral frontal horn and widening of contralateral frontal horn (Osborn, 1996; Loevner, 1999).

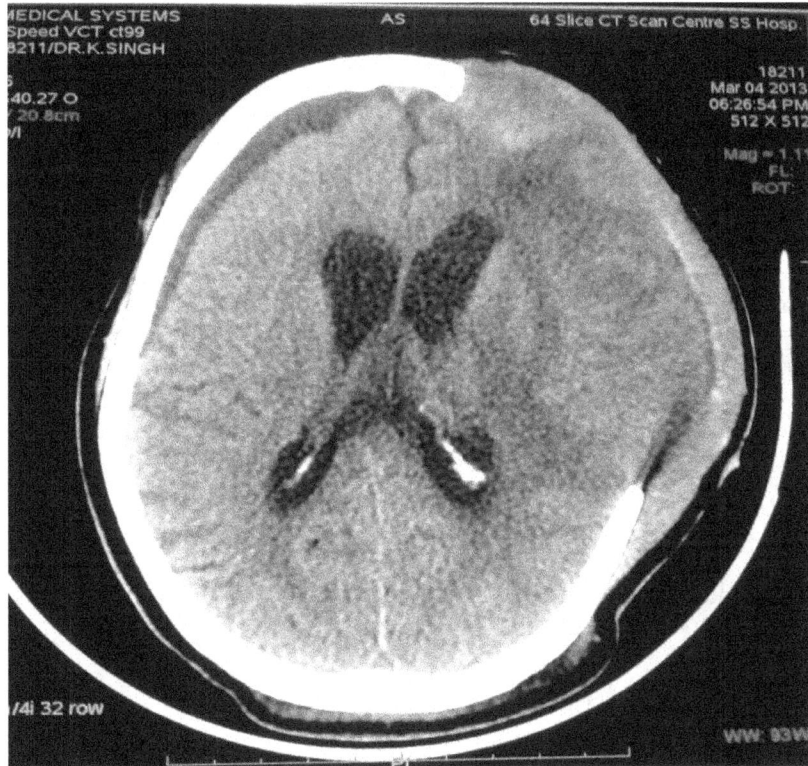

Figure 2: Transcalvarial Herniation

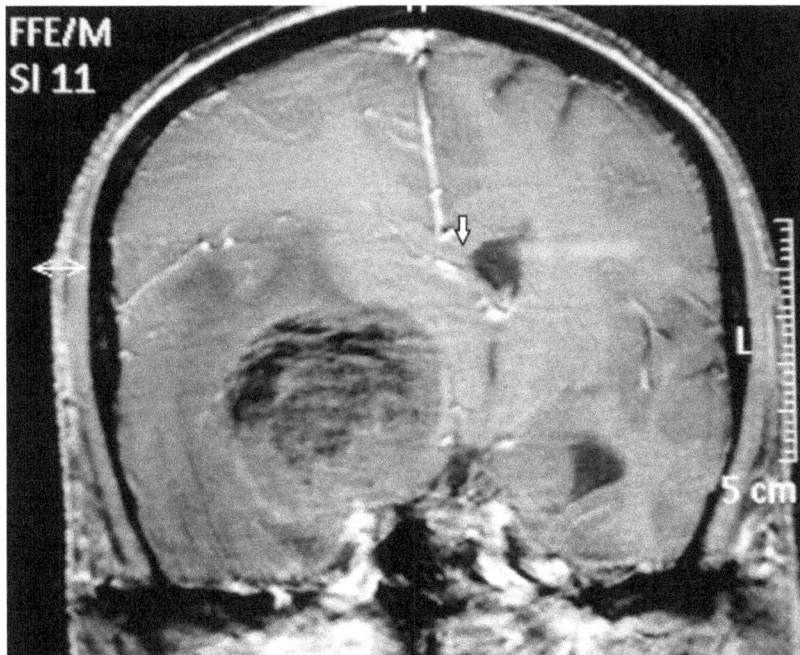

Figure 3: Subfalcine Herniation

4.2   Transtentorial herniation (Uncal)

Imaging findings include inferiomedial displacement of uncus across the tentorial edge, widening of ipsilateral cerebellopontine angle cistern, distortion of suprasellar cistern, compression of cerebral peduncle (ipsilateral or contralateral) and midbrain, acqueductal compression with consequent obstructive hydrocephalus, and PCA compression with occipital infarction (Taveras, 1996; Osborn, 1976) (Figure 4). Duret haemorrhages may also be seen.

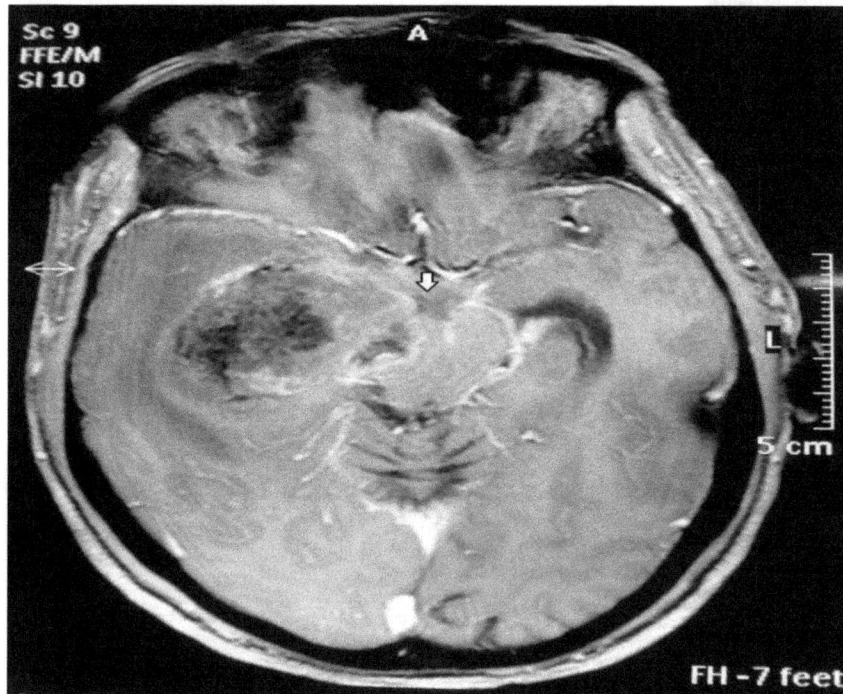

Figure 4: Uncal herniation

4.3   Transtentorial herniation (Descending)

Imaging findings include the downward displacement of the parahippocampal gyrus through the incisura, and widening of ipsilateral and obliteration of contralateral ambient and prepontine cisterns (Feldmann *et al.*, 1988; Osborn, 1976; Osborn, 1996). The contralateral temporal horn is also widened. There may be ipsilateral lateral ventricle compression with subsequent dilatation of the contralateral ventricle. Midbrain is twisted, and the cerebral peduncles become elongated and flattened (Feldmann *et al.*, 1988; Osborn, 1976). There is downward shift of pineal calcification and midline shift of brain parenchyma. Occipital lobe infarction and Duret haemorrhage can also be seen.

4.4   Transtentorial herniation (Ascending)

MR imaging is useful in early identification of upward herniation, prior to the development of severe neurological complications and can be used to monitor the course of progression or recovery of ascending herniation (Figure 5). Imaging findings include upward migration of cerebellar tissue through the tentorium cerebelli, flattening of smile shaped quadrigeminal cistern (termed as crooked smile), obliteration of

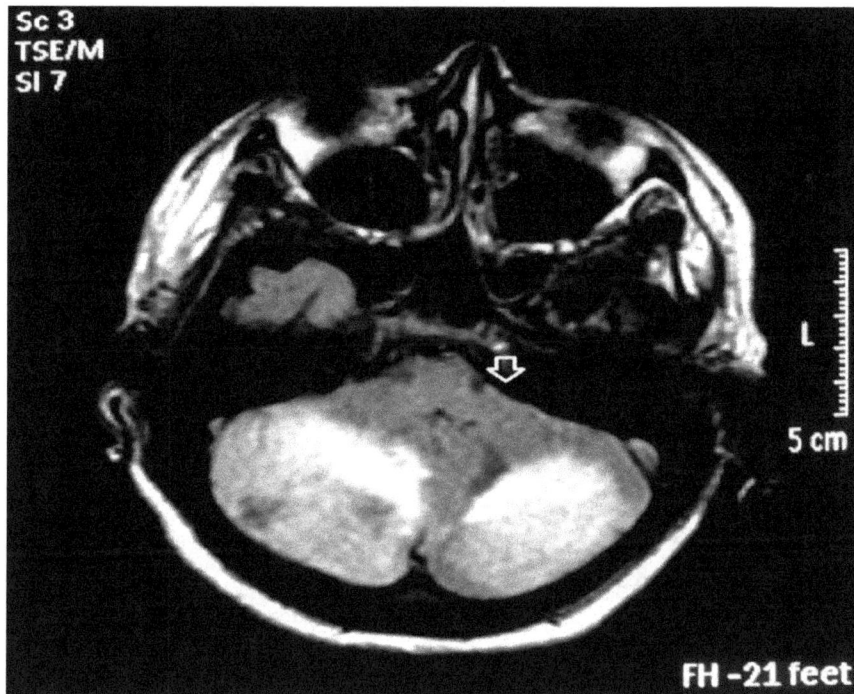

Figure 5: Ascending herniation

quadrigeminal cistern (termed as frown shape) and superior cerebellar cistern and in severe cases, 'spinning top appearance' of midbrain due to bilateral compression of posteriolateral aspect of midbrain (Osborn, 1978). It may be associated with infarct in the territory of PCA and SCA, obstructive hydrocephalus as a result of pressure upon aqueduct (Reich *et al.*, 1993). Rostral migration of the vermis into the tentorial apex is confirmed angiographically by elevation of superior vermian arteries and anterosuperior displacement of cistern segment of the ACHA (Osborn, 1978).

4.5 Tonsillar herniation

Radiological findings include downward displacement of cerebellar tonsil up to the level of odontoid process and lesser amount of CSF in the foramen magnum, on axial CT images (Grossman & Yousem, 1994). A sagittal MRI is however, more accurate method for determining the herniation (Reich *et al.*, 1993). Tonsillar herniation should be differentiated from low lying normal cerebellar tonsils. Radiologically, cerebellar tonsil should lie at least five millimetres below the level of foramen magnum in adults or seven millimetres in children, to categorize it as herniation (Reimer *et al.*, 2010).Cisterna magna obliteration with associated PCA infarction and hydrocephalus are also common (Reimer *et al.*, 2010).

4.6 Transphenoidal (transalar) herniation

Imaging characteristics include anterior or posterior displacement of middle cerebral artery in anterior or posterior alar herniation, respectively (Taveras, 1996).

5   Clinical Symptomatology

Type	Early features	Late Features
Subfalcine	• Headache • Contralateral leg weakness	• Ipsilateral anterior cerebral artery infarction • Contralateral hydrocephalus
Transtentorial (Uncal)	• Anisocoria • Ipsilateral dilated pupil • Loss of light reflex • Altered consciousness • Contralateral hemiparesis • Ipsilateral hemiparesis	• Midpositioned fixed pupil • Ptosis • Downward and outward deviation of eye • Homonymous hemianopia • Pituitary infarction • Hydrocephalus • Hemiplegia • Coma
Transtentorial (descending)	• Constricted reactive pupils • Cheyne stokes breathing • Decorticate posturing • Altered consciousness	• Midpositioned fixed pupils • Loss of oculocephalic reflex • Decerebrate posturing • Coma, Apnoea, cardiac arrest
Transtentorial (ascending)	• Nausea, vomiting • Constricted minimal reactive pupil (pontine pupils) • Loss of vertical eye movement • Altered consciousness	• Hydrocephalus • Coma
Sphenoidal	• Subtle	• Subtle
Tonsillar	• Bilateral arm dysesthesia • Pontine pupils • Loss of lateral eye movement (Ocular bobbing) • Altered consciousness	• Hydrocephalus • Coma • Apnoea, cardiac arrest

Table 2: Symptoms of brain herniation

6   Management

Management of brain herniation begins with initial resuscitative measures like airway, breathing and hemodynamic concerns, followed by therapies aimed at reduction of ICP while maintaining cerebral perfusion pressure (CPP), minimizing oxygen demand while maximizing oxygen delivery and prevention of hypercarbia and acidosis/alkalosis (Figure 4) (Lidofsky *et al.*, 1992; Stevens *et al.*, 2012; Andrews, 2003). If the initiating cause is uncertain, a cranial CT scan should be performed as an emergency measure just after initial resuscitation, for early identification of a treatable mass lesion. Prolonged unattended herniation may lead to permanent brain injury, having devastating consequences in the form of permanent neurological sequel or death. These interventions help to tolerate the pressure effect of an expanding intracranial mass lesion temporarily, until final diagnosis and treatment is initiated.

6.1   Initial Resuscitation and Management

Resuscitative measures began with assessment of airway patency, ventilation and adequate circulation.Loss of consciousness diminishes the normal neuromuscular tone and reflexes of upper airway (cough and gag), endangering the airway further through aspiration and its sequel (Colquhoun et al., 2004). This may be corrected by various maneuvers including head tilt with chin lift or jaw thrust technique or use of adjuncts, such as an oropharyngeal or nasopharyngeal airway. Though, the use of head tilt alone will itself relieve the obstruction in 80% of patients, it should be avoided in cases of suspected cervical spine injury. If injuries are visible on upper half of the body, trauma to cervical spine should be considered by default, unless excluded by its radiography (Colquhoun et al., 2004). Such cases should be managed by chin lift and jaw thrust alone, if possible. Furthermore, head and neck should be maintained in a neutral position by manual inline immobilization, semi-rigid collars, sandbags, spinal board, and securing straps. If the patient needs to be turned, "log rolled" rotation should be there into a true lateral position, avoiding any movement in the spine (Colquhoun et al., 2004). In the field, non-invasive ventilation with 100% oxygen through an integrated mask and reservoir bag, may act as a temporary maneuver to prevent hypoxemia. However, endotracheal intubation remains the gold standard for securing an airway, so it should be provided as early as possible. Regardless of a negative cervical radiograph, excessive movement over the cervical spine should be avoided during intubation, as there are 20% chances of significant cervical injury despite a normal screening radiograph (Bivins, 1988). This could be better achieved by use of flexible fibreoptic bronchoscope, McCoy laryngoscope, supraglottic airway or combitube etc. Surgical approaches like needle cricothyroidotomy or tracheostomy may be necessary, if other means of securing an airway fail. Once the airway has been secured, controlled ventilation should be started at the earliest in order to maximize oxygen delivery, reverse hypercarbia and to prevent acidosis/alkalosis (Andrews, 2003).

Once the airway, oxygenation and ventilation are adequate, circulation should be assessed and supportive measures should be rapidly initiated. Isolated head injury rarely causes hypotension, although associated scalp lacerations or multisystem injuries may cause significant blood losses (Colquhoun et al., 2004; Haddad & Arabi, 2012). Hypotension may also be due to systemic vasodilation due to spinal cord injury.Wherever possible, any on-going bleeding should be controlled and fluid resuscitation should be started, if the losses appear to be significant. If the initial blood pressure is normal, fluid resuscitation should be modest, as overhydration may aggravate cerebral/pulmonaryoedema (Colquhoun et al., 2004; Haddad & Arabi, 2012). Most vital parameters change little in adults until more than 30% blood volume has been lost; children compensate even more effectively. Any patient who is hypotensive through blood loss should be, therefore, considered to have lost a significant volume. Choice of resuscitative fluid is usually balanced salt solution such as ringer lactate, although hypertonic saline has also been tried in such situations (Prougn, 2005). Though hypertonic saline could additionally reduce ICP, there is associated risk of severe hypernatremia; it should be considered in refractory cases only, who no longer respond to mannitol or developing uremia (Prougn, 2005; De Vivo et al., 2001).

6.2   Control of Intracranial pressure

Various studies indicate that sustained rise in ICP over 20 mm Hg results in a poor outcome (Marshall et al., 1983; Howard et al., 1988; Narayan et al., 1982). Jiang JY et al (2002) showed that mortality rates were 14% if ICP rise was less than 20 mm Hg, but 34% if ICP was greater than 30 mm Hg at 48 hrs. For this reason, the brain trauma foundation recommends for initiating decrease in ICP, at a threshold rise of

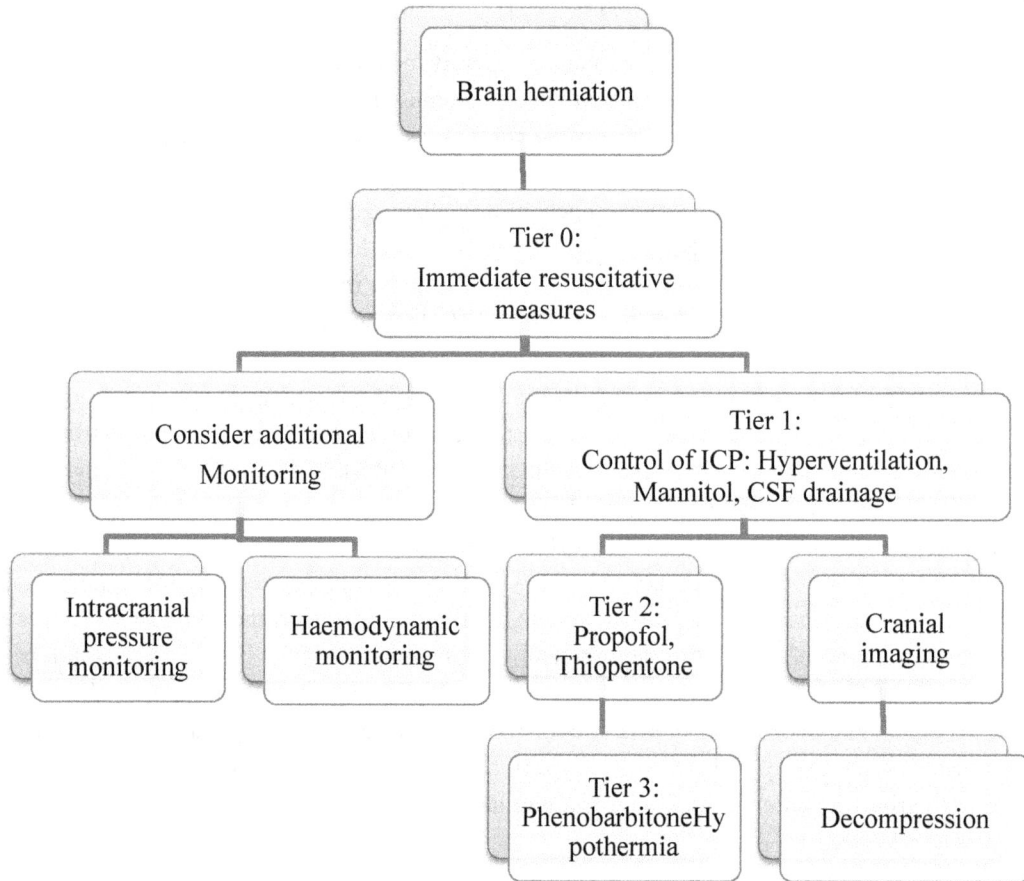

Figure 6: Protocol for management of intracranial herniation

20 mm Hg with level II recommendation (Bratton *et al.*, 2007). Various researches have documented that CPP levels of less than 60-70 mm Hg adversely affect the cerebral oxygenation and metabolism; what is the safe range of CPP still remains controversial, with the consensus that it should be 60-70 (Unterberg *et al.*, 1997; Vespa *et al.*, 1998, Bullock *et al.*, 1996). However, CPP levels of less than 50 mm Hg should always be avoided, as recommended by brain trauma foundation (Bratton *et al.*, 2007). Various manoeuvres used for lowering of ICP include head end elevation of bed, hyperventilation, and use of osmotic agents, diuretics, barbiturates, CSF drainage and hypothermia. Other agents like procaine derivatives, indomethacin, propofol, hyperbaric oxygen and tromethamine have been tried in the past, but in absence of convincing results, not used in routine clinical practice. Role of sedatives still remain controversial, with no clear advantage in absence of anxiety or agitation. Moreover, use of sedatives or paralytics is associated with increased ICU stay and added complications (Hsiang *et al.*, 1994).

6.2.1   Hyperventilation

Hyperventilation is known to lower arterial carbon dioxide tension, resulting in diffuse cerebral vasoconstriction (approximately 3% for every 1 mm Hg decrease in $PaCO_2$), decreasing cerebral vascular volume and lowering ICP (Robertson, 2004; Kochanek *et al.*, 2012). Thus, hyperventilation can temporarily revert the constellation of symptoms observed in acute rise in ICP, until investigations are performed and the definitive treatment is initiated (Robertson, 2004; Kochanek *et al.*, 2012). However, cerebral vasoconstriction is only effective in unaffected areas of the brain; therefore hyperventilation may be less effective in patients with diffuse brain injury than in those with focal lesions. Cerebral vasoconstriction in hyperventilation could result in brain ischemia (Andrews, 2003). Therefore, hyperventilation should only be instituted for short periods where immediate control of ICP is necessary and the target PaCO2 levels should be maintained between 30-35 mm Hg (Cruz, 1993). In some situations, hyperventilation may be necessary for longer periods in patients with persistently high ICPs, who do not respond to other treatment modalities. However, these patients should be regularly monitored for adequate cerebral oxygenation and tissue perfusion by utilizing various neuromonitoring modalities such as jugular bulb venous oxygen saturation, brain tissue oxygen tension, transcranial doppler ultrasonography and near infrared spectroscopy assessments, with level III recommendation (Cruz, 1993; Robertson, 1995; Lewis, 1996; Cruz, 1998; Dosemeci *et al.*, 2004; Robertson, 2004; Stiefel *et al.*, 2005; De Freitas & Andre, 2006; Rosenthal *et al.*, 2008; Kochanek *et al.*, 2012). Hyperventilation is highly controversial, with the 2012 Cochrane database concluding that hyperventilation should not be used in the first 24 hours after TBI when cerebral blood flow (CBF) is generally lowest, with level III recommendation and prophylactic hyperventilation (PaCO2<25 mm Hg) is not recommended, with level II recommendations (Kochanek *et al.*, 2012).

6.2.2   CSF Drainage

Ventricular catheterization should be done wherever possible, if the ventricles are compressed or displaced. Drainage of even small amounts of CSF is sufficient to produce required fall in ICP and a rise in CPP (Gahjar *et al.*, 1993). However if the systolic blood pressure is dependent on continued stimulus by the Cushing response, then sudden decrease of ICP may precipitate hypotension. This can be precluded by IV fluid preloading and setting the CSF drainage pressure to about 20 cm H2O (Gahjar *et al.*, 1993). However, continuous CSF drainage is not recommended as it may lead to collapse of the ventricles and catheter malfunction.

6.2.3   Osmotic agents and Renal diuretics

From many decades, osmotic agents remained the primary means of controlling the raised ICP, yet their exact mechanism of action is still debated. Mannitol, a sugar alcohol solution, is an osmotic diuretic which causes increase in intravascular volume and reduction in blood viscosity (Muizelaar *et al.*, 1983; Burke *et al.*, 1981; Schrot & Muizelaar, 2005). To maintain a constant CBF, this leads to acute cerebral vasoconstriction with consequent rapid reduction in ICP (Muizelaar *et al.*, 1984, Leech & Miller, 1974). More prolonged reduction in ICP is due to osmotic effect, by drawing fluid into the vascular compartment. Mannitol reduces red blood cell rigidity, allowing them to pass through small blood vessels and areas of marginal perfusion (Burke *et al.*, 1981). It also acts as a free radical scavenger, which have been implicated in ischemic brain injury. Mannitol is not metabolized and remains in intravascular space, unless high concentrations or continuous infusion breaches the normal blood–brain barrier, allowing it to enter the interstitial space, taking fluid with it and causing a 'rebound' rise in ICP (Kaufmann & Cardoso, 1992). Conventionally, it is administered as a 20% solution in a bolus dose of 0.25–1.0 g/kg given over 10–20 min, to avoid the risk of hypotension from rapid and continuous infusion. ICP falls within 5–10 minutes. The maximum effect occurs in about 60 minutes and the total effect last for 3–4hours (James et al., 1977). Previous studies show that higher doses of mannitol (1.4 g/kg) are more effective in obtaining brain relaxation than conventional doses, in patients with brain herniation (Cruz *et al.*, 2001; Andrews, 2003). These observations support the use of higher dosage mannitol in patients with transtentorial herniation. However, it also has some limitations including progressive dehydration, hypotension, prerenal failure and expansion of an intracranial hemorrhage by brain shrinkage (Cottrell et al., 1977; Feig & McCurdy, 1977). To avoid the risk of hypotension, its use is prohibited in condition of haemorrhagic shock (Andrews, 2003). Central venous pressure, urine output, serum electrolytes and blood osmolality need to be carefully monitored, particularly if it is combined with the renal loop diuretics. In combination with mannitol, furosemide produces a synergistic effect in reduction in ICP and also increases the duration of its effect (Pollay *et al.*, 1983; Wilkinson & Rosenfeld, 1983). However, the considering the added risk of hypovolemia and renal failure, their combined use should be restricted for patients with associated cardiac failure or pulmonary edema.

6.2.4   Barbiturates

Barbiturate causes a decrease in cerebral metabolic rate; reduces CBF, decreases production of CSF, increases absorption of CSF, and causes burst suppression of EEG. This leads to a parallel fall in ICP (Michenfelder, 1974). To observe significant reduction in ICP, anesthetic equivalent doses are required and therefore cardiorespiratory and ICP monitoring is compulsory. Considering the risk of hypotension and respiratory depression, barbiturate therapy should be reserved as a step-down protocol therapy for ICP control, once other means of medical management have failed (Ward *et al*, 1985).

6.2.5   Corticosteroids

Corticosteroids lower ICP by decreasing vasogenic edema through inhibition of phospholipase A2, stabilization of lysosomal membranes, reduction of edema producing vascular endothelial growth factor expression, and improvement in microcirculation (Yamada *et al.*, 1989; Heiss *et al.*, 1996; Machein *et al.*, 1999). Corticosteroids play an important role in decreasing edema secondary to brain tumors, however not recommended for cytotoxic edema secondary to stroke or head injury (Yamada *et al*, 1989; Ruderman & Hall, 1965; Alderson & Roberts, 2005). In fact, systemic complications of steroids like gastrointestinal bleeding, and glucose intolerance (50% incidence) can further worsen the patient's condition (Gotzsche, 1994; Meyer, 2003; Conn & Poynard, 1994). Patients treated with systemic steroids are also at risk of infection with Pneumocystis carinii pneumonia; the reported incidence is about 2%. Prophylactic control with trimethoprim–sulfamethoxazole may prevent this complication, but is mainly utilized for immunocompromised patients (Kovacs, 2001). Patients with extensive brain edema may also develop withdrawal symptoms such as headache, lethargy, low-grade fever and adrenal insufficiency after rapid tapering of corticosteroids, thus leading to increased morbidity and mortality (Amatruda, 1965). The results of the large CRASH trial suggest that steroids should not be used in head injury, as they appear to increase mortality. However, the exact mechanism of this effect still remains unclear (CRASH Trial Collaborators, 2003). Current Cochrane review recommends for need to reassess the pathophysiologic understanding of the traumatic brain injury (TBI) and no need to start such future trials (Alderson & Roberts, 2005).

6.2.6   Hypothermia

Recent studies suggest that moderate hypothermia (32-34°C) can reduce ICP and is cytoprotective in cases of global ischemic injury. It is also known to prevent glutamate release and depletion of high-energy phosphate compounds (Chopp *et al.*, 1991; Busto *et al.*, 1989; Marion *et al.*, 1993). Although known to cause coagulopathy, there have been no reported significant complications with moderate hypothermia in the studies reported so far (Metz *et al.*, 1996; Resnick *et al.*, 1994). Thus, hypothermia could be a safe additional treatment in patients with high ICP.

6.3 Monitoring

Monitoring is a vital component in the optimal management of patient. It allows for early detection of intracranial mass lesion, guidance for therapy, early diagnosis of secondary complications, and determination of prognosis. Therefore, monitoring of patients with brain herniation, either traumatic or non-traumatic must comprise both general and specific neurologic monitoring.

6.3.1 General Monitoring

General parameters that should be repeatedly monitored include electrocardiography, arterial oxygen saturation, capnography, arterial blood pressure, central venous pressure, systemic temperature, urine output, arterial blood gases, and serum electrolytes and osmolality. Invasive or non-invasive cardiac output monitoring may be required in haemodynamically unstable patients who do not respond to fluid resuscitation and vasopressors therapy.

6.3.2 Neurological Monitoring

The brain trauma foundation guidelines recommends for ICP monitoring in all salvageable patients with severe TBI and an abnormal CT scan, and in patients with severe TBI with a normal CT scan, if two or more of the following features are noted at admission: age over 40 years, unilateral or bilateral motor posturing, or systolic blood pressure < 90 mm Hg (Bullock, 2007). Indications of ICP monitoring in patients with brain tumours are not clearly defined. It is mostly employed in cases with extensive cerebral oedema having brain herniation. Currently available methods of ICP monitoring include ventricular catheters, subdural-subarachnoid bolts or catheters, epidural transducers and intraparenchymal fiberoptic devices. The ventricular ICP catheter is the gold standard and preferred for ICP monitoring whenever possible. It is the most accurate, low-cost, and reliable technique of monitoring ICP. Additional benefits include provision for continuous ICP monitoring and therapeutic CSF drainage in the event of raised ICP (Marshman, 2001). ICP monitoring should be continued till the patient remains on intensive treatment or there is risk of secondary deterioration. This period usually last up to two weeks after injury. Advantages of ICP monitoring include early detection of intracranial mass lesion, guidance for therapy and prevention of irrational use of therapies to control ICP, CSF drainage with reduction of ICP and improvement of CPP, and determination of prognosis. Although ICP measurements have become an integral component of monitoring in patients with TBI, there is contradictory literature regarding improved outcome with this manoeuvre in acute coma, whether traumatic or non-traumatic (Saul & Ducker, 1982; Eisenberg *et al.*, 1988; Howells *et al.*, 2005; Aarabi *et al.*, 2006; Timofeev *et al.*, 2006; Bulger *et al.*, 2002; Lane *et al.*, 2000; Mauritz *et al.*, 2008; Stocchetti, 2001; Cremer *et al.*, 2005; Cremer, 2008; Shafi *et al.*, 2008; Randall *et al.*, 2012). Potential complications of ICP monitoring include infection, haemorrhage, and catheter malfunction or malposition. However, routine administration of prophylactic antibiotic after ventricular catheter placement is not recommended to reduce infection (Bullock, 2007).

6.4   Surgical Management

As soon as initial steps are over, a diagnostic brain CT should be performed immediately to identify the clinical cause; if not done so far because of hemodynamic instability (Andrews, 2003). CT scan is a vital tool for identification of intracranial mass lesions such as tumour, oedema, haemorrhage, or hydrocephalus. After obtaining the definitive diagnosis, if the patient has remained haemodynamically stable, exploratory burr-hole may be performed as an emergency measure on the same side of lateralizing signs such as dilated pupil, to explore the expanding mass lesion like epidural/subdural haemorrhage and immediate surgical evacuation should be done, if feasible (Andrews *et al.*, 1986; Chesnut *et al.*, 1994). In case of non-lateralizing signs of herniation, this procedure has to be considered bilaterally. Intraoperative ultrasonic brain imaging can further improve the utility of exploratory burr-holes, allowing for accurate identification and management of intracranial hematomas (Andrews *et al.*, 1990). In patients with haemodynamic instability, it is prudent to start ICP monitoring rather than performing exploratory burr holes, considering the lower probability of intracranial mass lesions in such patients. If the ICP is low, then no further intervention is required except for general stabilization of the patient. However, if the ICP is elevated, then further diagnostic imaging may be required, to decide for surgical exploration for such patients. If craniectomy is performed, it should be targeted to fully decompress the brain parenchyma. In case of non-traumatic mass lesion, immediate surgical decompressive craniotomy may be indicated for extensive cerebral oedema secondary to upward transtentorial or tonsillar herniation. For an external cerebral herniation, urgent surgical repair is mandatory to avoid any serious complications. The primary goal of surgery is to disconnect the encephalocele and perform dural repair. Various materials have been used for the dural repair includes fascia lata, temporalis fascia, lyophilised dura, or a biosorbable polyglycolic acid sheet (Jackson *et al.*, 1997). Other potential management tools include insertion of vascular cushions adjacent to large draining veins at the bone margin to reduce risk of venous ischemia (Stiver, 2009). Repair of the bony defect with bone or cartilage has also been described (Feenstra *et al,* 1985). However, this is not always performed as removal of the herniated brain tissue and prevention of CSF leak will in itself allow the bony defect to heal and thereby preventing recurrence.

6.5   Prognosis

The prognosis of patients with brain herniation syndromes depends mainly upon the age of presentation, initial GCS scores, pupillary response and size, hypoxia, hyperthermia, high intracranial pressure, aetiology, site and severity of brain herniation and how soon it is being attended (Jiang *et al.*, 2002). Recovery is better in patients of younger age group and with initial high GCS scores. In patients with a treatable cause like acute epidural or subdural hematoma, there are high chances of survival, if initial resuscitation and corrective management are initiated rapidly (Duffy, 1982; Andrews *et al.*, 1986).However, patients with traumatic transtentorial herniation have an overall mortality rate of 70%. Patients with non-traumatic causes of herniation (acute hydrocephalus, tumour-related cerebral oedema, temporal lobar haemorrhage, hemispheric infarction or cerebello-tonsillar herniation from lumbar drainage) having intact brain functions carry better prognosis and functional recovery, if appropriate resuscitative measures and surgical decompression of mass effect are instituted in a timely fashion (Dagnew *et al.*, 2002; Muhonen & Zunkeler, 1994; Weinberg *et al.*, 2003; Ross *et al.*, 1989; Andrews, 2005). The brain herniation can itself cause massive stroke which can lead to compression of cardiorespiratory centres in the brain stem, and consequent mortality. Brain herniation into temporal lobe or the cerebellum always carries a grave prognosis. However, outcome patterns are variable for other areas of the brain.

References

Aarabi, B., Hesdorffer, D., Ahn, E.S., Aresco, C., Scalea, T.M., & Eisenberg, H.M. (2006). Outcome following decompressive craniectomy for malignant swelling due to severe head injury. Journal of Neurosurgery, 104(4), 469-479.

Adler, D.E., & Milhorat, T.H. (2002). The tentorial notch: anatomical variation, morphometric analysis, and classification in 100 human autopsy cases. Journal of Neurosurgery, 96(6), 1103-1112.

Alderson, P., & Roberts, I. (2009). Corticosteroids for acute traumatic brain injury. Cochrane Database of Systematic Reviews 2009, 1, 1-27.

Amatruda, T.T., Hurst, M.H., & D'Esopo, N.D. (1965). Certain endocrine and metabolic facets of the steroid withdrawal syndrome. Journal of Clinical Endocrinology, 25(9), 1207–1217.

Andrews, B.T., Pitts, L.H., Lovely, M.P., & Bartkowski, H. (1986). Is computed tomographic scanning necessary in patients with tentorial herniation? Results of immediate surgical exploration without computed tomography in 100 patients. Neurosurgery, 19(3), 408-413.

Andrews, B.T., Mampalam, T.J., Omsberg, E., & Pitts, L.H. (1990). Intraoperative ultrasound imaging of the entire brain through unilateral exploratory burr holes after severe head injury. Surgical Neurology, 33(4), 291-294.

Andrews, B.T. (2003). Head injury management: Intensive surgery in Neurosurgery. Thieme Medical Publishers, New York, 125-136.

Andrews, B.T. (2003). Intensive Care in Neurosurgery. Thieme Medical Publishers, New York, USA, 1-243.

Andrews, B.T. (2005). Does decompressive craniectomy really improve outcome after head injury? In: Neurotrauma: Evidence-based Answers to Common Questions. Thieme Medical Publishers, New York, USA, 163-166.

Barr, R., & Gean, AD. (1994). Trauma In: Brandt WE, Helms CA. Fundamentals of Diagnostic Radiology. Williams & Wilkins, Baltimore, USA, 65-68.

Bivins, H.G., Ford, S., Bezmalinovic, Z., Price, H.M., & Williams, J.L. (1988). The effect of axial traction during orotracheal intubation of the trauma victim with an unstable spine. Annals of Emergency Medicine, 17(1), 25-29.

Blinkov, S.M., Gabibov, G.A., & Tanyashin, S.V. (1992). Variations in location of the arteries coursing between the brain stem and the free edge of the tentorium. Journal of Neurosurgery, 76(6), 973-978.

Bratton, S.L., Chestnut, R.M., Ghajar, J., Hammond, M.F.F., Harris, O.A., Hartl, R., Manley, G.T., Nemecek, A., Newell, D.W., Rosenthal, G., Schouten, J., Shutter, L., Timmons, S.D., Ullam, J.S., Videtta, W., Wilberger, J.E., & Wright, D.W. (2007). Guidelines for the management of severe traumatic brain injury: intracranial pressure thresholds. Journal of Neurotrauma, 24(1), 1-106.

Bulger, E.M., Nathens, A.B., Rivara, F.P., Moore, M., MacKenzie, E.J., & Jurkovich, G.J. (2002). Management of severe head injury: institutional variations in care and effect on outcome. Critical Care Medicine, 30(8), 1870-1876.

Bullock, R., Chesnut, R., Clifton, G., Ghajar, J., Marion, D.W., Narayan, R.K., Newell, D.W., Pitts, L.H., Rosner, M.J., & Wilberger, J.W. (1996). Guidelines for the management of severe head injury. European Journal of emergency medicine, 3(2), 109-127.

Burke, A.M., Quest, D.O., Chien, S., & Cerri C. (1981). The effects of mannitol on blood viscosity. Journal of Neurosurgery, 55(4), 550-553.

Busto, R., Globus, M.Y., Dietrich, W.D., Martinez, E., Valdés, I., & Ginsberg, M.D. (1989). Effect of mild hypothermia on ischemia-induced release of neurotransmitters and freefatty acids in rat brain. Stroke, 20(7), 904-10.

Chesnut, R.M., Gautille, T., Blunt, B.A., Klauber, M.R., & Marshall, L.E. (1994). The localizing value of asymmetry in pupil size in severe head injury: relation to lesion type and location. Neurosurgery, 34(5), 840-846.

Chesnut, R.M., Temkin, N., Carney, N., Dikmen, S., Rondina, C., Videtta, W., Petroni, G., Lujan, S., Pridgeon, J., Barber, J., Machamer, J., Chaddock, K., Celix, J.M., Cherner, M., & Hendrix, T. (2012). A Trial of Intracranial-Pressure Monitoring in Traumatic Brain Injury. The New England journal of medicine, 367, 2471-2481.

Chopp, M., Chen, H., Dereski, M.O., & Garcia, J.H. (1991). Mild hypothermic intervention after graded ischemic stress in rats.Stroke, 22(1), 37-43.

Collier, J. (1904). The false localizing signs of intracranial tumour. Brain, 27(4), 490-508.

Colquhoun, M.C., Handley, A.J., & Evans, T.R. (2004). ABC of Resuscitation. BMJ Publishing Group, London, 63-71

Conn, H.O., & Poynard, T. (1994). Corticosteroids and peptic ulcer: meta-analysis of adverse events during steroid therapy. Journal of Internal Medicine, 236(6), 619–632.

Cottrell, J.E., Robustelli, A., Post, K., & Turndorf, H. (1977). Furosemide- and mannitol-induced changes in intracranial pressure and serum osmolality and electrolytes. Anesthesiology, 47(1), 28–30.

CRASH Trial Collaborators. (2004). Effect of intravenous corticosteroids on death within 14 days in 10008 adults with clinically significant head injury (MRC CRASH trial): randomised placebo-controlled trial. Lancet, 364, 1321–1328.

Cremer, O.L., Van Dijk, G., Van Wensen, E.,Brekelmans, G.J., Moons, K.G., Leenen, L.P., & Kalkman, C.J. (2005). Effect of intracranial pressure monitoring and targeted intensive care on functional outcome after severe head injury. Critical Care Medicine, 33(10), 2207-2213.

Cremer, O.L. (2008). Does ICP monitoring make a difference in neurocritical care? European Journal of Anaesthesiology, 25(42), 87-93.

Cruz, J. (1993). On-line monitoring of global cerebral hypoxia in acute brain injury.Relationship to intracranial hypertension. Journal of Neurosurgery, 79(2), 513-520.

Cruz, J. (1998). The first decade of continuous monitoring of jugular bulb oxyhemoglobin saturation: management strategies and clinical outcome. Critical Care Medicine, 26(2), 344-351.

Cruz, J., Minoja, G., & Okuchi, K. (2001). Improving clinical outcomes from acute subdural hematomas with the emergency preoperative administration of high doses of mannitol: a randomized trial. Neurosurgery, 49(4), 864-871.

Cuneo, R.A., Caronna, J.J., Pitts, L., Townsend, J., & Winestock, D.P. (1979). Upward transtentorial herniation: seven cases and a literature review. Archives of Neurology, 36(10), 618-623.

Dagnew, E., VanLoveren, H.R., & Tew, J.M. (2002). Acute foramen magnum syndrome caused by an acquired Chiari malformation after lumbar drainage of cerebrospinal fluid: report of three cases. Neurosurgery, 51(3), 823-828.

De Freitas, G.R., & Andre, C. (2006). Sensitivity of transcranial Doppler for confirming brain death: A prospective study of 270 cases. Acta Neurologica Scandinavica, 113(6), 426-432.

De Vivo, P., Del Gaudio, A., Ciritella, P., Puopolo, M., Chiarotti, F., & Mastronardi, E. (2001). Hypertonic saline solution: A safe alternative to mannitol 18 % in neurosurgery. Minerva Anesthesiologica, 67(9), 603-11.

Dosemeci, L., Dora, B., Yilmaz, M., Cenqiz, M., Balkan, S., & Ramazanoqlu, A. (2004). Utility of transcranial Doppler ultrasonography for confirmatory diagnosis of brain death: Two sides of the coin. Transplantation, 77(1), 71-75.

Duffy, G.P. (1982). Lumbar puncture in spontaneous subarachnoid hemorrhage.British Medical Journal, 285(6349), 290-97.

Ecker, A. (1948). Upward transtentorial herniation of the brainstem and cerebellum due to tumor of the posterior fossa: With a special note on tumors of acoustic nerve. Journal of Neurosurgery, 5(1), 51-61.

Eisenberg, H.M., Frankowski, R.F., Contant, C.F., Marshall, L.F., & Walker, M.D. (1988). High-dose barbiturate control of elevated intracranial pressure in patients with severe head injury. Journal of Neurosurgery, 69(1), 15-23.

Elguera, M. (1962). Transtentorial Herniation, Finney LA, Walker AE. Springfield, IL.

Feenstra, L., Sanna, M., Zini, C., Gamoletti, R., & Delogu, P. (1985). Surgical treatment of brain herniation into the middle ear and mastoid. American Journal of Otology, 6, 311–315.

Feig, P.U. & McCurdy, D.K. (1977). The hypertonic state.New England Journal of Medicine, 297(26), 1444-1454.

Feldmann, E., Gandy, S.E., Becker, R., Zimmerman, R., Thaler, H.T., Posner, J.B., & Plum F. (1988). MRI demonstrates descending transtentorial herniation. Neurology, 38(5), 697-701.

Fisher, C.M. (1972). The arterial source of secondary brain stem hemorrhages (abstr). Journal of Pathology, 66, 9.

Gahjar, J.B., Hariri, R.J. & Patterson, R.H. (1993). Improved outcome from traumatic coma using only ventricular CSF drainage for ICP control. Advances in Neurosurgery, 21, 173-177.

Gotzsche, P.C. (1994). Steroids and peptic ulcer: an end to the controversy. Journal of Internal Medicine, 236(6), 599–601.

Gray, H. (1974). Gray's Anatomy, Philadelphia, Running Press, PA, 512-523.

Grossman, R.I., & Yousem, D.M. (1994). Neuroradiology- The Requisites., Mosby-Year Book, St.Louis, 161-162.

Haddad, S.H., & Arabi, Y.M. (2012). Critical care management of severe traumatic brain injury in adults. Scandinavian Journal of Trauma, Resuscitation and Emergency Medicine, 20(12), 1-15.

Hahn, F., & Gurney, J. (1985). CT signs of central descending transtentorial herniation. American Journal of Neuroradiology, 6(5), 844-845.

Hassler, O. (1967). Arterial pattern of human brainstem: Normal appearance and deformation in expanding supratentorial conditions. Neurology, 17(4), 368-375.

Heiss, J.D., Papavassiliou, E., Merrill, M.J., Nieman, L., Knightly, J.J., Walbridge, S., Edwards, N.A., & Oldfield, E.H. (1996). Mechanism of dexamethasone suppression of brain tumor-associated vascular permeability in rats. Involvement of the glucocorticoid receptor and vascular permeability factor. The Journal of Clinical Investigation, 98(6), 1400-1408.

Hill, L. (1896). The physiology and pathology of the cerebral circulation. Churchill Publishers, London, England, 208.

Howell, D.A. (1959). Upper brain-stem compression and foraminal impaction with intracranial space-occupying lesions and brain swelling. Brain, 82(4), 525-550.

Howells, T., Elf, K., Jones, P., Ronne-Engström, E., Piper, I., Nilsson, P., Andrews, P., & Enblad, P. (2005). Pressure reactivity as a guide in the treatment of cerebral perfusion pressure in patients with brain trauma. Journal of Neurosurgery, 102(2), 311-317.

Hsiang, J.K., Chesnut, R.M., Crisp, C.B., Klauber, M.R., Blunt, B.A., & Marshall, L.F. (1994). Early, routine paralysis for intracranial pressure control in severe head injury: is it necessary? Critical Care Medicine, 22(9), 1471-1476.

Jackson, C.G., Pappas, D.G., Manolidis, S., Glasscock, M.E., Von Doersten. P.G., Hampf. C.R., Williams J.B., Storper, I.S. (1997). Brain herniation into the middle ear and mastoid: concepts in diagnosis and surgical management. American Journal of Otolaryngology, 18, 198–206.

James, H.E., Langfitt, T.W., Kumar, V.S., & Ghostine, S.Y. (1977). Treatment of intracranial hypertension.Analysis of 105 consecutive, continuous recordings of intracranial pressure. Acta Neurochirurgica, 36(3-4), 189–200.

Jiang, J.Y., Gao, G.Y., Li, W.P., Yu, M.K., & Zhu, C. (2002). Early indicators of prognosis in 846 cases of severe traumatic brain injury. Journal of Neurotrauma, 19(7), 869-874.

Jefferson, G. (1938). The tentorial pressure cone. Archives of Neurology and Psychiatry, 40(5): 857-876.

Jennett, W.B., & Stern, W.E. (1960). Tentorial herniation, the mid brain and the pupil. Experimental studies in brain compression. Journal of Neurosurgery, 17, 598-609.

Kaufmann, A.M., & Cardoso, E.R. (1992). Aggravation of vasogenic cerebral edema by multiple-dose mannitol.Journal of Neurosurgery, 77(4), 584-589.

Kernohan, J.W., & Woltman, H.W. (1929). Incisura of the crus due to contralateral brain tumor. Archives of Neurology and Psychiatry, 21(2), 274-287.

Kochanek, P.M., Carney, N., Adelson, P.D., Ashwal, S., Bell, M.J., Bratton, S., Carson, S., Chesnut, R.M., Ghajar, J., Goldstein, B., Grant, G.A., Kissoon N., Peterson, K., Selden, N.R., Tasker, R.C., Vavilala, M.S., Wainwright, M.S., & Warden, C.R. (2012). Guidelines for the acute medical management of severe traumatic brain injury in infants, children and adolescents: second edition. Pediatric critical care medicine, 13(1), 1-82.

Komaki, S., & Handel, S. (1974). Molding of the posterior communicating artery in downward transtentorial herniation. Radiology, 113, 107-110.

Kovacs, J.A., Gill, V.J., Meshnick, S., & Masur, H. (2001). New insights into transmission, diagnosis, and drug treatment of Pneumocystis cariniipneumonia.The Journal of American medical association, 286(19), 2450–2460.

Lane, P.L., Skoretz, T.G., Doig, G., & Girotti, M.J. (2000). Intracranial pressure monitoring and outcomes after traumatic brain injury. Canadian Journal of Surgery, 43(6), 442-448.

Leech, P., & Miller, J.D. (1974). Intracranial volume-pressure relationships during experimental brain compression in primates, III: The effect of mannitol and hyperventilation. Journal of Neurology, Neurosurgery and Psychiatry, 37(10), 1105-1111.

Lewis, S.B., Myburgh, J.A., Thornton, E.L., & Reilly, P.L. (1996). Cerebral oxygenation monitoring by near-infrared spectroscopy is not clinically useful in patients with severe closed-head injury: A comparison with jugular venous bulb oximetry. Critical Care Medicine 1996, 24(8), 1334-1338.

Lidofsky, S.D., Bass, N.M., Prager, M.C., Washington, D.E., Read A.E., Wright T.L., Ascher, N.L., Roberts, J.P., Scharschmidt, B.F., & Lake, J.R. (1992). Intracranial pressure monitoring and liver transplantation for fulminant hepatic failure.Hepatology, 16(1), 1-7.

Loevner, L.A. (1999). Case review, brain imaging. Mosby Inc., St. Louis, USA, 1-266.

Machein, M.R., Kullmer, J., Ronicke, V., Machein, U., Krieg, M., Damert, A., Breier, G., Risau, W., & Plate, K.H. (1999). Differential downregulation of vascular endothelial growth factor by dexamethasone in normoxic and hypoxic rat glioma cells. Neuropathology and Applied Neurobiology, 25(2), 104–112.

Marion, D.W., Obrist, W.D., Carlier, P.M.,Penrod, L.E., & Darby, J.M. (1993). The use of moderate therapeutic hypothermia for patients with severe head injuries: a preliminary report. Journal of Neurosurgery, 79(3), 354-362.

Marshall, L.F., Barba, D., Toole, B.M., & Bowers, S.A. (1983). The oval pupil: clinical significance and relationship to intracranial hypertension. Journal of Neurosurgery, 58(4), 566-568.

Marshman, L.A., Polkey, C.E., & Penney, C.C. (2001). Unilateral fixed dilation of the pupil as a false-localizing sign with intracranial hemorrhage: case report and literature review. Neurosurgery, 49(5), 1251-1255.

Mauritz, W., Steltzer, H., Bauer, P., Dolanski-Aghamanoukjan, L., & Metnitz, P. (2008). Monitoring of intracranial pressure in patients with severe traumatic brain injury: an Austrian prospective multicenter study. Intensive Care Medicine, 34(7), 1208-1215.

Metz, C., Holzschuh, M., Bein, T., Woertgen, C., Frey, A., Frey, I., Taeger, K., & Brawanski, A. (1996). Moderate hypothermia in patients with severe head injury: cerebral and extracerebral effects. Journal of Neurosurgery, 85(4), 533–541.

Meyer, A. (1920). Herniation of the brain. Archives of Neurology & Psychiatry, 4, 387-400.

Meyer, G., & Badenhoop, K. (2003). Glucocorticoid-induced insulin resistance and diabetes mellitus.Receptor-, postreceptor mechanisms, local cortisol action, and new aspects of antidiabetic therapy.MedizinischeKlinik, 98(5), 266–270.

Michenfelder, J.D. (1974). The interdependency of cerebral functional and metabolic effects following massive doses of thiopental in the dog.Anesthesiology, 41(3), 231-236.

Muhonen, M.G., & Zunkeler, B. (1994). Management of acute hydrocephalus (landmarks and techniques): Neurosurgical emergencies: Neurosurgical Topics. AANS Publications Committee, Chicago, USA, 29-41.

Muizelaar, J.P., Wei, E.P., Kontos, H.A., & Becker, D.P. (1983). Mannitol causes compensatory vasoconstriction and vasodilation in response to blood viscosity changes. Journal of Neurosurgery, 59(5), 822-828.

Muizelaar, J.P., Lutz, H.A., & Becker, D.P. (1984). Effect of mannitol on ICP and CBF and correlation with pressure autoregulation in severely head injured patients. Journal of Neurosurgery, 61(4), 700-706.

Nakstad, P., Nornes, H., & Hauge, H.N. (1986). Traumatic aneurysms of the pericallosal arteries. Neuroradiology, 28(4), 335-338

Narayan, R.K., Kishore, P.R., Becker, D.P., Ward, J.D., Enas, G.G., Greenberg, R.P., Domingues Da Silva, A., Lipper, M.H., Choi, S.C., Mayhall, C.G., Lutz, H.A. & Young, H.F. (1982). Intracranial pressure: to monitor or not to monitor? A review of our experience with severe head injury. Journal of Neurosurgery, 56(5), 650-659.

Nguyen, J.P., Djindjian, M., Brugières, P., Badiane, S., Melon, E., & Poirier, J. (1989). Anatomy-computerized tomography correlations in transtentorial brain herniation. Journal of Neuroradiology, 16(3), 181-196.

Osborn, A.G. (1976). Diagnosis of descending transtentorial herniation by cranial computed tomography. Radiology, 123(1), 93-96.

Osborn, A.G. (1991). Secondary effects of intracranial trauma. Neurosurgery Clinics of North America, 1, 461-474.

Osborn, A.G. (1996). Handbook of Neuroradiology: Brain and Skull. Mosby Inc., St. Louis, USA, 222-30.

Osborn, A.G., Heaston, D.K., & Wing, S.D. (1978). Diagnosis of Ascending Transtentorial Herniation by Cranial Computed Tomography. American Journal of Roentgenology, 130(4), 755-760.

Pollay, M., Fullenwider, C., Roberts, P.A. & Stevens, F.A. (1983). Effect of mannitol and furosemide on blood–brain osmotic gradient and intracranial pressure.Journal of Neurosurgery, 59(6), 945–950.

Prough, U.S. (2005). Should I use hypertonic saline to treat high intracranial pressure? In; Neurotrauma; Evidence-based Answers to Common Questions.Thieme Medical Publishers, New York, 148-151.

Ramsden, R.T., Latif, A., Lye, R.H., Dutton, J.E.M. (1985). Endaural cerebral hernia. Journal of Laryngology & Otolaryngology, 99, 643–651.

Ramsey, R.G. (1994). Disorders of the spine: Neuroradiology. WB Saunders, Philadelphia, USA, 476, 42-43.

Reich, J.B., Sierra, J., Camp, W., Zanzonico, P., Deck, M.D., & Plum, F. (1993). Magnetic resonance imaging measurements and clinical changes accompanying transtentorial and foramen magnum brain herniation. Annals of Neurology, 33(2), 159-170.

Reimer, P., Parizel, P.M.,Meaney, J.F.M., & Stichnoth, F.A. (2010). Clinical MR Imaging: A practical approach, Springer-Verlag, Heidelberg, Berlin, 107, 114.

Resnick, D.K., Marion, D.W., & Darby, J.M. (1994). The effect of hypothermia on the incidence of delayed traumatic intracerebral hemorrhage.Neurosurgery, 34(2), 252-256.

Robertson, C. (2004). Every breath you take: Hyperventilation and intracranial pressure. Cleveland clinic journal of medicine, 71(1), 14-15.

Robertson, C.S., & Cormio, M. (1995).Cerebral metabolic management. New Horizons, 3(3), 410-422.

Ropper, A.H. (1986). Lateral displacement of the brain and level of consciousness in patients with an acute hemispheric mass. New England Journal of Medicine, 314(15), 953-958.

Rosenthal, G., Hemphill, J.C., Sorani, M., Martin, C., Morabito, D., Obrist, W.D., & Manley, G.T. (2008). Brain tissue oxygen tension is more indicative of oxygen diffusion than oxygen delivery and metabolism in patients with traumatic brain injury. Critical Care Medicine, 36(6), 1917-1924.

Ross, D.A., Olsen, W.L., Ross, A.M., Andrews, B.T., & Pitts, L.H. (1989). Brain shift, level of consciousness, and restoration of consciousness in patients with acute intracranial hematoma. Journal of Neurosurgery, 71(4), 498-502.

Ruderman, N., & Hall, T. (1965). Use of glucocorticoids in the palliative treatment of metastatic brain tumors. Cancer, 18, 298–306.

Saul, T.G., & Ducker, T.B. (1982). Effect of intracranial pressure monitoring and aggressive treatment on mortality in severe head injury. Journal of Neurosurgery, 56(4), 498-503.

Saul, T.G., & Ducker, T.B. (1982). Intracranial pressure monitoring in patients with severe head injury. The American Surgeon, 48(9), 477-480.

Scheinker, I.M. (1945). Transtentorial herniation of the brainstem; A characteristic clinicopathologic syndrome; Pathogenesis of hemorrhages in the brainstem. Archives of Neurology & Psychiatry, 53(4), 289-298.

Schrot, R.J., & Muizelaar, J.P. (2005). Is there's "best" way to give mannitol? In Neurutrauma: Evidence-based Answers to Common Questions. Thieme Medical Publishers, New York, USA, 142-147.

Schwarz, G.A., & Rosner, A.A. (1941). Displacement and herniation of the hippocampal gyrus through the incisuratentorii. Archives of Neurology and Psychiatry, 46(2), 297-321.

Shafi, S., Diaz-Arrastia, R., Madden, C., & Gentilello, L. (2008). Intracranial pressure monitoring in brain-injured patients is associated with worsening of survival. Journal of Trauma, 64(2), 335-340.

Smyth, G.E., & Henderson, W.R. (1938). Observations on the cerebrospinal fluid pressure on simultaneous ventricular and lumbar punctures. Journal of Neurology and Psychiatry, 1(3), 226-238.

Sohn, D., & Levine, S. (1967). Frontal lobe infarcts caused by brain herniation: Compression of anterior cerebral artery branches. Archives of Pathology, 84(5), 509-512.

Speigelman, R., Hadani, M., Ram, Z., Faibel, M., & Shacked, I. (1989). Upward transtentorial herniation: A complication of postoperative edema at the cervicomedullary junction. Neurosurgery, 24(2), 284-288.

Stevens, R.D., Huff, J.S., Duckworth, J., Papangelou, A., Weingart, S.D., & Smith, W.S. (2012). Emergency neurological life support: Intracranial hypertension and herniation. Neurocritical care, 17(1), 60-65.

Stiefel, M.F., Spiotta, A., Gracias, V.H., Garuffe, A.M., Guillamondegui, O., Maloney- Wilensky, E., Bloom, S., Grady, M.S., & LeRoux, P.D. (2005). Reduced mortality rate in patients with severe traumatic brain injury treated with brain tissue oxygen monitoring. Journal of Neurosurgery, 103(5), 805-811.

Stiver, S. I. (2009). Complications of decompressive craniectomy for traumatic brain injury. Neurosurgery focus, 26(6),7.

Stocchetti, N., Pennym, K.I., Dearden, M., Braakman, R., Cohadon, F., Iannotti, F., Lapierre, F., Karimi, A., Maas, A., Murray, G.D., Ohman, J., Persson, L., Servadei, F., Teasdale, G.M., Trojanowski, T., & Unterberg, A. (2001). Intensive care management of head-injured patients in Europe: a survey from the European brain injury consortium. Intensive Care Medicine, 27(2), 400-406.

Stovring, J. (1977). Descending tentorialherniations: Findings on computed tomography. Neuroradiology, 14(3), 101-105.

Sunderland, S. (1958). The tentorial notch and complications produced by herniations of the brain through that aperture. British Journal of Surgery, 45(193), 422-438.

Sunderland, S., & Hughes, E.S.R. (1946). The pupillo-constrictor pathway and the nerves to the ocular muscles in man. Brain, 69(4), 301-309.

Taveras, J.M. (1996). Neuroradiology. Williams & Wilkins, Baltimore, USA, 111-115.

Thompson, R.K., & Salcman, M. (1988). Brain stem hemorrhages: historical perspective. Neurosurgery, 22(4), 623-628.

Timofeev, I., Kirkpatrick, P., Corteen, E., Hiler, M., Czosnyka, M., Menon, D.K., Pickard, J.D., & Hutchinson, P.J. (2006). Decompressivecraniectomy in traumatic brain injury: outcome following protocol-driven therapy. ActaNeurochirurgica supplement, 96, 11-16.

Toutant, S.M., Klauber, M.R., Marshall, L.F., Toole, B.M., Bowers, S.A., Seelig, J.M., & Varnell, J.B. (1984). Absent or compressed basal cisterns on first CT scan: ominous predictors of outcome in severe head injury. Journal of Neurosurgery, 61(4), 691-694.

Unterberg, A.W., Kiening, K.L., Härtl, R., Bardt, T., Sarrafzadeh, A.S., &Lanksch, W.R. (1997). Multimodal monitoring in patients with head injury: evaluation of the effects of treatment on cerebral oxygenation. Journal of Trauma, 42(5), 32-37.

Vespa, P., Prins, M., Ronne-Engstrom, E., Caron, M., Shalmon, E., Hovda, D.A., Martin, N.A., & Becker, D.P. (1998). Increase in extracellular glutamate caused by reduced cerebral perfusion pressure and seizures after human traumatic brain injury: a microdialysis study. Journal of Neurosurgery, 89(6), 971-982.

Ward, J.D., Becker, D.P., Miller, J.D. Choi, S.C., Marmarou, A., Wood, C., Newlon, P.G., & Keenan, R. (1985). Failure of prophylactic barbiturate coma in the treatment of severe head injury.Journal of Neurosurgery, 62(3), 383-388.

Weinberg, J.S., Rhines, L.D., Cohen, Z.R., Langford, L., & Levin, V.A. (2003). Posterior fossa decompression for life-threatening tonsillar herniation in patients with gliomatosiscerebri: report of three cases. Neurosurgery, 52(1), 216-223.

Wilkinson, H.A. & Rosenfeld, S.R. (1983). Furosemide and mannitol in the treatment of acute experimental intracranial hypertension.Neurosurgery, 12(4), 405-410.

Yamada, K., Ushio, Y., & Hayakawa, T. (1989). Effects of steroids on the blood–brain barrier.Implications of the Blood–Brain Barrier and Its Manipulation. Plenum Press, New York, USA, 53–76.

Yang, X.F., Wen, L., Shen, F., Li, G., Lou, R., Liu, W.G., & Zhan, R.Y. (2008). Surgical complications secondary to decompressive craniectomy in patients with a head injury: a series of 108 consecutive cases. Acta Neurochirurgica, 150(12), 1241-1247.

Posterolateral Debridment and Anterior Reconstruction By Limited Spinal Shortening In Spinal Infections

Mohamed El-Sayed Abdel-Wanis
Sohag Faculty of Medicine
Sohag University, Egypt

1   Introduction

In severe osteomyelitis of the spine, open debridement and anterior fusion by anterior bone grafting offers the advantage of eradication of the focus of infection and improvement of conditions for bony fusion of the affected vertebral bodies (Benli *et al.* 1997, Dai *et al.* 2005, Korovessis *et al.* 2006, Krodel *et al.* 1999). In last few years a shift occurred in the preferred surgical approach for management of thoracic and lumbar spinal infections with a lot of research works reported good results with posterior surgical approach (Abdel-Wanis2006, Abdel-Wanis 2012, Chanplakorn *et al.* 2011, El-Sharkawi & Said 2011, Guzey *et al.* 2005, Zhang *et al.* 2012). In 2006, I reported the results of 12 patients of spinal infections of the thoracic and lumbar spine treated through a single posterior circumspinal exposure (Abdel-Wanis 2006). El-Sharkawi and Said compared the results of one stage circumferential fusion and anterior debridment and fusion followed 10-14 days later by posterior stabilization and posterolateral fusion for treatment of dorsolumbar spine tuberculosis. They reported that one-stage surgery is advantageous because it has a lower complication rate, shorter hospital stay, less operative time and blood loss (El-Sharkawi & Said 2011). Zhang *et al.* retrospectively reviewed 36 cases of thoracic spinal tuberculosis treated by two different surgical procedures: 20 cases in Group A underwent single-stage posterior debridement, transforaminal fusion and instrumentation, and 16 cases in Group B underwent posterior instrumentation, anterior debridement and bone graft in a single- or two-stage procedure. They concluded that the posterior approach only procedure obtained better clinical outcomes than combined posterior and anterior surgeries. They considered that single-stage posterior debridment is a better surgical treatment for thoracic spinal tuberculosis in aged patients with poor health status, especially for cases in early phase of bone destruction and/or mild and moderate kyphosis (Zhang *et al.* 2012).

The first report of removal of a portion of the spine to correct a deformity was by Roile in 1928 (Roile 1928). A two stage procedure was reported by von Lackum and Smith in 1933. This procedure involved the removal of the vertebral body through an anterior approach in the first stage and removal of the posterior elements and performance of fusion in the second stage (von Lackum and Smith 1933). The Hodgson convex side closing wedge osteotomy for correction of fixed kyphosis is actually a spinal shortening operation allows straightening of the spine while preserving the neurological function (Hodgson 1965). Spinal column shortening may be used in spinal fractures (Reyes –Sanchez *et al.* 2002), congenital spinal deformities (Lazar & Hall 1999, Nakamura *et al.* 2002, Ruff & Harms 2003, Ruff *et al.* 2005, Shono *et al.* 2001 Smith *et al.* 2005), primary or secondary malignant tumors (Abdel-Wanis 2002,Grunenwald *et al.* 1996, Heary *et al.* 1998, Kawahara *et al.* 1997, Magerl & Costia 1998, Murakami *et al.* 2001, Tomita *el al* 1994, Tomita *et al.* 1997), kyphotic deformities (Kawahara *et al.* 2001, Smith *et al.* 2005), fixed sagittal and coronal imbalance (Bradford & Clifford 1997, Bridwell *et al.* 2004), tethered cord syndrome (Hsieh *et al.* 2010), and flatback deformity of the spine (Kawahara *et al.* 2001, Potter *et al.* 2004).

The first case of use of limited spinal shortening for anterior spinal reconstruction in spinal infection was reported by the current author in 2006. The paper published was entitled "Single- stage posterior circumspinal debridment and reconstruction for thoracic and lumbar spinal infections". In this work I reported on 12 patients, 5 of whom received spinal shortening for anterior reconstruction of the spine (Abdel-Wanis 2006). In 2011, I reported 10 patients of infections of the thoracic spine treated by single posterolateral exposure and the anterior reconstruction was achieved in all patients by spinal shortening (Abdel-Wnis 2011, Abdel-Wanis 2012). Also, in 2011, Chanplakorn et al. reported treatment of 3 patients with acute tuberculous spondylitis by spinal shortening osteotomy (Chanplakorn *et al.* 2011).

2   My Technique

Patients are operated under general anesthesia in the prone position through a single posterior exposure. No intraoperative neuromonitoring was used during the operation. The incision is a straight vertical midline incision extended for one level above and below the planed instrumentation levels. The paraspinal muscles are dissected and laterally retracted. Lateral dissection is performed till the tip of the transvers process in the lumbar spine and about 5 cm of the rib is exposed in the thoracic spine. Posterior stabilization by trans-pedicular screw fixation is performed usually for one level above and one level below the affected vertebra. A rod is inserted in one side (usually the right side) while the rod in the other side is not inserted to give space sufficient for laminectomy and anterior dissection. Laminectomy is carried out. For full exposure of the anterior aspect of the vertebral bodies, excision of the medial 5 cms of one or two ribs is performed in one side (Figure 1 A). We prefer anterior circumspinal dissection on the left side because the wall of the aorta is strong and resistant to injury by the blunt dissection contrary to the wall of the vena cava that might be injured easily. The intercostal artery and nerve are ligated and divided. The stump of the intercostal nerve is used for gentle indirect manipulation of the spinal cord. Blount anterior dissection using the finger and gauze is carried out. Then, spatual-originally developed for posterior total en bloc spondylectomy operation by Tomita (Abdel-Wanis *et al.* 2002, Murakami *et al.* 2001, Tomita *et al.* 1994, Tomita *et al.* 1997) – is then inserted anterior to the vertebral body or bodies (Figure 1 B). In the lumbar spine, dissection around the vertebral body is not needed as retraction of the cauda equine usually gives good space sufficient for curettage of the disc and debridment of the infected tissues and the technique should be a modification of posterior lumbar interbody fusion (PLIF) (Lee & Suh 2006). Also, in the thoracic spine, when there is no much debris or pus to be evacuated lying anterior to the vertebral column, curettage of the disc infection might be possible from the space available lateral to the spinal cord. Then, reconstruction of the anterior column is performed by limited spinal shortening. Care must be given during shortening to avoid kinking of the cord or compression on the nerve roots by the pedicles. Then, posterior fusion is performed. Bone graft used is local graft from the ribs and laminae (Figure 1 C). Postoperatively, a brace is used during walking or sitting for 3 months. Patients were followed up by monthly radiographs.

3   Results of the Technique

I treated 10 patients with infection of the thoracic spine (Figure 2) and 22 patients of infections of lumbar spine by this technique (Figure 3). Causative organisms were TB in 20 patients, Staph aureus in 4 patient, salamonella typhi 1 patient, brucella in 1 patient and bacteriologic testing of intraoperative samples did not find germs in 6 patients. Operative time ranged between 100-190 (mean 135) minutes for thoracic spine operations, and between 110-180 minutes for the lumbar spine operations. For thoracic spine infections, local kyphosis angle ranged between 0 ° to 40 ° and (mean 17.5°), while post-operatively ranged between 0° and 19° (mean 10.9°). For the lumbar spine infections preoperative local lordotic angle ranged between 30° to -10° (mean 2.5°), improved post-operatively to a mean of 10.04° (range; 35° to -10°) (lordotic angle is expressed as + while kyphotic angle is expressed as -). Only3 patients received antibiotic medication pre-operatively; one caused by brucellla and 2 caused by pyogenic infections. However, in the 3 patients as there was no response for full course of antibiotics, surgery was indicated.

(a)   (b)

(c)

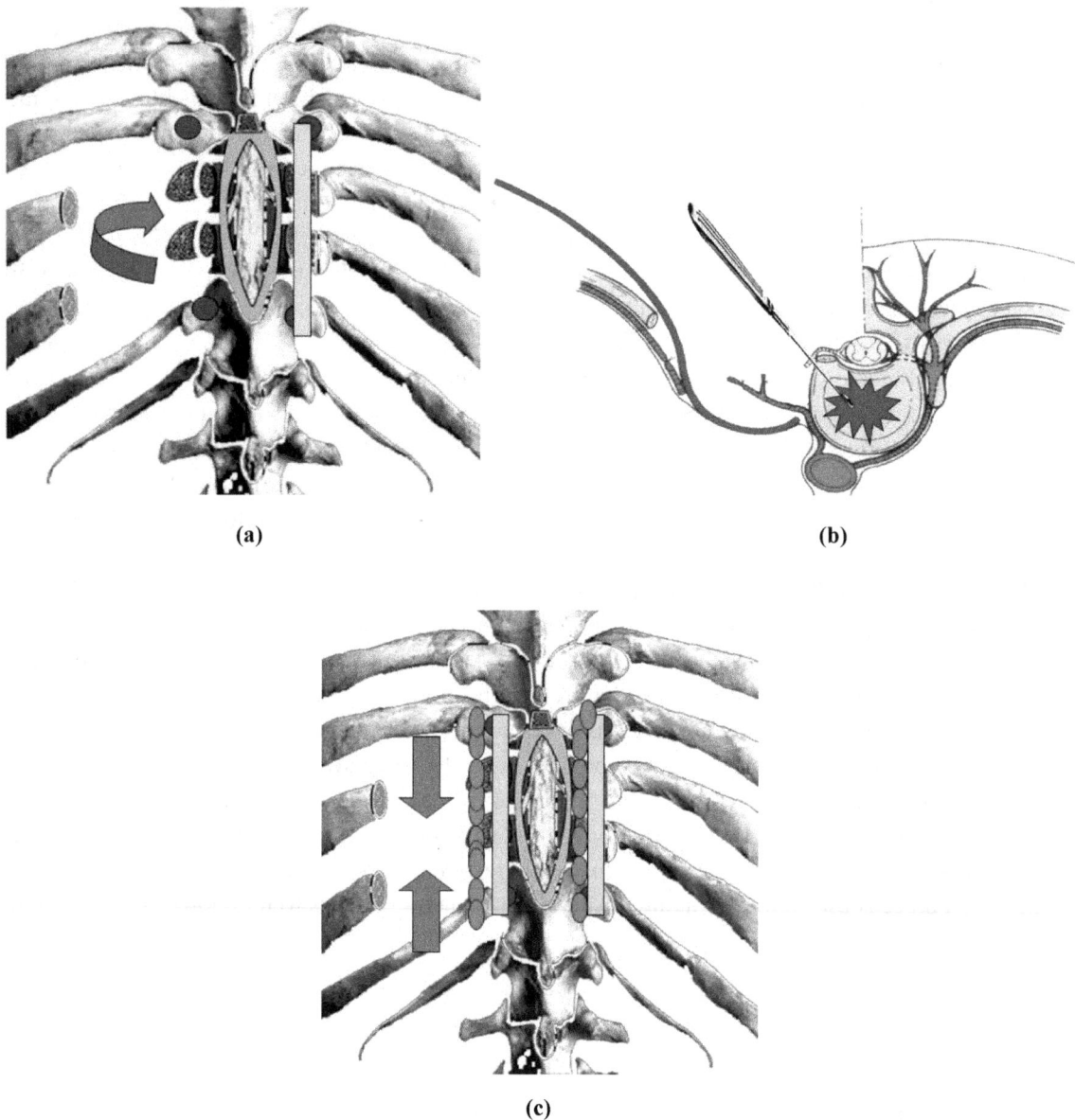

Figure 1: Technique (A) Posterior stabilization by trans-pedicular screw fixation is performed for one level above and one level below the affected vertebra. A rod is inserted in the right side. Laminecto-my is carried out. Then, excision of the medial 5 cms of one or two ribs is performed in one side. We prefer anterior circumspinal dissection on the left side (B) Blount anterior dissection using the finger and gauze is carried out. Ligation of the intercostal nerve and artery is done. Then, a spatuala is in-serted anterior to the vertebral. The space developed is sufficient for evacuation of the abscess and cu-rettage of the lesion. (C) Left-side rod is inserted. Anterior reconstruction is achieved by spinal short-ening and local bone graft obtained from the laminae and ribs is used for achieving posterior spinal fusion.

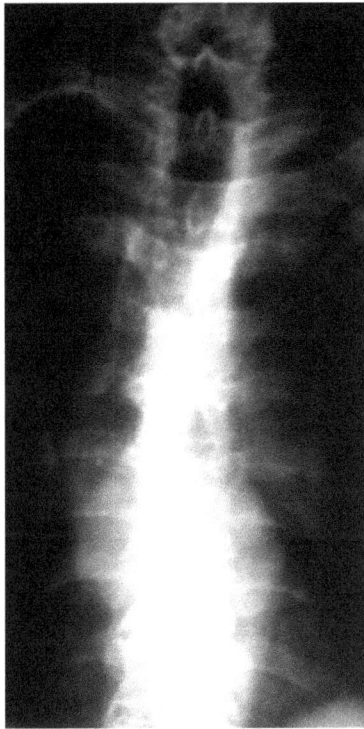 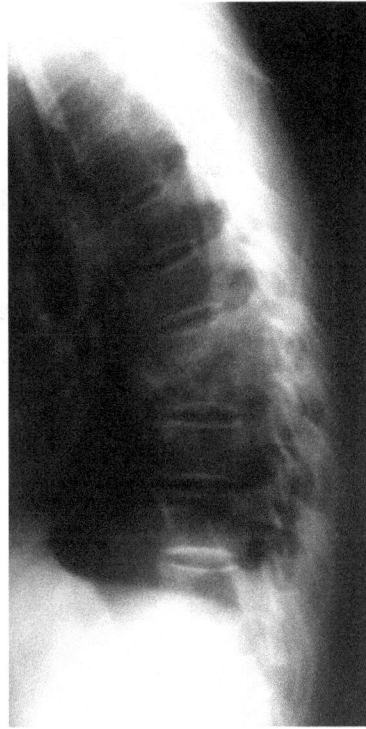

(a)   (b)

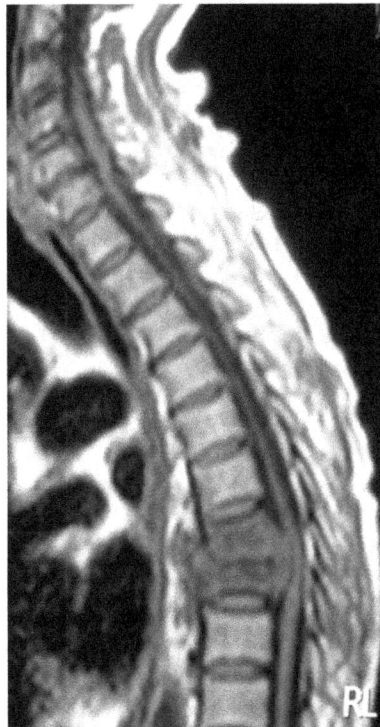 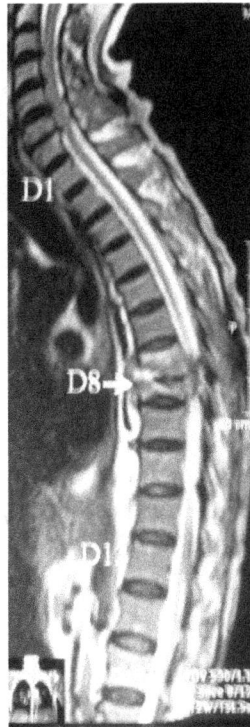

(c)   (d)

(e)   (f)

(g)   (h)

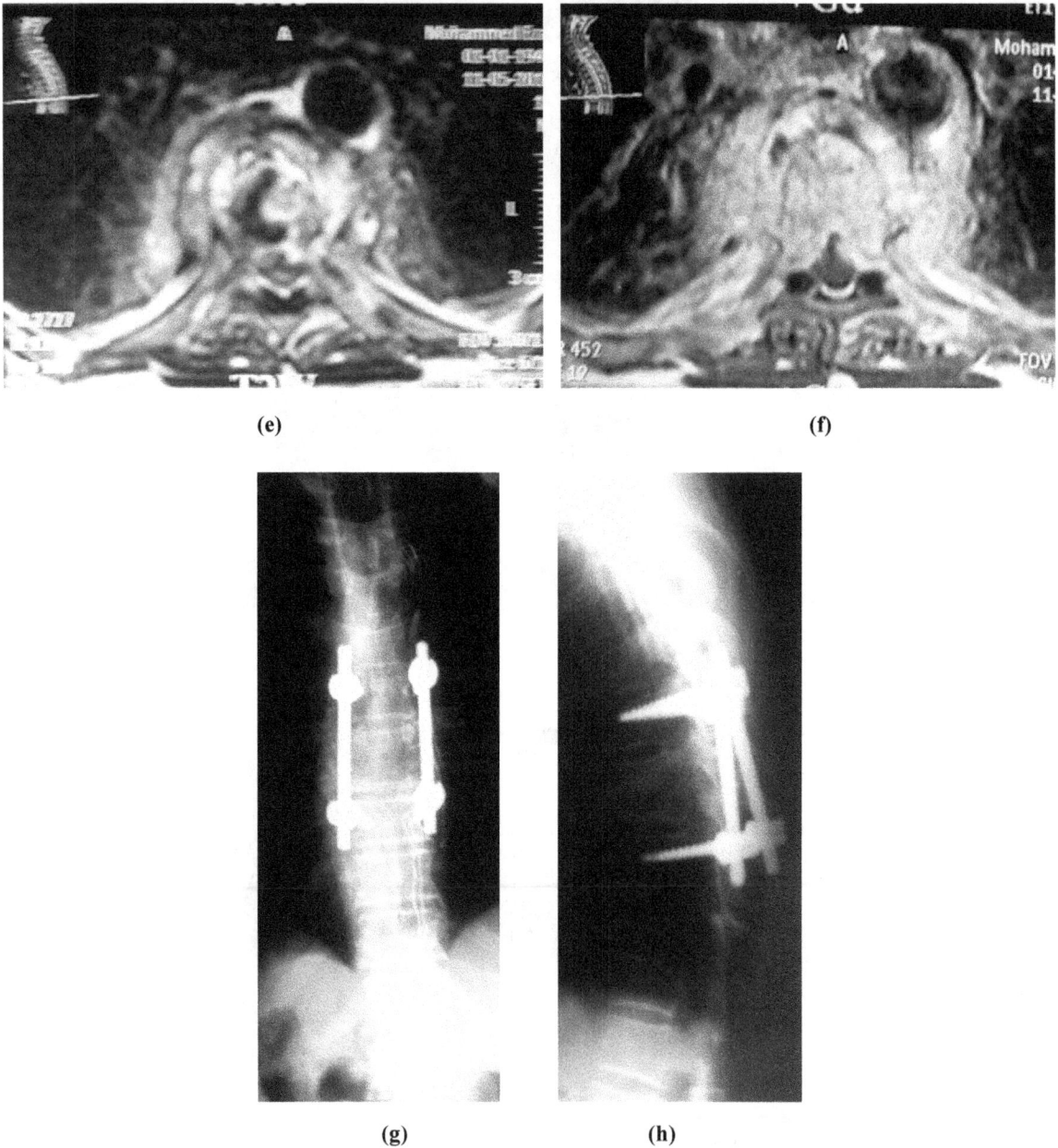

Figure 2: Male patient 50 years old presented with spasticity of both lower limbs although the motor power of muscles were normal. The patient had liver impairment due to infection by hepatitis C virus. A and B: Plain radiographs of the thoracic spine showing destruction of Th7 and 8 including the intervertebral disc C: MRI sagittal T1-weighted image and D: MRI sagittal T2-weighted image showing severe destruction with abscess formation and compression on the spinal cord at the level of Th7-8. E: MRI axial T2-weighted image at the level of Th7-8 disc and F: MRI gadolinium enhanced axial image at the level of Th7-8 disc showing big paraspinal abscess and spinal cord compression. G and H: Post-operative plain radiographs showing instrumentation to the pedicles of Th 6 and 9 vertebrae with anterior reconstruction achieved by spinal shortening and the lower border of Th7 comes to contact to the upper border of Th8.

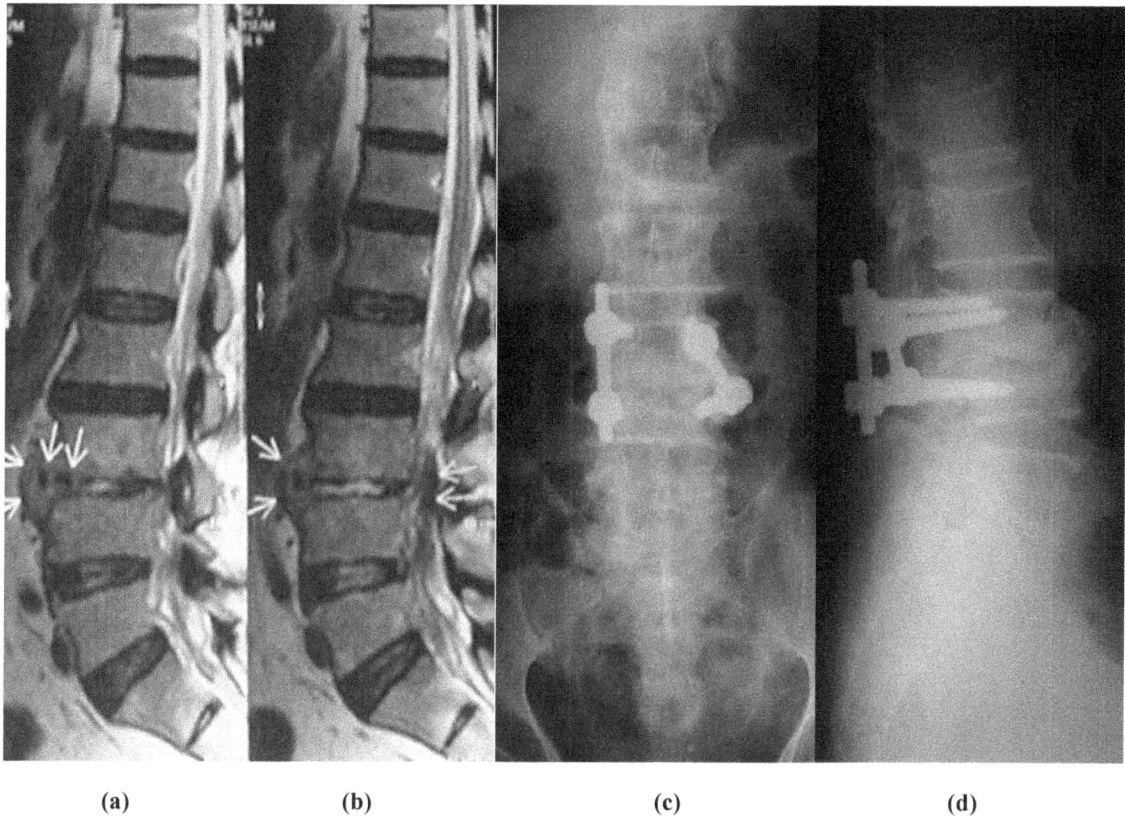

| (a) | (b) | (c) | (d) |

Figure 3: Male patient -69 years old- presented with agonizing low back pain and rapid neurological deterioration (Frankel grade C). (A) and (B): pre-operative sagittal MRI T2- weighted image of the lumbar spine showing the abscess and neural compression. The patient was treated by PLIF with anterior reconstruction achieved by spinal shortening. Specimen obtained during the operation showed no growth of micro-organisms on the culture media. (C) and (D): plain AP and lateral radiographs 1 year post-operative showing good bone healing of the affected level. The patient was followed up for 72 months with no reactivation of infection or occurrence of any complication.

Five complications were encountered; mal-positioned pedicle screw, deep venous thrombosis (DVT), delayed wound healing, kyphosis progression and temporary neurological deterioration. No active infection occurred tell the end of follow up. The temporary neurological dysfunction was related to malpositioned screw inside the thoracic spinal canal and was discovered intra-operative. The screw was repositioned inside the corresponding pedicle. However, post-operatively there was clear neurological deterioration from Frankel grade D to Frankel grade C. The patient got full neurological recovery to Frankel grade E within 3 months.

4   Advantages

In my opinion and based in my experience in management of my patients, the posterolateral exposure of the spine used as a sole approach has a lot of advantages over the anterior exposure in treatment of infections of the spine. It carries less morbidity, spine surgeons are more familiar with the posterior exposure than the anterior one (Saita *et al.* 2005), it gives access to both the vertebral body and neural arch and for multiple levels, it gives access to all levels from the first thoracic to fifth lumbar vertebrae and complications are less serious. It does not present risks to the chest or abdomen, which might induce serious hazards for extremely elder patients (Saita *et al.* 2005). Another main advantage of posterior spinal exposure is that the spinal cord or the cauda equina is always under surgeon's vision during debridment and reconstruction. This is contrary to the situation in case of anterior spinal debridment because the dura lies behind the vertebral body. If dural tear to complicate anterior debridment, dural reconstruction through the anterior exposure is extremely difficult. Reconstruction of the anterior column by limited spinal shortening, has a lot of advantages; avoiding the complications of bone graft harvesting and insertion. The operative time is short. A very wide anterior cancellous bone contact can be achieved so that the stability of the construct is high, so that early mobilization can be allowed with remote possibility of failure of instrumentation or dislodgment of anterior cage or bone graft.

5   Risks

For sure there are some risks that must be noted and avoided.

5.1   Neurological Deficit

The great concern in this technique is neurological deficit that might occur as a result of 4 causes: excessive shortening causing kinking of the cord or cauda equina, anterior compression of the spinal cord by any bone fragment or debris pushed into the spinal canal during spinal shortening, kinking of the nerve root in its canal or impingement on the nerve root by the pedicle.

   It is clear that the safety of spinal shortening might depend on the spinal level of shortening. The safe range of spinal shortening might be more at the cauda equina levels than at the spinal cord level. This may be related to the fact that the nerves in the cauda equina may be capable of responding to spinal shortening by increasing their redundancy. In an experimental study morphometric changes of the spinal cord and dura, influence on spinal cord evoked potentials (SCEPs) and spinal cord blood flow (SCBF) and postoperative function of hind limbs were studied in various degrees of acute spinal column shortening in dogs. Total spondylectomy of T13 was performed in dogs after spinal instrumentation placed 2 levels above and 2 levels below the spondylectomy level. Spinal column was gradually shortened until the lower endplate of T12 contacted the L1 upper endplate (maximum of 20 mm) come into contact. No morphometric changes occurred in the dural sac and the spinal cord until shortening of 7.2+1.7 mm. From 7.2 ± 1.7 to 12.5 ± 1.1 mm shortening, the dural sac was deformed while the spinal cord maintained its shape. Shortening more than 12.5 ± 1.1 mm buckled the dural sac and the spinal cord was kinked itself and compressed by the buckled dura in its concave side. No changes could be detected in SCEPs in 5 or 10 mm of shortening. SCEPs changes were recorded in the 2 of 6 dogs with 15 mm of shortening. At 20 mm of shortening, SCEPs abnormality was observed in 4 of 6 dogs. At shortening of 5, 10, 15 and 20 mm, spinal cord blood flow was 146 ± 10 %, 160 ± 21 %, 102 ± 17 % and 93 ± 7 % of the control (29.2 ± 7.9 ml/100g/min), respectively. All 3 dogs with 10 mm of shortening had normal hind limbs function after operation. One of the 3 dogs with 15 mm of shortening had paraparesis. Three of the 4 dogs with 20 mm of shortening had also paraparesis after operation. From this work it was concluded that acute spinal column shortening can be characterized into three phases: Phase 1; safe range: occurred during shortening within one-third of the vertebral segment and is characterized by no deformity of the dural sac or the spinal cord. Phase 2; warning range: occurs during spinal shortening between one and two-thirds of the vertebral segment and is characterized by shrinking and buckling of the dural sac and no deformity of the spinal cord. Phase 3; dangerous range: occurred after shortening in excess of two-thirds of the vertebral segment and is characterized by spinal cord deformity and compression by the buckled dura. Spinal shortening within the safe range increases spinal cord blood flow (Kawahara *et al.* 2005).

Other experimental paper was published by Alemdaroğlu *et al.* (2007) and described the mechanism of the sliding and kinking of the cord due to gradual shortening of the spine. Total vertebrectomy of T12 was applied to ten sheep models after spinal instrumentation. Measurements were taken at different laminectomy lengths to record kinking of the spinal cord with gradual shortening. The mean sliding of the spinal cord was 9 mm cranially and 7.8 mm caudally. T11 spinal nerves became more vertical caudally, and T12 spinal nerves achieved an ascending position with gradual shortening. Both T11 and T12 spinal nerves were sharply bent in the foramen and on the pedicle of T13, respectively. In full-length shortening, the mean kink of the spine in the sagittal plane was 92.4° for two levels of hemi-laminectomies, 24.6 ° for complete laminectomy of T11 with hemilaminectomy of T13, and 20.2° for two levels of complete laminectomies. Increasing the laminectomy length by only a half or one level prevents excessive kinking and compressions at the upper and lower margins of the laminectomy. In the later stages of shortening, the spinal nerves near the vertebrectomy site are at risk because of the sharp bending of the nerves. This study concluded that it is possible to avoid excessive kinking by planning the appropriate technique of laminectomy style in full-length shortening.

To avoid neurological complications, we insist on the following points:

a-   Shortening in the thoracic spine must be limited to one third of the height of one vertebra.

b-   Spinal cord must be carefully observed during shortening to avoid kinking. If kinking is noticed, release the shortening, widen the laminectomy and then re-shorten the spine

c-   The anterior aspect of the cord must be carefully examined after achieving full shortening to be sure that there is no anterior compression to the cord

d-   The whole course of the nerve roots tell neural foramen must be checked after achieving full shortening to ensure no kinking or compression on the root by the pedicle of the upper vertebra .

5.2   Scarification of Motion Segments

Posterior surgery for spinal infections might be criticized by causing loss of motion segments more than the anterior surgery. Lee and Suh reported on 18 patients with lumbar spine pyogenic infection treated by PLIF with an autogenous iliac crest bone graft. They considered that the main disadvantage of PLIF in comparison with anterior debridment is the need for fixation of one, two or more segments when vertebral body destruction is severe (Lee and Suh 2006). In general, our policy in the lumbar spine infection was that transpedicular screws be placed in the upper part of the infected vertebral body if it is not massively destroyed by infection. This would decrease the extent of fixation and help us to save motion segments in cases with limited vertebral body destruction (Figure 3). This advantage may be lost in cases with severe vertebral body destruction where multiple motion segments must be immobilized. In 16 out of 22 patients of lumbar spine infection (73%) insertion of the pedicle screws was in the affected vertebrae with one level fusion. In 6 patients (27%), we sacrificed an additional single monition segment.

5.3 Possibility of Reactivation of Infection

The subject of using metallic implants in the setting of spinal infection remains controversial, although more and more surgeons acknowledge that instrumentation can help the body to combat the infection rather than to interfere with it. The combination of radical debridement and instrumentation has lots of merits such as, restoration and maintenance of the sagittal alignment of the spine, stabilization of the spinal column and reduction of bed rest period (Chen *et al.* 2007). Korovessis *et al.* reported 14 patients with thoracolumbar spondylitis treated with anterior surgery with insertion of titanium mesh cage and posterior instrumented fusion. Most patients had also systemic diseases as lung tuberculosis, hepatic cirrhosis, diabetes mellitus, or chronic renal failure. There was one complication, an anterior wound abscess culminating in an abdominal hernia. They concluded that the presence of the mesh cage anteriorly at the site of spondylitis had no negative influence on the course of infection healing, and additionally it stabilized the affected segment maintaining sufficient sagittal profile (Korovessis *et al.* 2006). Other authors reported safety of instrumentation in spinal infections (Masuda *et al.* 2006, Rayes *et al.* 2010). I have the same experience in my patients. Among 32 patients treated by my technique, I did not get any case of activation of infection.

5.4 Injury to the Anteriorly Located Blood Vessels

In our technique, there is a possibility to injure the aorta or the vena cava while performing circumspinal dissection for anterior debridment. We prefer dissection from the left side because the wall of the aorta is strong and might not be injured by blunt dissection. Dissection in the right side is better to be avoided unless highly indicated because the wall of the vena cavae is thin and liable to injury. Insertion of the spatula anterior to the vertebral body actually adds more protection to the anteriorly located anatomical structures. In all of my patients, no injury of anterior structures was encountered.

References

Abdel-Wanis, M. E., Kawahara, N., Murata, A., Nambu, K., Murakami, H., Ueda, Y.& Tomita, K (2002). *Surgical treatment of thyroid cancer spinal metastases: report on 25 operations in 14 patients. Anticancer Research 22 (4), 2509-2516.*

Abdel-Wanis, M. E. (2006). *Single-Stage Posterior Circumspinal Debridment and Reconstruction for Thoracic and Lumbar Spinal Infections. Journal of Musculoskeletal Research 10, 173-180.*

Abdel-Wanis, M. E. (2011). *Posterolateral Debridment and Anterior Reconstruction By Limited Spinal Shortening In Thoracic Spine Infections. Presented at SICOT 2011 XXV Triennial World Congress, September 6-9, Prague, Czech Republic.*

Abdel-Wanis, M. E. (2012). *Treatment of Acute Tuberculous Spondylitis by the Spinal Shortening Osteotomy: A Technical Notes and Case Illustrations. Letter to editor. Asian Spine Journal, 6 (3), 219.*

Alemdaroğlu, K. B., Atlihan, D., Cimen, O., Kilinç, C. Y. & Iltar, S. (2007). *Morphometric effects of acute shortening of the spine: the kinking and the sliding of the cord, response of the spinal nerves. European Spine Journal, 16, 1451-1457.*

Benli, I. T., Alanay, A., Akalin, S., Kis, M., Acaroglu, E., Ates, B. & Aydin, E. (2004). *Comparison of anterior instrumentation systems and the results of minimum 5 years follow-up in the treatment of tuberculosis spondylitis. Kobe Journal of Medical Science, 50 (5-6), 167-180.*

Bradford, D. S. & Clifford, B. T. (1997). *Vertebral column resection for the treatment of rigid coronal decompensation, Spine 22, 1590-1599.*

Bridwell, K. H., Lewis, S. J., Rinella, A., Lenke, L. G., Baldus, C.& Blanke, K. (2004). Pedicle subtraction osteotomy for the treatment of fixed sagittal imbalance. Surgical technique. Journal of Bone and Joint Surgery, 86-A, 44–49.

Chanplakorn, P., Chanplakorn, N., Kraiwattanapong, C., Wajanavisit, W.& Laohacharoensombat, W. (2011) Treatment of Acute Tuberculous Spondylitis by the Spinal Shortening Osteotomy: A Technical Notes and Case Illustrations. Asian Spine Journal, 5 (4), 237-244.

Chen, W.H., Jiang, L. S. & Dai, L. Y. (2007). Surgical treatment of pyogenic vertebral osteomyelitis with spinal instrumentation. European Spine Journal, 16(9), 1307-1316.

Dai, L.Y., Jiang, L. S., Wang, W.& Cui, Y. M. (2005). Single-stage anterior autogenous bone grafting and instrumentation in the surgical management of spinal tuberculosis. Spine, 30 (20), 2342-2349.

El-Sharkawi, M. M, Said, G. K. (2011). Instrumented circumferential fusion for tuberculosis of the dorso-lumbar spine. A single or double stage procedure? International Orthopedics, 36, 315-324.

Grunenwald, D., Mazel, C., Girard, P., Berthiot, G., Dromer, C. & Baldeyrou, P. (1996). Total vertebrectomy for en-bloc resec-tion of lung cancer invading the spine. Annals of Thoracic Surgery, 61, 723–726.

Guzey, F. K., Emel, E., Bas, N. S., Hacisalihoglu, S., Seyithanoglu, M. H., Karacor, S. E., Ozkan, N., Alatas, I. & Sel B. (2005) Thoracic and lumbar tuberculous spondylitis treated by posterior debridement, graft placement, and instrumentation: a retrospective analysis in 19 cases. Journal of Neurosurg Spine, 3 (6):450-458.

Heary, R. F., Vaccaro, A. R., Benevenia, J. & Cotler, J. M. (1998). "En-bloc" vertebrectomy in the mobile lumbar spine. Surgical Neurology, 50, 548–556.

Hodgson, A. R. (1965). Correction of fixed spinal curves. Journal of Bone and Joint Surgery, 47-A, 1221-1227.

Hsieh, P. C., Stapleton, C. J., Moldavskiy, P., Koski, T. R., Ondra, S. L., Gokaslan, Z. L. & Kuntz, C. (2010). Posterior vertebral column subtraction osteotomy for the treatment of tethered cord syndrome: review of the literature and clinical outcomes of all cases reported to date. Neurosurgical Focus, 29 (1), E6.

Kawahara, N., Tomita, K., Fujita, T., Maruo, S., Otsuka, S. & Kinoshita, G. (1997). Osteosarcoma of the thoracolumbar spine: total en bloc spondylectomy. A case report. Journal of Bone and Joint Surgery, 79-A, 453–458.

Kawahara, N., Tomita, K., Baba, H., Kobayashi, T., Fujita, T. & Murakami, H. (2001). Closing-opening wedge osteotomy to correct angular kyphotic deformity by a single posterior approach. Spine, 26:391–402.

Kawahara, N., Tomita, K., Kobayashi, T., Abdel-Wanis, M. E., Murakami, H. & Akamaru, T. (2005). Influence of Acute Shortening on the Spinal Cord: An Experimental Study. Spine, 30 (6), 613-620.

Korovessis, P., Petsinis, G., Koureas, G., Iliopoulos, P. & Zacharatos, S. (2006) Anterior surgery with insertion of titanium mesh cage and posterior instrumented fusion performed sequentially on the same day under one anesthesia for septic spondylitis of thoracolumbar spine: is the use of titanium mesh cages safe? Spine, 31(9), 1014-1019.

Krodel, A., Kruger, K., Loscheidt, M., Pfahler, M. & Refior, H. J. (1999). Anterior debridment, fusion and extrafocal stabilization in the treatment of osteomyelitis of the spine. Journal of Spinal Disorders, 12, 17-26.

Lazar, R. D. & Hall J. E. (1999). Simultaneous anterior and posterior hemivertebra excision. Clinical Orthopedics and Related Research, 364, 76–84.

Lee, J. S. & Suh, K. T. (2006). Posterior lumbar interbody fusion with an autogenous iliac crest bone graft in the treatment of pyogenic spondylodiscitis. Journal of Bone and Joint Surgery, 88-B, 765-770.

Magerl, F. & Costia, M. F. (1998). Total posterior vertebrectomy of the thoracic or lumbar spine. Clinical Orthopedics and Related Research, 232, 62– 69.

Masuda, T., Miyamoto, K., Hosoe, H., Sakaeda, H., Tanaka, M. & Shimizu, K. (2006) Surgical treatment with spinal instrumentation for pyogenic spondylodiscitis due to methicillin-resistant Staphylococcus aureus (MRSA): a report of five cases. Archives of Orthopaedics and Trauma Surgery, 126(5), 339-345.

Murakami, H., Kawahara, N., Abdel-Wanis, M. E. & Tomita, K. (2001). Total En Bloc Spondylectomy. Seminars in Musculoskeletal Radiology, 5, 189-194.

Nakamura, H., Matsuda, H., Konishi, S. & Yamano, Y. (2002). Single stage excision of hemivertebrae via the posterior approach alone for congenital spine deformity. Spine, 27, 110–115.

Potter, B. K., Lenke, L.G. & Kuklo T. R. (2004). Prevention and management of iatrogenic flatback deformity. Journal of Bone and Joint Surgery, 86-A, 1793–1808.

Rayes, M., Colen, C. B., Bahgat, D. A., Higashida, T., Guthikonda, M., Rengachary, S. & Eltahawy, H. A. (2010) Safety of instrumentation in patients with spinal infection. J Neurosurg Spine, 12(6), 647-659.

Reyes-Sanchez, A., Rosales, L. M., Miramontes, V. P. & Garin, D. E. (2002). Treatment of thoracolumbar burst fractures by vertebral shortening. European Spine Journal, 11, 8–12.

Roile, N. D. (1928) The operative removal of an accessory vertebra. Medical Journal of Australia, 1, 467-451.

Ruf, M. & Harms, J. (2003). Posterior hemivertebra resection with transpedicular instrumentation: early correction in children aged 1 to 6 years. Spine, 28, 2132–2138.

Ruf, M., Jensen, R. & Harms J. (2005). Hemivertebra resection in the cervical spine. Spine, 30, 380–385.

Saita, K., Hoshino, Y., Kikkawa, I. & Nakamura, H. (2000) Posterior Spinal Shortening for Paraplegia After Vertebral Collapse Caused by Osteoporosis. Spine, 25 (21), 2832–2835.

Shono, Y., Abumi, K. & Kaneda, K. (2001). One-stage posterior hemivertebra resection and correction using segmental posterior instrumentation. Spine, 26, 752–757.

Smith, J. T., Gollogly, S., Dunn, H. K. (2005). Simultaneous anterior–posterior approach through a costotransversectomy for the treatment of congenital kyphosis and acquired kyphoscoliotic deformities. Journal of Bone and Joint Surgery, 87-A, 2281–2289.

Tomita, K., Kawahara, N., Baba, H., Tsuchiya, H., Nagata, S. & Toribatake, Y. (1994). Total en bloc spondylectomy for solitary spinal metastases. International Orthopedics, 18, 291-298.

Tomita, K., Kawahara, N., Baba, H., Tsuchiya, H., Fujita, T., Toribatake, Y. (1997). Total en bloc spondylectomy- a new surgical technique for primary malignant vertebral tumors. Spine, 22 (3), 324-333.

Von Lackum, Le, R. H. & Smith, A. D. (1933). Removal of vertebral bodies in the treatment of scoliosis. Surgery Gynecology and Obstetrics, 57, 250-256.

Zhang, H. Q., Li, J. S., Zhao, S. S., Shao, Y. X., Liu, S. H., Gao, Q., Lin, M. Z., Liu, J. Y., Wu, J. H. & Chen, J. (2012). Surgical management for thoracic spinal tuberculosis in the elderly: posterior only versus combined posterior and anterior approaches. Archives of Orthopaedics and Trauma Surgery, 132(12), 1717-1723.

Relationship between EEG Alpha3/Alpha2 Ratio and the Impulsive Disorders Network in Subjects with Mild Cognitive Impairment

Davide Vito Moretti, Donata Paternicò, Giuliano Binetti
Orazio Zanetti, Giovanni Battista Frisoni
IRCCS S. Giovanni di Dio Fatebenefratelli, Brescia; Italy

1   Introduction

EEG have been demonstrated a reliable diagnostic tool in dementia research (Stam *et al.*, 2003; Rossini *et al.*, 2008). The increase of high alpha relative to low alpha power has been recently demonstrated a reliable EEG marker of hippocampal atrophy as well as conversion of patients with mild cognitive impairment (MCI) in Alzheimer's disease (AD; Moretti *et al.*, 2009c).

Impulsive behaviors are frequently described in brain-damaged patients, including patients with AD. More specifically, a significant increase in urgency, lack of premeditation, and lack of perseverance was noted, whereas a decrease in sensation seeking was observed in these patients (Rochat *et al.*, 2008). Furthermore, this increase of impulsivity on urgency, lack of premeditation, and lack of perseverance was not associated with global cognitive impairment as assessed by the Mini Mental State Examination (MMSE; Folstein *et al.*, 1975) or the Mattis Dementia Rating scale (Mattis, 1976), whereas lower sensation seeking was associated with a lower score on the MMSE (Rochat *et al.*, 2008, 2013).

The nucleus accumbens (NAc) is a key component of the neural processes regulating impulsivity (Basar *et al.*, 2010). Data from imaging studies (Basar *et al.*, 2010) suggest the involvement of the ventral striatum/NAc in impulsive choice. In particular an increase in the activity of ventral striatum network has been associated with decisions involving immediate outcome (McClure *et al*, 2004, 2007; Boettinger *et al.*, 2007), with decisions including intertemporal differences (Weber and Huettel, 2008), with choices of shorter delays (Wittmann *et al.*, 2007) as well as with switching to risk-seeking choices (Kuhnen and Knutson, 2005).

Recently, it has been demonstrated that the increase of high alpha relative to low alpha power is a reliable EEG marker of hippocampal atrophy and amigdalo-hippocampal complex atrophy. Furthermore, the increase in alpha3/alpha2 power ratio has been demonstrated predictive of conversion of patients with MCI in AD, but not in non-AD dementia. The same increase of alpha3/alpha2 power ratio was found to be correlated with hippocampal atrophy in subjects with AD. (Moretti *et al.*, 2009a; 2009b; 2009c; 2011; 2012).

In the present study the association of EEG indexes with grey matter (GM) changes in basal ganglia has been studied in subjects with MCI. The working hypothesis was that modifications of alpha3/alpha2 power ratio could be underpinned by different deep brain structures. Results show that subjects with higher a3/a2 ratios showed minor atrophy in the ventral striatum-nucleus accumbens network bilaterally when compared to subjects with lower and middle a3/a2 ratios. The results are discussed in the light of possible relationship with impulsive behavior in prodromal Alzheimer's disease patients.

2   Materials and Methods

2.1   Subjects

For the present study, 74 subjects with MCI was recruited from the memory Clinic of the Scientific Institute for Research and Care (IRCCS) of Alzheimer's and psychiatric diseases 'Fatebenefratelli' in Brescia, Italy. All experimental protocols had been approved by the local ethics committee. Informed consent was obtained from all participants or their caregivers, according to the Code of Ethics of the World Medical Association (Declaration of Helsinki).

2.2   Diagnostic criteria

Patients were selected from a prospective study on the natural history of cognitive impairment (the translational outpatient memory clinic—TOMC study) carried out in the outpatient facility of the National Institute for the Research and Care of Alzheimer's Disease (IRCCS Istituto Centro San Giovanni di Dio Fatebenefratelli, Brescia, Italy).

The project was aimed to study the natural history of non-demented persons with apparently primary cognitive deficits, i.e., deficits not due to psychic (anxiety, depression, etc.) or physical (hypothiroidism, vitamin B12 and folate deficiency, uncontrolled heart disease, uncontrolled conditions (diabetes, etc.) in the absence of functional impairment. The selection criteria has the aim to include as much as possible primary prodromal dementia due to neurodegenerative disorders. Demographic and cognitive features of the subjects in study are summarized in Table 1.

	All	Alpha3/Alpha2			
		High	*Middle*	*Low*	*p*
Number of subjects	74	18	38	18	
Age, years	69.4 ± 7.6 [52-85]	70.4 ± 6.7 [60-85]	68.4 ± 8.2 [52-83]	70.4 ± 7.4 [57-80]	.55
Sex, female	51 (%)	13 (%)	24 (%)	14 (%)	.51
Education, years	7.6 ± 3.9 [3-18]	6.6 ± 3.6 [4-18]	7.6 ± 3.7 [3-17]	8.3 ± 4.7 [3-18]	.42
Mini mental state exam	27.2 ± 1.7 [23-30]	26.9 ± 1.3 [23-29]	27. ± 1.7 [24-30]	27.4 ± 1.2 [23-30]	.46
Alpha3/alpha2	1.09 ± 0.15 [0.77-1.52]	1.29 ± 0.1*† [1.17-1.52]	1.08 ± 0.0* [#] [1-1.16]	0.9 ± 0.1[#]† [0.77-0.98]	.000

*significant different then Low; [#] significant different then High; † significant different then Middle.

Table 1: Demographic and cognitive characteristics in the whole sample, disaggregated for increased levels of Alpha3/ Alpha2 ratio. Numbers denote mean ± standard deviation, number and [range]. *p* denotes significance on ANOVA (continuous variables) and chi-square test (dichotomous variables).

Patients were rated with a series of standardized diagnostic and severity instruments, including the Mini-Mental State Examination (MMSE; Folstein *et al.*, 1975), the Clinical Dementia Rating Scale (CDRS; Hughes *et al.*, 1982), the Hachinski Ischemic Scale (HIS; Rosen *et al.*, 1980) and the Instrumental and Basic Activities of Daily Living (IADL, BADL; Lawton and Brodie, 1969). In addition, patients underwent diagnostic neuroimaging procedures (magnetic resonance imaging, MRI), and laboratory testing to rule out other causes of cognitive impairment. These inclusion and exclusion criteria for MCI were based on previous seminal studies (Petersen *et al.*, 2001; Portet *et al.*, 2006; Dubois *et al.*, 2007). Inclusion criteria of the study were all of the following: (i) complaint by the patient, or report by a relative or the general practitioner, of memory or other cognitive disturbances; (ii) Mini-Mental State Examination (MMSE) score of 24–27/30, or MMSE of 28 and higher plus low performance (score of 2–6 or higher) on the clock drawing test (Lezak *et al.*, 2004); (iii) sparing of instrumental and basic activities of daily living or functional impairment steadily due to causes other than cognitive impairment, such as physical impairments, sensory loss, gait or balance disturbances, etc. Exclusion criteria were any one of the following: (i) patients aged 90 years and older (no minimum age to participate in the study), because of the risk of major cerebrovascular load that could blur the detection of EEG markers due to degenerative cognitive decline; (ii) history of depression (from mild to moderate or major depression) or juvenile-onset psychosis; (iii) history or neurological signs of major stroke; (iv) other psychiatric diseases, overt dementia, epilepsy, drug addiction, alcohol dependence; (v) use of psychoactive drugs, including acetylcholinesterase inhibitors or other drugs enhancing brain cognitive functions or biasing EEG activity; and (vi) current or previous uncontrolled or complicated systemic diseases (including diabetes mellitus), or traumatic brain injuries. All subjects were right-handed.

All patients underwent: (i) semi-structured interview with the patient and – whenever possible – with another informant (usually, the patient's spouse or a child of the patient) by a geriatrician or neurologist; (ii) physical and neurological examinations; (iii) performance-based tests of physical function, gait and balance; (iv) neuropsychological battery assessing memory (Babcock Story Recall – Rey–Osterrieth Complex Figure, Recall – Auditory-Verbal Learning Test, immediate and delayed recall; Lezak *et al.*, 2004) verbal and non-verbal memory, attention and executive functions (Trail Making Test B, A and B-A; Inverted Motor Learning-Clock Drawing Test; Lezak *et al.*, 2004), abstract reasoning thinking (Raven Colored Progressive Matrices; Lezak *et al.*, 2004), frontal functions (Inverted Motor Learning); language (Phonological and Semantic fluency-Token test, Lezak *et al.*, 2004), and apraxia and visuo-constructional abilities (Rey–Osterrieth Complex Figure, Rey figure copy, Clock Drawing Test; Lezak *et al.*, 2004); (v) assessment of depressive symptoms by means of the Center for Epidemiologic Studies Depression Scale (CES-D; Radloff, 1977). All the neuropsychological tests were standardized on Italian population, thus scores were compared to normative values with age, education and gender corrections in an Italian population.

As the aim of our study was to evaluate the reliabilityin a clinical and diagnostic setting of the EEG alpha3/alpha2 frequency ratio as a screening marker for degenerative cognitive decline and its relationship with GM loss in MCI subjects, we did not consider the clinical subtype of MCI, i.e., amnesic, or non-amnesic, single or multiple domains.

2.3   EEG Recordings

The EEG activity was recorded continuously from 19 sites by using electrodes set in an elastic cap (Electro-Cap International, Inc.) and positioned according to the 10–20 international systems (Fp1, Fp2, F7, F3, Fz, F4, F8, T3, C3, Cz, C4, T4, T5, P3, Pz, P4, T6, O1, and O2). In order to keep constant the level of vigilance, an operator controlled on-line the subject and the EEG traces, alerting the subject any time there were signs of behavioural and/or EEG drowsiness. The ground electrode was placed in front of Fz. The left and right mastoids served as reference for all electrodes. The recordings were used off-line to re-reference the scalp recordings to the common average. Re-referencing was done prior to the EEG artifact detection and analysis. Data were recorded with a band-pass filter of 0.3–70 Hz, and digitized at a sampling rate of 250 Hz (BrainAmp, BrainProducts, Germany). Electrodes-skin impedance was set below 5 khz. Horizontal and vertical eye movements were detected by recording the electrooculogram (EOG). The recording lasted 5 min, with subjects with closed eyes. Longer recordings would have reduced the variability of the data, but they would also have increased the possibility of slowing of EEG oscillations due to reduced vigilance and arousal. EEG data were then analyzed and fragmented off-line in consecutive epochs of 2 s, with a frequency resolution of 0.5 Hz. The average number of epochs analyzed was 140, ranging from 130 to 150. The EEG epochs with ocular, muscular and other types of artifact were preliminary identified by a computerized automatic procedure (Moretti *et al.*, 2003, 2004, 2007a,b, 2008a,b, 2009a,b, 2011). Two expert electroencephalographists manually double-checked and confirmed the automatic selections. The epochs with ocular, muscular and other types of artifacts were discarded.

2.4   Analysis of Individual Frequency Bands

All recordings were obtained in the morning with subjects resting comfortably. Vigilance was continuously monitored in order to avoid drowsiness. A digital FFT-based power spectrum analysis (Welch technique, Hanning windowing function, no phase shift) computed – ranging from 2 to 45 Hz – the power density of EEG rhythms with a 0.5 Hz frequency resolution. Two anchor frequencies were selected according to the literature guidelines (Klimesch, 1997, 1999), that is, the theta/alpha transition frequency (TF) and the individual alpha frequency (IAF) peak. These anchor frequencies were computed on the power spectra averaged across all recording electrodes. The TF marks the transition frequency between the theta and alpha bands, and represents an estimate of the frequency at which the theta and alpha spectra intersect. TF was computed as the minimum power in the alpha frequency range, since our EEG recordings were performed at rest. The IAF represents the frequency with the maximum power peak within the extended alpha range (5–14 Hz). Based on TF and IAF, we estimated the frequency band range for each subject, as follows: delta from TF-4 to TF- 2, theta from TF-2 to TF, low alpha band (alpha1 and alpha2) from TF to IAF, and high alpha band (or alpha3) from IAF to IAF + 2. The alpha1 and alpha2 bands were computed for each subject as follows: alpha1 from TF to the middle point of the TF-IAF range, and alpha2 from such middle point to the IAF peak (Moretti *et al.*, 2004, 2007; 2008; 2009a,b). Moreover, individual beta and gamma frequencies were computed. Three frequency peaks were detected in the frequency range from the individual alpha 3 frequency band and 45 Hz. These peaks were named beta1 peak (IBF 1), beta2 peak (IBF 2) and gamma peak (IGF). Based on peaks, the frequency ranges were determined. Beta1 ranges from alpha 3 to the lower spectral power value between beta1 and beta2 peak; beta2 frequency ranges from beta 1 to the lower spectral power value between beta2 and gamma peak; gamma frequency ranges from beta 2 to 45 Hz, which is the end of the range considered. Moreover, within theta frequency the frequency peak (individual theta frequency, ITF) was also individuated. The mean frequency range computed in MCI subjects considered as a whole are: delta 2.9–4.9 Hz; theta 4.9–6.9 Hz; alpha1 6.9–8.9 Hz; alpha2 8.9–10.9 Hz; alpha3 10.9–12.9 Hz; beta1 12.9–19.2 Hz; beta2 19.2–32.4; gamma 32.4–45. Finally, in the frequency bands determined on an individual basis, we computed the relative power spectra for each subject. The relative power density for each frequency band was computed as the ratio between the absolute power and the mean power spectra from 2 to 45 Hz. The relative band power at each band was defined as the mean of the relative band power for each frequency bin within that band. The alpha3/alpha2 was computed in all subjects and three groups were obtained according to increasing tertiles values of alpha3/alpha2: low (a3/a2 < 1;) middle (1 < a3/a2 < 1.16) and high (a3/a2 > 1.17). The three groups of MCI has been demostrated in previous studies to be different in nature. In particular, the high alpha3/alpha 2 EEG power ratio MCI group is at major risk to convert to Alzheimer's disease (Moretti *et al.*, 2011,), as well as to have different pattern of hippocampal atrophy (Moretti *et al.*, 2009b) and basal ganglia and thalamus gray matter lesions (Moretti *et al.*,2011, 2012) as compared to the other alpha3/alpha2 power ratio MCI groups. Moreover, this group subdivision has been chosen for reason of homogeneity and comparability with the previous studies

2.5   MRI Scans

For each subject, a high-resolution sagittal T1 weighted volumetric MR scan was acquired by using a 1.0 T Philips Gyroscan scanner, with a gradient echo 3D technique: TR = 20 ms, TE = 5 ms, flip angle = 30_, field of view = 220 mm, acquisition matrix 256 · 256, slice thickness 1.3 mm. The pattern of gray matter atrophy was studied using the Voxel Based Morphometry technique (Ashburner, 2007).

2.6   Voxel-based Morphometry

3D images were processed through SPM5 software package (Statistical Parametric Mapping, Version 5; Wellcome Department of Imaging Neuroscience, London, UK; http://www.fil.ion.ucl.ac.uk/spm), running on Matlab 7.0.1 (Math-Works, Natick, MA, USA). DICOM files were converted in ANALYZE format image, the extra-cranial voxels were removed and the anterior commissure (AC) was manually set for all images as the origin of the spatial coordinates for an anatomical normalization algorithm implemented in SPM. Converted files were then segmented into gray and white matter and normalized to the GM population templates, generated from the complete image set, using the Diffeomorphic Anatomical Registration using Exponentiated Lie algebra (DARTEL) registration method (Ashburner, 2007). This non-linear warping technique minimizes between-subject structural variations.

Spatially normalized images were modulated by the Jacobian determinants derived from the spatial normalization, to ensure that the overall amount of each tissue class was not altered by the spatial normalization procedure. The final voxel resolution after DARTEL was 1.5X1.5X1.5 mm. Finally each modulated, warped GM image was transformed to MNI space and smoothed with a 8-mm full-width at half-maximum (FWHM) Gaussian kernel filter. The experimenter performing the MRN computations was blinded to the results of previous EEG works, so that there were not biases in the analysis.

2.7   Statistical Analysis

VBM results were assessed at an uncorrected threshold of $p \leq 0.001$. This threshold has an important limit in that it allows the tipe I statistical error. Anyway, a more permissive threshold could be more adequate, given the explorative nature of the study, in order to avoid the beta (or type II) statistic error, with the risk to neglect interesting results. Anyway, the power of the study was allowed by size of the sample, and by the robust results of the subsequent analyses. The sample was disaggregated into three groups according to three increasing values of alpha3/alpha2 ratio: low-a3/a2 (a3/a2 < 1), middle-a3/a2 (1 < a3/a2 < 1.16), high-a3/a2 (a3/a2 > 1.17).

Voxel-based analyses were carried out comparing the three patient groups with increasing values of the alpha3/alpha2 ratio (high-a3/a2; middle-a3/a2; low-a3/a2).

Between-group regional differences in GM volumes were assessed by using the two sample t-tests between GM difference maps (High vs Middle; High vs Low; Middle vs Low) entering age, gender, education and MMSE scores. Moreover, the total intracranial volume was introduced in the statistical analysis as a covariate, to avoid the confounding item of the global cortical atrophy. The total intracranial volume (TIV) was computed by manually tracing the entire intracranial cavity on 7-mm thick coronal slices, by the use of the software DISPLAY 1.3 tools. Correlation or regression analyses were not performed. The reason is that the EEG markers represents different patients population (MCI who will convert and MCI who will not), as previously demonstrated (Moretti *et al.*, 2009c). So, the population in study is not expected as homogeneous. As a consequence, it is not correct to use the correlation or regression analysis because significant results should have masked by the possible different nature of the subjects in the whole groups. It should be possible only within each of the three groups individuated by the tertile subdivisions, but the small size of each group does not allow a powerful correlation or regression analysis.

All the analyses were restricted to the basal ganglia as regions of interest in order to focus the relationship between there brain areas and EEG markers. It should be possible to perform a computation encompassing other brain areas, but this was beyond the scope of the present work. Moreover, the relationship of EEG markers with hippocampus and amygdala was faced in previous papers (Moretti *et al.*, 2009b). To this purpose, a mask including Caudate Nucleus, Putamen, Globus Pallidus, and NAc was entered into the models as explicit mask. It was manually traced, through the software MRIcroN, on the previous template generated from the complete image set. The detection of the anatomical regions was based on the localization of the thalamic nuclei and basal ganglia in histological sections from a human atlas (Mai *et al.*, 1997).

3   Results

Table 1 shows the sociodemographic and neuropsychological characteristics of MCI subgroups defined by the tertile values of alpha3/alpha2. The ANOVA analysis showed that there was not statistically significant differences between groups which resulted well paired for age, sex, white matter hyperintensities (WMHs) burden, education and global cognitive level. Anyway, age, sex, education, global cognitive level (MMSE score) and WMHs were introduced as covariates in the subsequent analsysis to avoid confounding factors. Alpha3/alpha2 ratio levels were significant at Games-Howell post hoc comparisons (p=0.000).

3.1   EEG alpha3/alpha2 ratio

* Low-a3/a2 group: Subjects with low a3/a2 ratio exhibited a region of GM more atrophic than subjects with high a3/a2 ratios located in the head of Caudate, specifically in the ventral part bilaterally and slightly wider on the right side (see Figure 1). No regions of GM tissue loss were found when patients with low a3/a2 ratio were compared to those with Middle a3/a2 ratio.

* Middle-a3/a2 group: Subjects with middle a3/a2 ratio, contrasted to individuals with high a3/a2 ratios, showed more atrophy in the bilateral Accumbens nuclei, though the atrophic area was minimal in the left hemisphere (see Figure 2). No regions of significant GM tissue loss were found in other comparisons in this group.

4   Discussion

4.1   Preliminary remarks

In this study we have considered the GM changes of deep brain structures, basal ganglia and NAc based on brain electrical activity markers. As a consequence, the analysis of anatomical structural changes in MCI patients was EEG markers-driven. This is a crucial point for considering the results of the present study. Indeed, it is not a simple detection of atrophy pattern between two clinically different populations of subjects, but it would investigate the association of EEG markers with specific GM changes in the

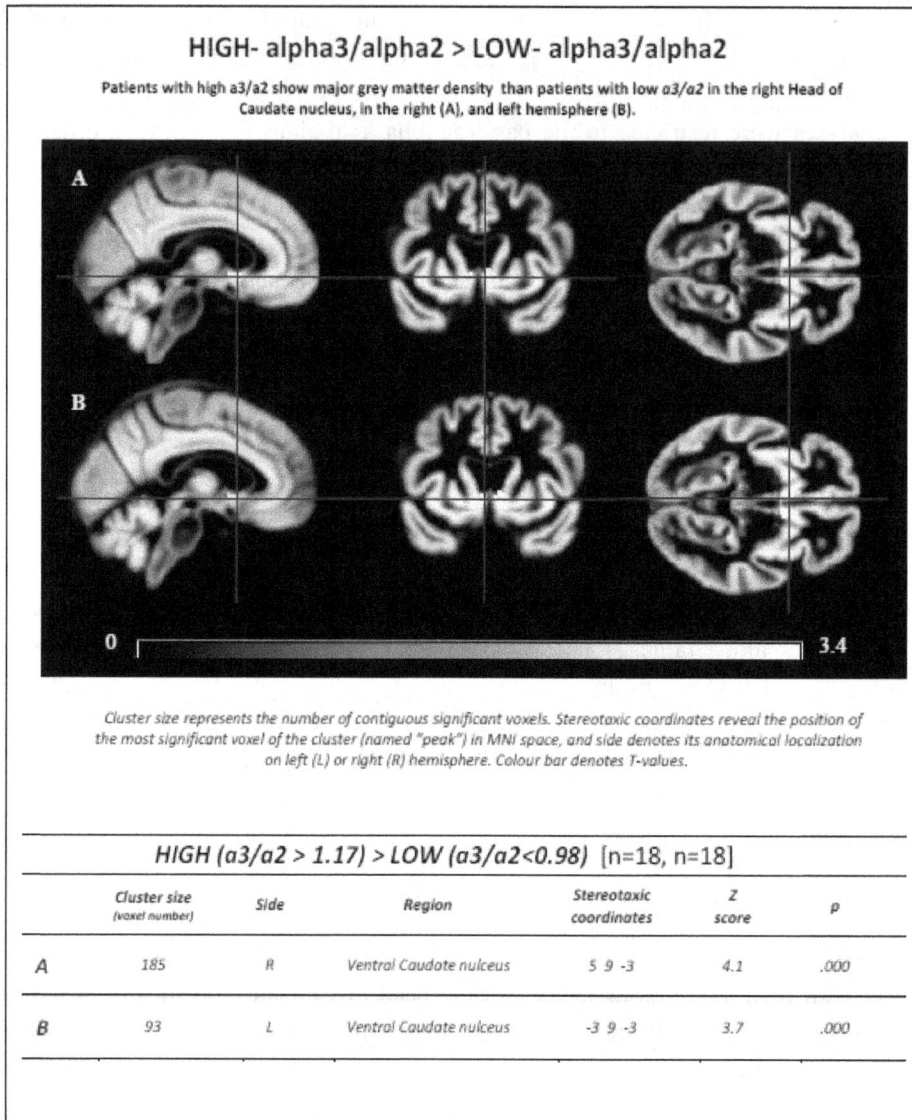

HIGH- alpha3/alpha2 > LOW- alpha3/alpha2

Patients with high a3/a2 show major grey matter density than patients with low *a3/a2* in the right Head of Caudate nucleus, in the right (A), and left hemisphere (B).

Cluster size represents the number of contiguous significant voxels. Stereotaxic coordinates reveal the position of the most significant voxel of the cluster (named "peak") in MNI space, and side denotes its anatomical localization on left (L) or right (R) hemisphere. Colour bar denotes T-values.

HIGH (a3/a2 > 1.17) > LOW (a3/a2<0.98) [n=18, n=18]

	Cluster size (voxel number)	Side	Region	Stereotaxic coordinates	Z score	p
A	185	R	Ventral Caudate nulceus	5 9 -3	4.1	.000
B	93	L	Ventral Caudate nulceus	-3 9 -3	3.7	.000

Figure 1 : T-map showing greater regional grey matter density in patients with high a3/a2 ratio contrasted to patients with low a3/a2 ratio ($p \leq 0.001$ uncorrected, the symbol '>' denotes 'major grey matter density then', see also table).

basal ganglia-nucelus accumbens ntework in subpopulations of subjects with MCI. The alpha3/alpha2 frequency ratio has been chosen for two principal reasons: 1) previous studies demonstrated their association with different anatomical substrates atrophy, namely the hippocampus for alpha3/alpah2 frequency ratio (Moretti *et al.* 2009b); 2) a recent study have demonstrated that this EEG index has peculiar diagnostic and prognostic value: the increase in alpha3/alpha2 ratio is associated with the conversion of MCI subjects in AD (Moretti *et al.*, 2009c). Moreover, the increase the same index has been previously correlated with impairment in psychometric tests in MCI subjects (Moretti *et al.*, 2009a;

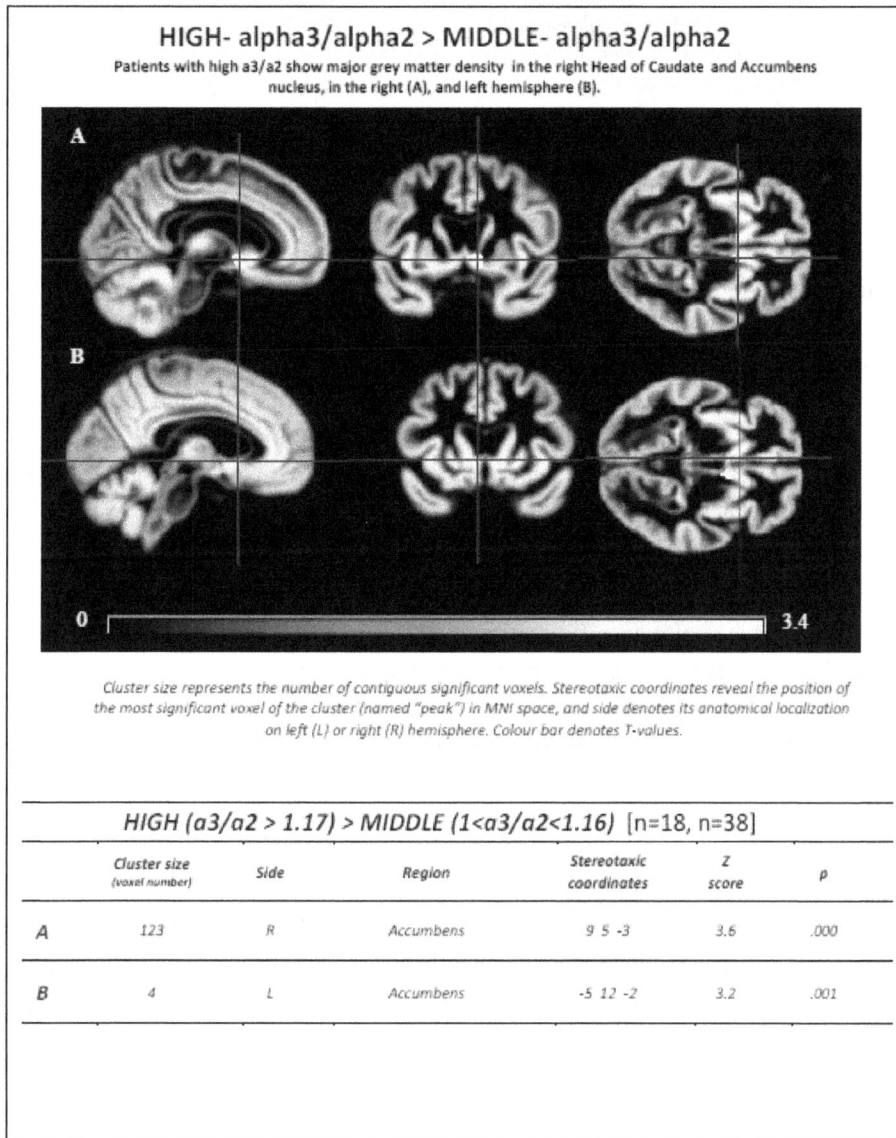

HIGH- alpha3/alpha2 > MIDDLE- alpha3/alpha2

Patients with high a3/a2 show major grey matter density in the right Head of Caudate and Accumbens nucleus, in the right (A), and left hemisphere (B).

Cluster size represents the number of contiguous significant voxels. Stereotaxic coordinates reveal the position of the most significant voxel of the cluster (named "peak") in MNI space, and side denotes its anatomical localization on left (L) or right (R) hemisphere. Colour bar denotes T-values.

HIGH (a3/a2 > 1.17) > MIDDLE (1<a3/a2<1.16) [n=18, n=38]

	Cluster size (voxel number)	Side	Region	Stereotaxic coordinates	Z score	p
A	123	R	Accumbens	9 5 -3	3.6	.000
B	4	L	Accumbens	-5 12 -2	3.2	.001

Figure 2 : T-map showing greater regional grey matter density in patients with high a3/a2 ratio contrasted to patients with midlle a3/a2 ratio ($p \leq 0.001$ uncorrected, the symbol '>' denotes 'major grey matter density then', see also table).

2009b). Of note, the present results derive from comparisons within masked regions along with relatively liberal statistical thresholds. This implies that these findings need to be confirmed by further studies with larger size patients population. On the other hand, the presence of a peculiar pattern of association between EEG and MRI markers in a subgroup of MCI subjects useful in the comprehension of anatomo-physiological underpinning of the MCI entity. Indeed, in the previous studies published by our group, the increase of alpha3/alpha2 ratio was associated to a decrease (or atrophy) of the hippocampal volume. On the contrary, in the present study the alpha3/alpha3 ratio is associated with a bigger volume (or minor atrophy) in basal ganglia and NAc.

4.2   Association between EEG Markers and GM Changes

Results show that the increase of alpha3/alpha2 ratio is mostly associated with minor atrophy of caudate nuclei and accumbens nuclei. These results confirm previous studies on AD patients, showing basal ganglia involvement in AD (deJong *et al.*, 2008; Canu *et al.*, 2010; Cherubini *et al.*, 2010; Zarei *et al.*, 2010). The principal difference with the most of other studies is that they reported a greater atrophy of basal ganglia. There some possible explanations: 1) the EEG-driven evaluation of atrophy, focusing on specific morpho-structural features of patients, have magnified only some GM patterns; 2) previous observed atrophy patterns could be linked to aspecific regressive processes due to aging (Cabeza *et al.*, 2004; Logan *et al.*, 2002; Park *et al.*, 2003, Grady *et al.*, 2006; 3) previous studies were most performed on AD patients whereas subjects with MCI could have different, perhaps compensatory, mechanism as compared to AD patients (Dickerson *et al.*, 2004, 2005; Golob *et al.* 2007).

4.3   Anatomo-physiological Relationship between EEG Markers and GM Changes

Our results show the presence of a specific pattern of GM changes associated with an EEG marker. We suggest an interesting, although speculative, hypothesis that could explain the novelty emerging from our results. A ventral stream, encompassing striatum (ventral caudate nuclei), and accumbens nuclei seems to be less affected in MCI patients who will develop AD. The relatively preserved anatomical structure could suggest a state of compensatory hyperfunction of this circuitry, determining both cognitive and psychiatric symptoms of prodromal AD (Spalletta *et al.*, 2010). Indeed, the ventral caudate and accumbens nuclei are related to the regulation of emotional control function, in particular with the impulsivity and fear behaviour control (Basar *et al.*, 2010). The brain electrical activity marker of these structural changes is represented by the increase of alpha3/alpha2 ratio. This could be due to the prevalence of an anterior circuit impinging on anterior cingulate cortex, ventral (limbic) striatum and orbito-frontal cortex, relatively spared (in the initial time of disease) in pre-AD patients. The well-known disrupture of the posterior circuit, encompassing hyppocampal cortex, posterior cingulate, precuneus, posterior parietal cortices, will give rise to the decrease of low alpha (alpha 2 in our analysis) rhythm, whereas the dominance of an anterior circuit give rise to the increase of high alpha.

4.4   Clinical and Anatomo-phyisiological Implications

Our results shows a clear association between the increase of alpha3/alpha2 power ratio and bigger volume inside the ventral striatum network in subjects with MCI, suggesting that this network could be hyperactive in patients at major risk to develop AD. These findings confirm a large body of previous literature. Recent factor analyses conducted on the Neuropsychiatric Inventory (Cummings *et al.*, 1994) collected from a large sample of AD patients have all identified factors called "behavioural dyscontrol" (Hollingworth *et al.*, 2006), "hyperactivity" (Aalten *et al.*, 2007), or "psychomotor syndrome" (Spalletta *et al.*, 2010) that globally encompass the same symptoms (e.g., agitation, irritability, aggressivity, disinhibition, euphoria, appetite disturbances, aberrant motor behaviors). These symptoms are frequently described even in the early phase of the disease and explain a substantial part of variance of the total behavioral and psychological symptoms of dementia.

The ventral stiatum network (ventral caudate and accumbens nuclei) is a key entry point structure for afferent information from the periphery as well as for afferents and efferents of wider cortico-striatal-pallido-thalamo-cortical functionally segregated loops (CSPTC; Steriade, 2006; Kopell and Grindberg, 2008; Haber and Calzavara, 2009). The ventral striatum is primarily characterized by its strong inputs from limbic structures such as the amygdala, hippocampus, midline thalamus and certain regions of the prefrontal cortex, as well as from the mesolimbic dopamine system originating in the ventral tegmental area (VTA). Impulsive acts and decisions are related to individual differences in the neural representations of stimuli/events (Chambers and Potenza, 2003). The NAc plays an important regulatory role in the neural representation of response options, as shown by functional neuroimaging studies in healthy individuals (Rochat et al., 2008). A voluminous literature on decision-making in humans provides imaging evidence of the involvement of a variety of brain structures in impulsive choice; different subregions of the human prefrontal cortex, cingulate cortex, insula, and the amygdala are the most prominent ones (Ernst and Paulus, 2005; Knutson and Bossaerts, 2007; Rushworth and Behrens, 2008). These structures are known to either have direct anatomical connections to the NAc, or are indirectly connected (Rochat et al., 2008). The selection of immediate reinforcement has been repeatedly reported to be associated with increased activity in the ventral striatum (McClure et al., 2004). Imaging studies with various task have implied an association between increased ventral striatal activity and selection of less safe option (Ernst et al., 2004; Matthews et al., 2004; Kuhnen and Knutson, 2005; Weber and Huettel, 2008). Another possible explanation of increase in NAc and ventral striatum hyperactivity could be related to exposure associated to novel environments. A recent study has convincingly demonstrated that a modifications in glutamatergic transmission with an increase of glutamatergic receptorial subtypes occurrs in NAc after novelty exposure (Rothwell et al., 2011). A modification in the shape of ventral striatum and NAc has been demonstrated also in patients with AD showing sensation-seeking behavior (deJong et al., 2011). In this optic the alpha3/alpha2 power ratio could a physiological network marker, related to a specific behavioral disorder, useful to screen out MCI subjects that could develope AD.

5   Study Limitations

There are some limitations due to the obvious explorative nature of the present study: 1) further studies are needed to confirm our result on larger samples; 2) need to applicate an appropriate multiple comparison correction, considering that the results derive from comparisons within masked regions; 3) the present study is not prospective so future research is needed in order to know if these EEG markers and grey matter changes corresponded to MCI patients at higher risk of conversion to dementia; 4) the present results have to be compared with a control group analysis; 5) correlations with clinical and behavioral data are mandatory to confirm the association between the the impusive disorders network and psychiatric symptoms. Anyway, given the exploratve nature of the study it is plausible a permissive approach in order to avoid to reject possibly interesting results.

6   Conclusion

The integrated analysis of EEG and morpho-structural markers could be useful in the comprehension of anatomo-physiological underpinning of the MCI entity.

References

Aalten P, Verhey FR, Boziki M, Bullock R, Byrne EJ, Camus V, et al. Neuropsychiatric syndromes in dementia. Results from the European Alzheimer disease consortium: Part I. Dementia and Geriatric Cognitive Disorders, 24(6): 457-463, 2007.

Ashburner J., 2007. A fast diffeomorphic image registration algorithm. Neuroimage. Oct 15;38(1):95-113.

Basar K, Sesia T, Groenewegen H, Steinbusch HW, Visser-Vandewalle V, Temel Y. Nucleus accumbens and impulsivity. Prog Neurobiol. 2010 Dec;92(4):533-57. Doi: 10.1016/j.pneurobio.2010.08.007.

Boettiger, C.A., Mitchell, J.M., Tavares, V.C., Robertson, M., Joslyn, G., D'Esposito, M., Fields, H.L., 2007. Immediate reward bias in humans: fronto-parietal networks and a role for the catechol-O-methyltransferase 158(Val/Val) genotype. J. Neurosci. 27, 14383–14391.

Cabeza R, Daselaar SM, Dolcos F, Prince SE, Budde M, Nyberg L., 2004. Task-independent and task specific age effects on brain activity during working memory, visual attention and episodic retrieval. Cereb Cortex; 14: 364-375.

Canu E, McLaren DG, Fitzgerald ME, Bendlin BB, Zoccatelli G, Alessandrini F, Pizzini FB, Ricciardi GK, Beltramello A, Johnson SC, Frisoni GB., 2010. Microstructural diffusion changes are independent of macrostructural volume loss in moderate to severe Alzheimer's disease. J Alzheimers Dis.;19(3):963-76.

Chambers, R.A., Potenza, M.N., 2003. Neurodevelopment, impulsivity, and adolescent gambling. J. Gambl. Stud. 19, 53–84.

Cherubini A, Péran P, Spoletini I, Di Paola M, Di Iulio F, Hagberg GE, Sancesario G, Gianni W, Bossù P, Caltagirone C, Sabatini U, Spalletta G., 2010. Combined volumetry and DTI in subcortical structures of mild cognitive impairment and Alzheimer's disease patients. J Alzheimers Dis. 19(4):1273-82.

Cummings JL, Mega M, Gray K, Rosenberg-Thompson S, Carusi DA, and Gornbein J. The Neuropsychiatric Inventory: Comprehensive assessment of psychopathology in dementia. Neurology, 44(12): 2308-2314, 1994.

de Jong LW, van der Hiele K, Veer IM, Houwing JJ, Westendorp RG, Bollen EL, de Bruin PW, Middelkoop HA, van Buchem MA, van der Grond J., 2008. Strongly reduced volumes of putamen and thalamus in Alzheimer's disease: an MRI study. Brain. 131(Pt 12):3277-85. Epub 2008 Nov 20.

de Jong LW, Ferrarini L, van der Grond J, Milles JR, Reiber JH, Westendorp RG, Bollen EL, Middelkoop HA, van Buchem MA. Shape abnormalities of the striatum in Alzheimer's disease. J Alzheimers Dis. 2011; 23(1):49-59. doi: 10.3233/JAD-2010-101026.

Dickerson BC, Salat DH, Bates JF, Atiya M, Killiany RJ, Greve DN, Dale AM, Stern CE, Blacker D, Albert MS, Sperling RA. 2004. Medial temporal lobe function and structure in midl cognitive impairment. Ann Neurol; 56: 27-35.

Dickerson BC, Salat DH, Greve DN, Chua EF, Rand-Giovannetti E, Rentz DM, Bertram L, Mullin K, Tanzi RE, Blacker D, Albert MS, Sperling RA. 2005. Increased hippomcapal activation in midl cognitive impairment compared to normal aging and AD. Neurology; 65: 404-411.

Dubois B, Feldman HH, Jacova C, Dekosky ST, Barberger-Gateau P, Cummings J, Delacourte A, Galasko D, Gauthier S, Jicha G, Meguro K, O'brien J, Pasquier F, Robert P, Rossor M, Salloway S, Stern Y, Visser PJ, Scheltens P., 2007. Research criteria for the diagnosis of Alzheimer's disease: revising the NINCDS-ADRDA criteria. Lancet Neurol. Aug;6(8):734-46. Review.

Ernst, M., Nelson, E.E., McClure, E.B., Monk, C.S., Munson, S., Eshel, N., Zarahn, E., Leibenluft, E., Zametkin, A., Towbin, K., Blair, J., Charney, D., Pine, D.S., 2004. Choice selection and reward anticipation: an fMRI study. Neuropsychologia 42, 1585–1597.

Ernst, M., Paulus, M.P., 2005. Neurobiology of decision making: a selective review from a neurocognitive and clinical perspective. Biol. Psychiatry 58, 597–604.

Folstein MF, Folstein SE, McHugh PR.,1975. 'Mini mental state': a practical method for grading the cognitive state of patients for clinician. J Psychiatr Res;12:189–98.

Golob EJ, Irimajiri R. Starr A., 2007. Auditory cortical activity in amnestic mild cognitive impairment: relationship to subtype and conversion to dementia. Brain; 130:740-752.

Grady CL, Springer MV, Hongwanishkul D, McIntosh AR, Winocur G., 2006. Age-related changes in brain activiy across the adult lifespan. J. Cogn Neurosci; 18: 227-241.

Haber SN, Calzavara R., 2009. The cortico-basal ganglia integrative network: the role of the thalamus. Brain Res Bull. Feb 16;78(2-3):69-74. Epub 2008 Oct 23. Review.

Hollingworth P, Hamshere ML, Moskvina V, Dowzell K, Moore PJ, Foy C, et al. Four components describe behavioral symptoms in 1,120 individuals with late-onset Alzheimer's disease. Journal of the American Geriatrics Society, 54(9): 1348-1354, 2006.

Hughes CP, Berg L, Danziger WL, Cohen LA, Martin RL., 1982. A new clinical rating scale for the staging of dementia. Br J Psychiatry. 140: 1225–30.

Klimesch W., 1997. EEG-alpha rhythms and memory processes, Int J Psychophysiol. 26: 319– 340.

Klimesch W., 1999. EEG alpha and theta oscillations reflect cognitive and memory performance: a review and analysis. Brain Res Rev. 29: 169–95.

Knutson, B., Bossaerts, P., 2007. Neural antecedents of financial decisions. J. Neurosci. 27, 8174–8177.

Kopell BH, Greenberg BD., 2008. Anatomy and physiology of the basal ganglia: implications for DBS in psychiatry. Neurosci Biobehav Rev.;32(3):408-22.

Kuhnen, C.M., Knutson, B., 2005. The neural basis of financial risk taking. Neuron 47, 763–770.

Lawton MP, Brodie EM., 1969. Assessment of older people: self maintaining and instrumental activity of daily living. J Gerontol. 9:179–86.

Lezak, M., Howieson, D., & Loring, D. W., 2004. Neuropsychological Assessment, fourth edition. Oxford: University Press.

Logan JM, Sanders AL, Snyder AZ, Morris JC, Buckner RL., 2002. Underrecruitment and non-selective recruitment: dissociable neural mechanisms associated with aging. Neuron. 33: 827-840.

Mai JK, Assheuer J, Paxinos G., 1997. Atlas of the Human Brain. Academic Press, San Diego

Matthews, S.C., Simmons, A.N., Lane, S.D., Paulus, M.P., 2004. Selective activation of the nucleus accumbens during risk-taking decision making. Neuroreport 15, 2123–2127.

Mattis M. Mental status examination for organic mental syndrome in the elderly patient. In Bellack L (Ed), Geriatric Psychiatry: A Handbook for Psychiatrists and Primary Care Physicians. New York: Grune and Stratton, 1976: 77-121.

McClure, S.M., Laibson, D.I., Loewenstein, G., Cohen, J.D., 2004. Separate neural systems value immediate and delayed monetary rewards. Science 306, 503– 507.

McClure, S.M., Ericson, K.M., Laibson, D.I., Loewenstein, G., Cohen, J.D., 2007. Time discounting for primary rewards. J. Neurosci. 27, 5796–5804.

Moretti DV, Babiloni F, Carducci F, Cincotti F, Remondini E, Rossini PM, Salinari S, Babiloni C.,2003. Computerized processing of EEG-EOG-EMG artifacts for multi-centric studies in EEG oscillations and event-related potentials. Int J Psychophysiol. 47(3):199-216.

Moretti D.V., Babiloni C., Binetti G., Cassetta E., Dal Forno G., Ferreri F., Ferri R., Lanuzza B., Miniussi C., Nobili F., Rodriguez G., Salinari S., Rossini P.M., 2004. Individual analysis of EEG frequency and band power in mild Alzheimer's disease. Clin. Neurophysiol. 115, 299–308.

Moretti D.V., Miniussi C. , Frisoni G., Zanetti O., Binetti G., Geroldi C., Galluzzi S., Rossini P.M., 2007a. Vascular damage and EEG markers in subjects with mild cognitive impairment. Clinical neurophysiology. 118, 1866-1876.

Moretti D.V., Miniussi C., Frisoni G.B., Geroldi C., Zanetti O., Binetti G., Rossini P.M., 2007b. Hippocampal atrophy and EEG markers in subjects with mild cognitive impairment. Clinical neurophysiology. 118, 2716-2729.

Moretti D.V., Frisoni G.B., Pievani M., Rosini S., Geroldi C., Binetti G., Rossini P.M., 2008a. Cerebrovascular disease and hippocampal atrophy are differently linked to functional coupling of brain areas: an EEG coherence study in MCI subjects. J. Alzheimers. Dis. 14(3), 285-99.

Moretti D.V., Pievani M., Fracassi C., Geroldi C., Calabria M., DeCarli C., Rossini P.M., 2008b. Brain vascular damage of cholinergic pathways and E.E.G. markers in mild cognitive impairment. J. Alzheimers. Dis. 15(3), 357-72.

Moretti D.V., Fracassi C., Pievani M., Geroldi C., Binetti G., Zanetti O., Sosta K., Rossini P. M. Frisoni G. B., 2009a. Increase of theta/gamma ratio is associated with memory impairment. Clin. Neurophysiol. 120(2), 295-303.

Moretti D.V.,Pievani M., Fracassi C., Binetti G., Rosini S., Geroldi C., Zanetti O., Rossini P.M., Frisoni G.B., 2009b. Increase of theta/gamma and alpha3/alpha2 ratio is associated with amygdalo-hippocampal complex atrophy. J. Alzheimer Disease, 120 (2), 295-303.

Moretti DV, Pievani M, Geroldi C, Binetti G, Zanetti O, Cotelli M, Rossini PM, Frisoni GB., . 2009c. Increasing hippocampal atrophy and cerebrovascular damage is differently associated with functional cortical coupling in MCI patients. Alzheimer Dis Assoc Disord. 23(4):323-32.

Moretti DV, Frisoni GB, Fracassi C, Pievani M, Geroldi C, Binetti G, Rossini PM , Zanetti O., 2011. MCI patients' EEGs show group differences between those who progress and those who do not progress to AD. Neurobiology of aging. 32(4):563-71.

Moretti DV, Prestia A, Fracassi C, Binetti G, Zanetti O, Frisoni GB.Specific EEG changes associated with atrophy of hippocampus in subjects with mild cognitive impairment and Alzheimer's disease.Int J Alzheimers Dis. 2012a;2012:253153.

Moretti DV, Paternicò D, Binetti G, Zanetti O, Frisoni GB.EEG markers are associated to gray matter changes in thalamus and basal ganglia in subjects with mild cognitive impairment.Neuroimage. 2012b Mar;60(1):489-96.

Park DC, Welsh RC, Marshuetz C, Gutchess AH, Mikels J, Polk TA, Noll DC, Taylor SF,. 2003. Working memory for complexes scenes: age differences in frontal and hippocampal activations. J. Cogn. Neuroscience; 15: 1122-1134.

Petersen RC, Doody R, Kurz A, Mohs RC, Morris JC, Rabins PV, Ritchie K, Rossor M, Thal L, Winblad B., 2001. Current concepts in mild cognitive impairment. Arch Neurol; 58(12):1985–92.

Portet F, Ousset P J, Visser P J, Frisoni G B, Nobili F, Scheltens Ph, Vellas B, Touchon J. and the MCI Working Group of the European Consortium on Alzheimer's Disease (EADC)., 2006. Mild cognitive impairment (MCI) in medical practice: a critical review of the concept and new diagnostic procedure. Report of the MCI Working Group of the European Consortium on Alzheimer's Disease. J. Neurol. Neurosurg. Psychiatry; 77;714-718.

Radloff, LS., 1977. The CES-D scale: A self-report depression scale for research in the general population. Applied Psychological Measurement; 1:385-401.

Rochat L, Delbeuck X, Billieux J, d'Acremont M, Juillerat Van der Linden AC, and Van der Linden M. Assessing impulsivity changes in Alzheimer disease. Alzheimer Disease and Associated Disorders, 2008; 22(3): 278-283.

Rochat L, Billieux J, Juillerat Van der Linden AC, Annoni JM, Zekry D, Gold G, Van der Linden M. A multidimensional approach to impulsivity changes in mild Alzheimer's disease and control participants: Cognitive correlates. Cortex. 2013 Jan;49(1):90-100. Doi: 10.1016/j.cortex. 2011.08.004.

Rosen WG, Terry RD, Fuld PA, Katzman R, Peck A., 1980. Pathological verification of ischemic score in differentiation of dementias. Ann Neurol;7(5):486–8.

Rossini PM, Buscema M, Capriotti M, Grossi E, Rodriguez G, Del Percio C, Babiloni C., 2008. Is it possible to automatically distinguish resting EEG data of normal elderly vs. mild cognitive impairment subjects with high degree of accuracy? Clin Neurophysiol. Jul;119(7):1534-45.

Rothwell PE, Kourrich S, Thomas MJ. Environmental novelty causes stress-like adaptations at nucleus accumbens synapses: implications for studying addiction-related plasticity. Neuropharmacology. 2011 Dec;61(7):1152-9. doi: 10.1016/j.neuropharm.2011.01.038.

Rushworth, M.F., Behrens, T.E., 2008. Choice, uncertainty and value in prefrontal and cingulate cortex. Nat. Neurosci. 11, 389–397.

Spalletta G, Musicco M, Padovani A, Rozzini L, Perri R, Fadda L, et al. Neuropsychiatric symptoms and syndromes in a large cohort of newly diagnosed, untreated patients with Alzheimer disease. American Journal of Geriatric Psychiatry, 18(11): 1026-1035, 2010.

Stam C.J., van der Made Y., Pijnenburg Y.A., Scheltens P., 2003. EEG synchronization in mild cognitive impairment and Alzheimer's disease. Acta Neurol. Scand; 108(2), 90-6.

Steriade M., 2006. Grouping of brain rhythms in corticothalamic systems. Neuroscience. 137(4):1087-106. Review.

Weber, B.J., Huettel, S.A., 2008. The neural substrates of probabilistic and intertemporal decision making. Brain Res. 1234, 104–115.

Wittmann M, Leland DS, Churan J, Paulus MP.Impaired time perception and motor timing in stimulant-dependent subjects. Drug Alcohol Depend. 2007 Oct 8;90(2-3):183-92.

Zarei M, Patenaude B, Damoiseaux J, Morgese C, Smith S, Matthews PM, Barkhof F, Rombouts SA, Sanz-Arigita E, Jenkinson M., 2010. Combining shape and connectivity analysis: an MRI study of thalamic degeneration in Alzheimer's disease. Neuroimage. 1;49(1):1-8. Epub 2009 Sep 8. Erratum in: Neuroimage. 2010 Jun;51(2):940.

The Art of Psychotherapy in Oman: Practice and Limitations

Zena Al-Sharbati
Department of Behavioural Medicine, Sultan Qaboos University Hospital
Sultan Qaboos University, Muscat, Oman

Marwan Al-Sharbati
Department of Behavioural Medicine, College of Medicine and Health Sciences
Sultan Qaboos University, Muscat, Oman

Ishita Gupta
Department of Genetics, College of Medicine and Health Sciences
Sultan Qaboos University, Muscat, Oman

1   Introduction

Mental illnessesare linked with distress and attributed to various genetic, biological, psychological and social factors (Akiskal & Benazzi, 2006). Mental health professionals utilize the Diagnostic and Statistical Manual of Mental Disorders (DSM-IV TR) and International Classification of Diseases and Related Health Problems (ICD-10) to diagnose mental disorders. Some of the common Axis I disorders in the DSM-IV TR include mood disorders, Attention Deficit Hyperactivity Disorder, autism spectrum disorders, and schizophreniawhile Axis II disorders include personality disorders (American Psychiatric Association,2012). The international classification of Diseases and Related Health Problems 10th Revision (ICD-10) is the World Health Organization coding system of diseases, signs, symptoms, abnormal findings and social circumstances (World Health Organization, 1992). Chapter V in the ICD-10 classifies mental and behavioral disorders as follows: organic, including symptomatic, mental disorders, mental and behavioral disorders due to psychoactive substance use, schizophrenia, schizotypal and delusional disorders, mood (affective) disorders, neurotic, stress-related and somatoform disorders, behavioral syndromes associated with physiological disturbances and physical factors, disorders of adult personality and behavior, mental retardation, disorders of psychological development, behavioral and emotional disorders with onset usually occurring in childhood and adolescence and unspecified mental disorder.It is quite common that a person may suffer from multiple psychological disorders (co morbidities) (Al-Sharbati *et al.*, 2011; Sivakumar *et al.*, 2013). Given that there is no fundamental difference and no agreed upon medical definition of mental illness, mental disorder or psychological disorders (Kendell, 1993; American Psychiatric Association, 2013), these three terms will be used interchangeably throughout the chapter.

1.1   Prevalence of Psychological Disorders

Various studies were conducted to estimate the prevalence of psychological disorders. According to the World Health Organization (WHO), 450 million people sufferfrom psychological disorders with one in four people meeting the criteria at some point in their life (Sherer, 2002). In addition, one third of people suffer from psychological disorders (WHO, 2000). A recent survey conducted by WHO, and based on the ICD-10 and DSM-IV TR criteria utilizing population samples, found that anxiety disorders were the most common mental disorders affecting more females(Demyttenaere *et al.*, 2004; Somers *et al.*, 2006; Jaju *et al.*, 2009). The prevalence of having any DSM-IV disorder in the previous year was not consistent, ranging from 4.3% in Shanghai to 26.4% in the United States. The next most prevalent category of mental disorders was mood disorders, with major depressive disorder being the most prevalent (4.1%), followed by dysthymic disorder (2%) and finally bipolar I disorder (0.72%). Mood disorders were most prevalent among females (Waraich, *et al.*, 2004). Personality disorderswere found to have prevalence of 6% worldwide (Huang *et al.*, 2009).

Researchers have explored prevalence of psychological disordersamong population samples worldwide. For example, the United States, Europe and Ukraine have higher lifetime and 12-month prevalence rates of psychological disorders compared to Nigeria, Italy and Asia where the rates were comparatively low (Demyttenaere *et al.*, 2004). Possible reasons for the higher prevalence in the West may include the increase complexity of materialistic life which may exaggerate the preponderance of psychological disorders in the population. Also, the diagnostic criteria adopted by Western communities may not be applicable to Eastern populations because of the difference in the clinical presentation of clinical disorders. According to the National Institute of Mental Health, approximately 26 % of individuals in the U.S. above the age of 18 suffer from a psychological disorder every year (Kessler *et al.*, 1994). Prevalence of anxiety and mood disorders were among the highest in the West, with the U.S having a prevalence rate of 28.8% and 20.8% (Kesler *et al.,* 2005) and Europe having a rate of 13.6% and 13.9% respectively (Alonso *et al.,* 2004). These prevalence rates are much higher than the previously reported rates by WHO. However, in Arab countries there is a dearth of research onthe prevalence of psychological disorders, especially those conducted in the community. However, even community studies show a discrepancy in the prevalence rates of mental disorders. For example, in a school-based study conducted in Oman, the prevalence rate of social phobia was around 36.6%(Al-Sharbati *et al.,* 2012). On the other hand, a high incidence of 70% for DSM-IV disorders was observed in Lebanon (Kessler *et al.,* 2007), while in Oman the prevalence rate is 17%, with the females being at a higher risk of Major Depression Disorder (MDD), any Mood Disorder (AMD) and specific phobia (Jaju *et al.,* 2009). Next section will discuss the importance of early and proper diagnosis of mental illness.

1.2   Diagnosis of Psychological Disorders

In general, people in the Middle East tend to avoid mental health services because of the social stigma. Cultural issues (Al-Sharbati *et al.,* 2012), economic and logistic challenges, and lack of awareness lead to the under-diagnosis of cases (Al Adawi *et al.,* 2002; Al-Farsi *et al.* 2011). However, a diagnosis can be an effective plan for better prognosis and treatment outcomes (Shear *et al.,* 2000).

Diagnosis of psychological disorders is done by a mental health professional based on a structured clinical interview,history taking, mental state exanimations and various personality tests (possibly neuropsychological tests) (Anastasi, 1996; Grant & Adams, 1996), and laboratory and radiological investigations to exclude organic causes if required (Tang *et al.*, 2013). The diagnosis is made based on the criteria set by ICD-10 or DSM-IV TR. The last lists 16 categories of maladjustment and it enables reliable diagnosis using observable behaviors. Based on the DSM-IV-TR, this method of diagnosis utilizes five axes or dimensions; Axis I (Clinical Syndromes), Axis II (Personality Disorders), Axis III (General Medical Conditions), Axis IV (Psychosocial and Environmental Problems) and Axis V (Global Assessment of Functioning) (American Psychiatric Association, 2012). Axes I and II characterize abnormal behavior while the remaining three axes provide supplementary information. The use of such classification system enables the mental health professional to make accurate decisions to allow better prognosis and effective treatment.

It is important to mention that the diagnostic system in mental health has undergone tremendous changes over the past 60 years. The DSM is published by the American Psychiatric Association and is mainly used in the United States and parts of the world (Dalal & Sivakumar, 2009). The DSM initially evolved from statistics obtained from psychiatric hospitals and United States army manual. It has undergone many revisions since its first publication in 1952. The first version of the DSM included (106) mental disorders (Grob, 1991), with more mental disorders on later versions reaching 279 mental disorders for the DSM-IV-TR (published in 2000) (American Psychiatric Association, 2000). The latest version was released on May 18, 2013 and is termed DSM-5 (Kinderman, 2013). Some of the major changes to DSM-5 are the exclusion of the multi-axial system (replaced by severity levels), incorporating the four previous separate disorders into a single condition (autism spectrum disorder), and the bereavement exclusion removal (Grohol, 2013).

The International Classification of Disease and Related Health Problems (ICD) produced by the World Health organization is another commonly used manual which also includes criteria for mental disorders (World Health Organization, 1992). Although, it is officially the diagnostic system for mental disorders in the United States, it is more widely used in Europe and other parts of the world. Although the

DSM and ICD seek to utilize the same codes in diagnosis, some major differences exist such as the categorization of personality disorders. The new version of the ICD (ICD-11) is scheduled on 2015.

1.3   Treatment of Psychological Disorders

Mental health professionals have to follow the code of ethics as set by the American Psychological Association, 2002 (Schacter *et al.*, 2010). In addition to the code of ethics, Kitchener (1984) has identified five moral principles which are considered the cornerstone of ethical guidelines (Kitchener, 1984). Given the fact that ethical guidelines cannot address all ethical dilemmas inherent within the field, the five moral principles help mental health professionals to appreciate complex ethical dilemmas. These principles are autonomy (allowing individuals the freedom of action and choice when deemed appropriate), nonmaleficense (not causing harm to others -considered the most critical of all principles) (Rosenbaum, 1982; Stadler, 1986), beneficence (contributing to the welfare of patients) (Forester-Miller & Rubenstein, 1992), justice (acting in a non-discriminatory manner to individuals or groups) and fidelity (honoring commitments within the professional setting) (Kitchener, 1984). A detailed discussion of each of the five moral principles is beyond the scope of this chapter.

Treatment of mental illnesses includes a number of modalities such as the use of psychotropic medications and various forms of psychotherapy. Psychiatrists use psychotropic medicationssuch as antidepressants (Furukawa *et al.*, 2001), anxiolytics (Barlow & Durand, 2009), mood stabilizers (Trevor *et al.*, 2003), antipsychotics (Kirk Morton & Zubek, 2013) and psycho-stimulants (Al-Sharbati *et al.*, 2003). Also, psychiatrists utilize Electro-Convulsive Therapy (ECT) under certain conditions (Weiner & Richard, 2001). In addition, patients can benefit from music, art or drama psychotherapies (Talwar *et al.*, 2006; Crawford *et al.*, 2012). Psychotropic medications intend to solve the acute stress and suffering of the patient to assist him/her solves life challenges and enhances the adaptation mechanisms. Therefore, medical treatment is not the sole method to treat psychological disorders, but it is a step toward a comprehensive therapy that should be complimented by other methods such as social support and psychotherapy. Psychotherapy, as a scientific field, was developed over the past century. Initially, Sigmund Freud introduced this technique recognized as psychoanalysis (Mitchell & Black, 1996).Psychotherapy is described as 'talk therapy' and is defined as the treatment of psychological disorders based on emblematic communications (Bloch, 2006). The therapeutic encounter allows the patient to interact with a qualified mental health care practitioner and explore challenging experiences. Psychotherapy aims to help patients gain an increased capacity for choice.Different types of psychotherapy exist for the treatment of various conditions such as depression, anxiety, marital problems, obsessive compulsive disorder, conduct disorder and other behavioral problems (Andrews & Harvey, 1981).

Psychotherapy encompasses various schools of thought which vary greatly in its emphasis. These schools of thoughts can be divided into four major types; Insight oriented psychotherapies; cognitive-behavioral therapies; existential psychotherapies and finally family therapies (Smith & Glass, 1977). Insight-oriented psychotherapy focuses on the unconscious emotional conflicts and helps clients to make those internal conflicts conscious (McGuire, 1965). Insight-oriented psychotherapies are effective in the treatment of complex mental disorders, chronic mental disorders and panic disorders (Leichsenring & Rabung, 2008). Behavior therapy is based on classical learning theories and aims to replace conditioned fearful stimulus with healthy responses. Cognitive therapy focuses on the individual's current thinking styles and replaces dysfunctional thoughts with balanced ones. Cognitive-behavioral therapy (CBT), on the other hand, integrates both the cognitive and behavioral aspects into the treatment (Wright *et al.*, 2006). Cognitive behavioral therapy is considered the gold treatment of a number of clinical mental disorders and personality disorders (Roth & Fonagy, 2005; Reis, 2007). Existentially oriented psychotherapies focuses on discovering new potentialities for clients' personal growth (Bloch, 2006). Family therapies, on the other hand, focus on helping family members to improve dysfunctional communication and resolve conflictual relationships (Goldenberg & Goldenberg, 2013). Research had demonstrated that adolescent clients respond better to family psychotherapy rather than supportive psychotherapy (Nordqvist, 2007).

1.3.1   The processes of Psychotherapy

Although many schools of thought exist within the psychotherapy tradition, all psychotherapy modalities aim to empower clients to satisfy their psychological needs (Lambert &Bergin, 1992).Through the utilization of various clinical skills, psychotherapists help people to satisfy their own needs by challenging and replacing unhelpful thoughts, emotions and behaviors (Longmore& Worrell, 2007;Wright *et al.*, 2006). These unhelpful thoughts and behaviors are barriers to achieve the client's therapy goals. In addition, all psychotherapies share common features such as the presence of a therapeutic contract, therapeutic conceptualization and intervention, therapeutic alliance, and therapeutic realization (Orlinsky & Kenneth, 1987). In addition, all psychotherapies emphasize change and the acquisition of new behaviors (Grencavage & Norcross, 1990).

1.3.2   The utilization of Psychotherapy Services Worldwide

The Caucasian-American populations and female clients are the most frequent users of psychotherapy compared to other ethnic groups/male clients (Olfson *et al.*, 2002; Dwairy, 2009; Wade & Good; 2010). However, the utilization of psychotherapy has declined suggesting an increase in the use of psychotropic medications (Olfson *et al.*, 2002). One of the factors that may have led to the decline in the use of psychotherapy include the increase in accessibility of over-the counter medications (Al-Rowais *et al.*, 2010; Furihata *et al.*, 2010; Man *et al.*, 2010).

Recently Eastern cultures have an increased interest in the use of psychotherapy given the rapid societal changes and associated emotional challenges, which render the populations more accepting of psychotherapy. This is despite the culturally interrelated healing practices that are widely used (Tseng 1999; Kirmayer, 2006). However, there is a dearth of data on the use of psychotherapy services within Eastern populations (Abel & Metraux, 1974). Generally speaking, people in the East prefer traditional support systems inherent within the extended family network (Dwairy, 2009).

1.4   Cultural Factors and Psychotherapy

The factors that prevent Arab people from engaging in psychotherapy include social stigma, fears of seeking professional help, self-disclosure and social norms (Ben-Porath, 2002).El-Islam (1994) has further discussed the term "associative stigma", which is a prevalent occurrence in Arabian Gulf countries. It describes the process by which social shame associated with a family member's abnormal behavior not only bring social shame to the patient but also to his/her family. Traditional people from Arab countries live in large extended families and tend to discuss their problems with their family members (Ben-Porath, 2002). That is why the majority of people depend on their family for support rather than professional personnel. In addition, seeking mental health consultation is largely dependent on the family as a "collective system" (El-Islam, 1994). Similar to other Arab Gulf states, the traditional Omani family serves many social functions such as arranging for marriages for both its healthy as unhealthy members. Interdependence rather than independence is the main theme in the traditional Omani Culture and family. As a result,it is crucial to consider the rights and opinions family members as well as those of patients in the treatment of mental illness given the nature of family relationships.

People avoid mental health treatment in fear of the ambiguity of the treatment modality (Kouyoumdijian *et al*.m, 2003). Individuals with drug/ alcohol abuse problems or people with academic difficulties tend to have more treatment fears compared to people with other emotional difficulties (Barrett *et al.,* 2008). Another withdrawing factor is the fear of emotional expression to a mental health professional (Barrett et al., 2008). Furthermore, in Arab countries, where the traditional and cultural values play a strong role, many individuals (specifically females) do not prefer disclosing personal information to strangers (Dwairy, 2009). Based on recent observations, the expression of physical pain is more accepted than the expression of emotional pain among Arab patients (Qasem, 2010). In addition, self-control, including the control of emotions, is largely reinforced within the Arab culture (Haj-Yahia, 1994).

Previous research studies have shown that women tend to have more positive attitudes as compared to men in terms of utilizing psychotherapy for depression (Fischer& Farina, 1995).Men, on the other hand, seek psychotherapy for severe conditions such as acute stress (Tomlinson & Cope, 1988). In Arab societies, males play a dominant role and hence seeking psychotherapy may reduce their self-esteem and is a threat to their masculine identity (White *et al.*, 1995). Some traditional individuals believe that such help should be considered only after they try other measures of support. Thus, men tend to avoid utilizing psychotherapy for certain psychological disorders as they fear social stigma.

Cultural beliefs, values and norms play a role in preventing people from utilizing psychotherapeutic services. Traditional Arab people tend to avoid psychotherapy as they believe that evil eye or supernatural powers cause mental illness (Al-Sharbati *et al.,* 2012). In some cultures, individuals do not seek psychotherapyas treatment outside the home is considered as a shame (Dwairy, 2009). Age and education are other factors that play a role in utilization of psychotherapy. Individuals who are 20 years-old with higher education tend to be open towards seeking professional help compared to people from other age groups (Vessey & Howard, 1993). On the contrary,the socio-cultural influence within the Arab population drives younger generations to avoid seeking psychotherapy(Al-Busaidi, 2010).

Within Arab countries, there is limited access and availability of mental health services and hence studies need to be conducted to determine the demographic and clinical characteristics of mental health users. Oman is a Gulf country covering an area of about 300,000 square kilometers with a population of 3 million catered by approximately 39 qualified registered mental health professionals. This indicates the dearth of mental health services to serve the population (Ministry of Health, 2009). Research showed the scarcity of Arabic speaking psychotherapists, which is critical given that Arabic, is the native language in Oman (Tseng, 1999). In addition to the language skills, professionals within the mental health field tend to lack essential communication and counseling skills; skills which are of high importance in the treatment of psychological disorders (Al-Busaidi, 2010).

With Oman being a developing country and undergoing rapid urbanization and acculturation, exploring trends with respect to socio-cultural context is of special interest. As compared to other Arab countries, Oman has its own distinctive collective cultural and religious teachings (Al Adawi, 2006; Al Riyami *et al.*, 2009). Traditional Omani people do not hold disparaging views about individuals diagnosed with mental disorders, and have unique beliefs about consulting mental health professionals (Al Adawi *et al.*, 2002). However, some of the Omani population, both young and old, have strong faith about the association of mental disorders with supernatural powers (*Jinn*), evil eye (*Al-Ain*), envy (*Hasad*) and sorcery (*Sihr*). This influences the use of psychotherapy services (Al Riyami *et al.,* 2009) as it has been reported that about 60-80 % of health care needs are met by traditional health care systems in many parts of the Eastern world, including Oman (Al-Adawi, 1993).

Some individuals believe in choosing the right 'Muttawa' (spiritual healer) to cure the illness (Al-Busaidi, 2010). In Arabic, Al-Muttawa refers to the person who has surrendered his life to Allah, and is therefore considered a highly religious and spiritual person. Typically, and from the name, the services he provides to people should be free; however, this is not always the case. From clinical and cultural experience, spiritual and religious means that Al-Muttawa utilize include reciting specific verses from the Holly Book (Qur'an) that tends to be associated with helping the ill person. Reading specific verses from the Qur'an is called (Ruqya). It is the spiritual treatment that was inherited in Islam from Sunnah (based on Prophet Muhammad's teachings).

As a part of the Ruqya, specific verses to help in the case of (Hasad) or (Ain) are recited to patient and may also be given as homework for the patient to read. In addition, (Maho) is the water that is given to patients to drink or wash themselves with. This water is different from normal water because, spiritually speaking; it has been blessed by Ruqya. In addition to the above mentioned spiritual aspect of the Omani culture, Al-Adawi *et al.* (2001) discussed the spiritual practice of (Zar) in Oman, which is associated with spirit possession (Jinn). Some of the functions that Zar serves include a form of cultural group psychotherapy. It is also compatible with religious mythology. The popularity of spiritual and religious techniques may be associated with its practices that are deeply ingrained in the local legends related to concepts of health and illness.

Based on the above discussion, it is crucial during the therapy process to be sensitive to clients' cultural, religious as well as spiritual needs. It been mentioned elsewhere that Arabian Gulf communities expect the mental health professional (considered as an authority figure) to offer patients a quick fix to remove their suffering, and therefore the use of techniques such as homework may be challenging in this context (El-Islam, 2005). However, based on clinical experience, clients showed interest and involvement in pursuing homework assignments as a part of cognitive behavioral therapy. It is also not uncommon for family members to be involved in encouraging and supporting clients in working on homework. Clinical experience in Oman supports El-Islam's (1994) observations that clients expect that the mental health professional to enter their own internal world to appreciate their symptoms. For Arab or Muslim clients, it is crucial to integrate their religious beliefs into the therapy process. For instance, it is clinically valuable if the therapist is familiar with the client's religion, to be able to help him/her find alternative ways of religious thinking. An interesting example discussed by Dwairy (2009) includes a client with difficulty asserting himself, and putting others needs first, is to be reminded of the importance Islam places for satisfying humans needs as evidenced by the verse:"Wabtagi fema Atak Allah aldar el aakhera wala tansa nasibak men addunia" (Al-Qusas] 77) (But seek, by means of that which God has given you, to attain the abode of the hereafter and do not forget your share in this world).

The following section will focus on the clinical and socio-demographic characteristics of a psychiatric population in Oman and highlight a study that was conducted in a university Hospital, using the only and newly developed psychotherapy service within the Omani public health care system (Al-Sharbati *et al.*, 2012).

2   Methods

The psychotherapy service was newly established within the Department of Behavioral Medicine. It consisted of two psychologists with post graduate training in health psychology and clinical psychology. The third member of the team was an assistant psychologist under training. Two of the team members we bilingual, while the third member was an English speaker, mainly seeing English speaking patients (English speaking Omani patients or Western patients), or Arabic speaking patients with the help of a translator. All team members had individual supervision once per week. Group supervision was also conducted on a regular basis once a month (Al-Sharbati *et al.*, 2012).Given the abundance of research on the efficacy of cognitive behavioral therapy in the treatment of various mental disorders, it was the main psychotherapeutic orientation utilized with the clients' population in this study (Roth & Fonagy, 2005).The first assessment session lasts 90 minutes, while follow up psychotherapy session lasts 50 minutes (Al-Sharbati *et al.*, 2012).

Consent was obtained from all the patients who were referred to the Psychotherapy Services within the Department of Behavioral Medicine at the tertiary care hospital in Oman, Sultan Qaboos University Hospital (SQUH), and were included in the study. Parental consent were obtained before the initiation of psychotherapy with minor patients. SQUH has 550 bed capacities. It was established in February 1992. It is considered as a major teaching hospital for students enrolled in College of Medicine and Health Sciences and College of Nursing.

Data were collected for both, inpatients and outpatients, making a total of 133 patients, during the period from September 2009 to March 2010. Progress notes of patients were obtained from the SQUH Hospital Information System, and were reviewed to attain the socio-demographic and clinical details of patients enrolled in the study. Psychiatrists within the department and physicians from other medical departments made referrals to psychotherapy. In addition, private health centers, Ministry of Health hospitals and Armed Forces Hospital made referrals to the Psychotherapy service. Mental health professionals used the referral forms to collect data on the patient's demographics, psychiatric diagnosis, and reasons of referral, medical diagnosis, medications and comorbidities (Al-Sharbati *et al.*, 2012).

Patients referred to the Psychotherapy service were categorized into ten ICD-10 diagnostic categories: schizophrenia, bipolar disorder, depression, phobias, obsessive compulsive disorder, other anxiety disorders, reactive stress and adjustment disorders, dissociative and somatoform disorders, non-organic sleep disorders, personality disorders and emotional disorders of childhood (Al-Sharbati *et al.*, 2012). Data was collected from the electronic medical record regarding psychotropic medication at the time of their first psychotherapy session. The information was classified according to the British Formulary System therapeutic classes (antipsychotics, benzodiazepines, mood stabilizers, anti-depressants and lithium) (Al-Sharbati *et al.*, 2012).

3   Results

The majority of cases were females (59.4%), the age ranged from 13 years to 65 years; most of them were between 18-34 years, (59.48%) for females and (51.4%) males. This finding is in accord with other studies which showed a greater preponderance of females in both clinical and community settings (Olfson *et al.*, 2002; Al Riyami *et al.*, 2009). About (46%) of patients had 13-16 years of education, followed by (33.96%) of them who had 12 years of education. The majority of cases were never married (53.01%).

About (38%) of the cases were employed, and about one-third were students (Al-Sharbati *et al.,* 2012) (Please see Table 1 for more information).

Characteristics		
Age (Years)	Percentage	
	Female	Male
<13	2.70	11.3
13–17	8.1	9.43
18–24	28.38	26.4
25–34	31.1	25
35–44	19	17
45–54	9.46	7.55
55–64	0	3.77
>65	1.35	0
Total	100	100
Characteristics	Percentage	
Sex		
Female	59.4	
Male	40.4	
Total	99.8	
Education (Years)		
<12		33.96
12		16.98
13–16		46.23
≥ 17		2.83
Total		100
Marital Status		
Never married	53.01	
Married	41.67	
Widowed	3.0	
Divorced/separated	2.4	
Total	100	
Employment Status		
Employed	38.84	
Student	33.88	
Unemployed(including housewives)	25.62	
Retired	1.65	
Total	99.99	

Table 1: Socio-demographic characteristics of the cases (both outpatients and inpatients) treated by psychotherapy from September 2009 to March 2010 at Sultan QaboosUnivesity Hospital, Oman (Al-Sharbati *et al.,* 2012).

Table 2 describes basic data on the referral sources and main reasons for referral to psychotherapy. About (87.30%) of cases were outpatients. Psychiatrists referred the majority (90.84%) of cases (whether inpatients or outpatients), while physicians from other SQUH medical departments/wards made the remaining referrals. Referral request included treatment of psychological adjustment difficulties

Characteristic	Percentage
Hospitalization	
Never hospitalized	87.30
Hospitalised	12.69
Total	99.99
Referral source	
Departmental (within psychiatry)	90.84
External	3.82
Internal (within hospital)	5.34
Total	100
Reason for visit	
Non-mental health condition (Migraine, seizures..etc)	15.1
Mental health condition	84.92
Total	100
Mental health conditions	
Depression	21.8
Phobias	13.53
Other anxiety disorders	13.53
Obsessive compulsive disorder and other comorbid conditions	10.05
Dissociative and somatoform disorders	6.77
Reactive stress and adjustment disorders	6.01
Obsessive compulsive disorder	5.0
Personality disorders	3.0
Emotional disorders of childhood (e.g. nonorganic separation anxiety disorder), enuresis, conduct disorders	2.0
Schizophrenia	1.5
Bipolar disorder	0.98
Non-organic sleep disorders	0.75
Total	84.92
Current psychotropic medication use	
Any medication	64.8
No medication	35.2
Total	100
Type of drugs used	
Antidepressant	83.75
Antidepressant and antipsychotic	6.25
Benzodiazepam	5
Antipsychotic	1.25
Mood stabilizers	1.25
Antidepressant and benzodiazepam	1.25
Lithium and antidepressants	1.25
Total	100

Table 2: Clinical characteristics of psychotherapy users between the period September 2009 and March 2010 in SQUH, Oman (Al-Sharbati *et al.,* 2012).

linked with other medical conditions such as neurological conditions (15.1%). Other regional hospitals or primary health care centers in Muscat referred a minority of cases (Al-Sharbati *et al.*, 2012). The clinical diagnosis of the majority of cases (78.67%) was mood disorders while other disorders (such as personality disorders, schizophrenia, and bipolar disorder) constituted (6.25%) of the total number of cases. Patients mainly used antidepressants, either alone (83.75%), or combined with other drugs (Al-Sharbati *et al.*, 2012).

4   Discussion

The possible cause of the excess of female patients may be attributed to various factors including the male-oriented culture which prevents men from seeking mental health services (Al-Sharbati, 2009). This will lead to the under-diagnosis of mental health problems among males and over-representation of females (Al-Sharbati, 2009). On the other hand, women are subjected to different socio-cultural stressors including familial, financial, occupational and marital stress therefore, they are more prone to develop mental distress and seek psychotherapy. However, this trend was not found to be highly predominant in this region (Eloul *et al.*, 2009).

Various factors play a role in the avoidance of psychotherapy. Some of the factors include nature of the problem (patients with personality disorders do not seek mental health consultation), gender (females are more prone to seek help and treatment), age (younger patients require more assistance and support as they lack life experience), as well as socio-cultural influences (social stigma, reluctance of males to ask for help as seeking help is considered a weakness and an insult to the masculine gender identity) (Rüsch, 2013). The data collected from the study has focused on the factors that contributed to the utilization of psychotherapy services in Oman.

Education plays a critical role in the utilization of psychotherapy. Individuals with little formal education were either hesitant or are less likely to utilize psychotherapy compared to those with higher levels of education (Qualls & Knight, 2007). However, results from the Omani study implied that education was not a determinant factor for the use of psychotherapy (Al-Sharbati *et al.*, 2012). Oman offers free health care service for all of its nationals which could be one of the reasons that allow people to benefit from a wide range of health services (Al-Sharbati *et al.*, 2012). Further, psychotherapy services offered in private clinics are costly as compared to the service provided at the hospital and hence is accessed predominantly by people with lower education and socio-economic status. However, a few studies have shown that the use of psychotherapy is not always dependent on the level of education or the socio-economic status of clients (Olfson & Pincus, 1994; Olfson *et al.*, 2002).

Generally, individuals who are single, separated or divorced tend develop psychological distress and seek psychotherapy at a higher rate compared to married people (Cohen, 2010). In this Omani study, only (41.67%) of the cases were married, while divorced or separated individuals constituted a small proportion of the referrals (2.4%). This suggests that divorced/separated individuals are stigmatized in an Arab society which deters them from seeking help. However, separated/divorced people could utilize family support systems to cope with emotional distress instead of seeking professional help (El-Islam, 2008).

The majority of cases (almost one third) suffer from anxiety disorders. A plausible reason for development of anxiety can be attributed to the societal transition or a cultural shock faced by this collectivist society for an individualistic approach (Al-Sharbati *et al.*, 2012). Only a few patients diagnosed with schizophrenia, bipolar disorders, dissociative and somatoform disorders and personality disorders were referred. This could indicate a predisposition by the referring psychiatrists who may be less motivated to refer patients in need of more regular long-term therapy or who may have (according to their beliefs) a less favorable outcome from psychotherapy.This is despite recent researches which show encouraging results of psychotherapy use with patients with psychosis (Passerieux, 2013). As the majority of patients were suffering from emotional disorders, it is not uncommon to find antidepressants as the most commonly used drugs either alone or with other psychotropic drugs.

The utilization of cultural sensitive psychotherapy in this service was evidenced by exploring the cultural meaning of illness as well as patients' spiritual as well as religious beliefs. As suggested by Dwairy (2009), given that Qur'an contains a lot of metaphors, such metaphors were utilized in therapy to provide possible new ways of understanding critical concepts for patients. The integration of patients' religious beliefs and practices into homework assignment was always utilized. For instance, if prayer was helpful to a patient's well-being, it was integrated into the treatment plan as a coping strategy.

Psychotherapy was generally utilized by the younger population as the Omani society is characterized by a wide base demographic pyramid with an excess of youth. On the other hand, the reduced use of psychotherapy by older individuals can be attributed to culturally specific beliefs contradicting the value of mental health services. Therefore, some people prefer traditional healers and spiritual/religious treatment (called Ruqqya). As mentioned in the earlier section, about more than half of the Omani population (60%) either visit a 'Muttawa' or use allopathic or non-allopathic treatment before seeing a psychiatrist (Al-Riyami et al., 2009). Traditional healers adopt a culturally-sensitive perspective to aid distressed people through the faith factor and spiritual means. This approach can be more convincing to traditional people given that stress is attributed to external forces, such as an evil eye or supernatural forces. However, with wide-spread education and influences from the West, individuals have started to realize the importance of psychotherapy over treatment from Muttawas. Another study conducted among Omani women, reflected their attitude in utilizing services for treating emotional distress and the views of their respective physician. Both the patient and the physician believed in the faith factor when coping with mental stress (Al Busaidi, 2010). The study showed that depending upon the doctor-patient relationship; women were in favor of seeking medical help in relation to psychological disorders (Al Busaidi, 2010).

5   Conclusion

The study exposed trends in the referral process to a Psychotherapy Service in Oman. This study is critical to highlight developing vicissitudes in the Omani society. With vast developments in the country over the last 4 decades, through the discovery of oil fields, traditional values have been eroded. These changes have consequences for the adjustment of the older Omani population. However, with the new generation, there is a broad mind of acceptance to change and accept the value of self-expression, thus accepting psychotherapy. The study conducted has paved way for further, more detailed research on the utilization of psychotherapy services in Oman. Psychiatrists should take into account these factors to understand the reasons behind the aversion of individuals to utilize psychotherapy. It is essential for the health care planners to initiate programs for the training and development of mental health practitioners. Furthermore, cultural issues can aid in paving a path to help teach communication skills and consultation methods, to enable an easy and approachable mode of treatment.

In addition, individuals who have reservations about psychotherapy may need additional information and hence, awareness programs should be initiated to focus on the benefits of seeking such services. These programs can explain about how psychotherapy works and possible expectations by both parties (psychotherapist and client). Awareness programs should not only be for the public, but also directed to the mental health professional. That way an increased awareness of the need for multidisciplinary treatment helps to increase quality of professional standards.

The study had several limitations which should be taken into account. First, referrals were generally made by hospital psychiatrists after obtaining the patient's consent; hence there were no self-referred cases (AL-Sharbati *et al.*, 2012). Secondly, the study could have had more severe psychiatric disorders in comparison to those individuals who attended other health care clinics. Thirdly, due to logistic and economic reasons, results cannot be generalized to the Omani people as the majority of patients were from the capital city (Al-Sharbati *et al.*, 2012). Psychological disorders and their treatment carry a well known social stigma, and hence, only those patients who were motivated and considered psychotherapeutic treatment over traditional healers and spiritual relief were engaged in the treatment. Under-reporting of male patients due to the reasons already mentioned could have also contributed to bias in the results. However, this study has proved to be beneficial as it identified issues that need amendment with reference to the psychiatric services in Oman, and can be considered as a baseline study for future research.

References

Abel, T.M. & Metraux, R. (1974). Culture and Psychotherapy. New Haven, CT: College and University Press.

Akiskal, H.S. & Benazzi, F. (2006). The DSM-IV and ICD-10 categories of recurrent [major] depressive and bipolar II disorders: evidence that they lie on a dimensional spectrum. Journal of Affective Disorders; 92 (1): 45–54.

Al Adawi S. (2006). Adolescence in Oman. In: Jeffrey JA, Eds. International Encyclopedia of Adolescence: A Historical and Cultural Survey of Young People Around the World (Vol. 2 Set). New York: Routledge.

Al Adawi, S., Dorvlo, A.S., Al Ismaily, S.S., Al Ghafry, D.A., Al Noobi, B.Z., & Al Salmi, A., et al. (2002). Perception of and attitude towards mental illness in Oman.International Journal of Social Psychiatry; 305–17.

Al Riyami, A., Al Adawi, S., Al Kharusi, H., Morsi, M.M., & Sanjay, SS. (2009). Health Service utilization by school going Omani adolescents and youths with DSM IV mental disorders and barriers to service use.International Journal of Mental Health Systems; 3:22.

Al-Adawi, S. (1993). A glimpse into traditional outlook towards health: A literature review. Journal of Medical Humanities; 14:67–79.

Al-Adawi, S.H, Martin, R.G., Al-Salmi, A., & Ghassani, H. (2001). Zar: Group distress and healing. Mental Health, Religion & Culture; 4 (1):47-61.

Al-Busaidi, Z.Q. (2010). A qualitative Study on the attitudes and beliefs towards help seeking for emotional distress in Omani women and Omani general practitioners: Implications for post-graduate training. Oman Medical Journal; 25:190–8.

Al-Farsi, Y.M, Al-Sharbati, M.M, Al-Farsi, O.A., Al-Shafaee, M.S., Brooks, D.R., & Waly, M.I. (2011). Brief report: Prevalence of autistic spectrum disorders in the Sultanate of Oman. Journal of Autism and Developmental Disorders; 41(6):821-5.

Alonso, J., Angermeyer, M.C., & Bernert, S., et al. (2004). Prevalence of mental disorders in Europe: results from the European Study of the Epidemiology of Mental Disorders (ESEMeD) project. Acta Psychiatrica Scandinavica Supplement; 109 (420): 21–7.

Al-Rowais, N., Al-Faris, E., Mohammad, A.G., Al-Rukban, M., & Abdulghanim, H.M. (2010). Traditional healers in Riyadh region: Reasons and health problems for seeking their advice. A household survey.Journal of Alternative and Complementary Medicine; 16:199–204.

Al-Sharbati, M.M, Al-Hussaini, A.A, & Antony, S.X. (2003). Profile of child and adolescent psychiatry in Oman.Saudi Medical Journal; 24(4):391-5.

Al-Sharbati, Z., Hallas, C., Al-Zadjali, H., & Al-Sharbati, M. (2012). Sociodemographic and Clinical Characteristics of Patients attending Psychotherapy in a Tertiary Care Hospital in Oman.Sultan Qaboos University Medical Journal; 12(1): 25-32.

Al-Sharbati, M., Zaidan, Z.A, Dorvlo, A.S, & Al-Adawi, S. (2011). Characteristics of ADHD among Omani school children using DSM-IV: descriptive study. Journal of attention Disorders; 15(2):139-46.

Al-Sharbati, Z. (2009). Re: Silent Epidemic of Depression in Women in the Middle East and North Africa Region. Sultan Qaboos University Medical Journal;9(3): 359–360.

Al-Sharbati ,M., Al-Adawi, S., Petrini, K., Bait Amer, A.,Al-Suleimani, A., Al-Lawatiya, S., & Al Hussaini,A. (2012). Two-phase survey to determine social anxiety and gender differences in Omani adolescents.Asia-Pacific Psychiatry; 4(2):131-139.

American Psychiatric Association. (2012). Diagnostic and statistical manual of mental disorders: DSM-IV-TR. American Psychiatric Publishing, Inc.

American Psychiatric Association. Summary of Practice-Relevant Changes to the DSM-IV-TR. Retrieved on 26/8/2013 from http://www.psych.org/practice/dsm/summary-of-practice-relevant-changes-to-the-dsm-iv-tr

Anastasi, A. (1996). Psychological Testing.7th edition. New York, NY: Macmillan.

Andrews, G., & Harvey R. (1981). Does psychotherapy benefit neurotic patients? A reanalysis of the Smith, Glass, and Miller data. Archives of General Psychiatry; 38(11) 1203-1208.

Barlow, D. H. & Durand, V. M. (2009). "Chapter 7: Mood Disorders and Suicide". Abnormal Psychology: An Integrative Approach (Fifth ed.). Belmont, CA: Wadsworth Cengage Learning. p. 239

Barrett, M.S., Chua, W.J., Crits-Christoph, P., Gibbons, M.B., Casiano, D., & Thompson, D. (2008). Early Withdrawal from Mental Health Treatment: Implications for Psychotherapy Practices. Psychotherapy (Chic);45 (2): 247-267.

Ben-Porath, D. D. (2002). Stigmatization of individuals who receive psychotherapy: An interaction between help-seeking behavior and the presence of depression. Journal of Social & Clinical Psychology; 21:400–413.

Bloch, S. (2006). An introduction to psychotherapies Oxford University Press. New York.

Cohen, S.N. (2010). Divorce Mediation: An Introduction. Routledge: Taylor and Francis Group.

Crawford, M.J., Killaspy, H., & Barnes, T.R., et al. (2012). Group art therapy as an adjunctive treatment for people with schizophrenia: multicentre pragmatic randomised trial. British Journal of Psychiatry; 28:344:e846.

Dalal, P.K, & Sivakumar, T. (2009) Moving towards ICD-11 and DSM-5: Concept and evolution of psychiatric classification.Indian Journal of Psychiatry; 51(4): 310-319.

Demyttenaere, K., Bruffaerts, R., & Posada-Villa, J., et al. (2004). Prevalence, severity, and unmet need for treatment of mental disorders in the World Health Organization World Mental Health Surveys. Journal of the American Medical Association; 291(21): 2581–90.

Dwairy, M. (2009). Culture analysis and metaphor psychotherapy with Arab-Muslim clients. Journal of Clinical Psychology; 65:199–209.

Dwairy, M. (2009).Culture Analysis and Metaphor Psychotherapy with Arab-Muslim Clients. Journal of Clinical Psychology: in session; 65(2), 199—209.

El-Islam, M. F. (1994). Collaboration with families: An alternative to mental health legislation. Care in Place, 1, 256–260.

El-Islam, M. F. (2005).Some cultural aspects of the Arab patient-doctor relationship.International Psychiatry, 7, 18–20.

El-Islam, M.F. (2008).Arab culture and mental health.Transcultural psychiatry; 45(4): 671–682.

Eloul, L., Ambusaidi, A., & Al-Adawi, S. (2009). Silent epidemic of depression in women in the Middle Eastand North Africaregion: Emerging tribulation or fallacy. Sultan Qaboos University Medical Journal; 9: 123-130.

Fischer, E., & Farina, A. (1995). Attitudes toward seeking professional help: A shortened form and considerations for research. Journal of College Student development; 36:368–373.

Forester-Miller, H. & Rubenstein, R.L. (1992). Group Counseling: Ethics and Professional Issues. In D. Capuzzi& D. R. Gross (Eds.) Introduction to Group Counseling (307-323).Denver, CO: Love Publishing Co.

Furihata R., Uchiyama M., Takahashi S., Konno C., Susuki M., & Osaki K., et al. (2010). Self-help behaviors for sleep and depression: A Japanese nationwide general population survey. Journal of Affective Disorders; 130:75–82.

Furukawa, T.A, Streiner, D., Young, L.T., & Kinoshita, Y. (2001). "Antidepressants plus benzodiazepines for major depression". In Furukawa, T.A. Cochrane Database of Systematic Reviews (2).

Goldenberg, H., & Goldenberg, I. (2013). Family therapy: an overview. Eight Edition, Brooks/Cole: Belmont.

Grant, I., & Adams, K.M. (1996). Neuropsychological Assessment of Neuropsychiatric Disorders.2nd Ed. New York, NY: Oxford University Press.

Grencavage, L.M., & Norcross, J.C. (1990). Where are the commonalities among the therapeutic common factors? Professional Psychology: Research and Practice; 21(5): 372-378

Grob, GN. (1991).Origins of DSM-I: a study in appearance and reality. American Journal Psychiatry. April; 148(4):421–31.

Grohol, J. (2013). DSM-5 Released: The Big Changes. Psych Central. Retrieved on August 26, 2013, from http://psychcentral.com/blog/archives/2013/05/18/dsm-5-released-the-big-changes/

Haj- Yahia, M. (1994). The Arab Family in Israel, its cultural values and their relevance to social work. Society Welfare; 14:249-64. Rebalance Focus Group: A position paper.

Health Organization's World Mental Health Survey Initiative.World Psychiatry; 6(3):168-176.

Huang, Y., Kotov, R., de Girolamo, G., Preti, A., Angermeyer, M., Benjet, C., Demyttenaere, K., de Graaf, R., Gureje, O., Karam, A. N., Lee, S., Lepine, J. P., Matschinger, H., Posada-Villa, J., Suliman, S., Vilagut, G.,& Kessler, R. C. (2009). DSM-IV personality disorders in the WHO World Mental Health Surveys. The British Journal of Psychiatry; 195 (1): 46–53.

Jaju, S., Al-Adawi, S., Al-Kharusi H., Morsi M., & Al-Riyami A. (2009). Prevalence and age-of-onset distributions of DSM IV mental disorders and their severity among school going Omani adolescents and youths: WMH-CIDI findings. Child and Adolescent Psychiatry and Mental Health 2009, 3:29.

Kendell, R. E. (1993).The nature of psychiatric disorders.In Companion to Psychiatric Disorders (5th edn) (eds R. E. Kendell& A. K. Zealley), pp. 1 -7. Edinburgh: Churchill Livingstone.

Kessler, R.C., Angermeyer, M., Anthony, J.C., De Graaf, R., Demyttenaere, K., & Gasquet, I., et al. (2007). Lifetime prevalence and age-of-onset distributions of mental disorders in the WorldHealth Organization's WorldMental Health Survey Initiative.World Psychiatry; 6(3):168-76.

Kessler, R.C., Berglund, P., Demler, O., Jin, R., Merikangas, K.R., & Walters, E.E. (2005). Lifetime prevalence and age-of-onset distributions of DSM-IV disorders in the National Comorbidity Survey Replication. Archives of Geneneral Psychiatry; 62 (6): 593–602.

Kessler, R.C., McGonagle, K.A., Zhoa, S., Nelson, C.B., Hughes, M., & Eshleman, S., et al. (1994). Lifetime and 12-month prevalence of DSM-III-R psychiatric disorders in the United States: Results from the National Comorbidity Survey (NCS). Archives of General Psychiatry; 51: 8-19.

Kirk Morton, N., & Zubek, D. (2013). Adherence challenges and long-acting injectable antipsychotic treatment in patients with schizophrenia.Journal of Psychosocial Nursing and Mental Health Services; 51(3):13-8.

Kirmayer, L.J. (2006). Cultural and psychotherapy in a creolizing world.Transcultural Psychiatry; 43:163-168.

Kitchener, K.S. (1984). Intuition, critical evaluation and ethical principles: The foundation for ethical decisions in counseling psychology. The Counseling Psychologist, 12(3), 43-55.

Kouyoumdjian, H., Zamboanga, B.L., & Hansen, D.J. (2003). Barriers to community mental health services for Latinos: Treatment considerations. Clinical Psychology Science and Practice; 10:394 – 422.

Lambert, M.J., & Bergin, A.E. (1992) Achievements and limitations of psychotherapy research. Freedheim, Donald K. (Ed); Freudenberger, Herbert J. (Ed); Kessler, Jane W.(Ed); Messer, Stanley B. (Ed); Peterson, Donald R. (Ed); Strupp, Hans H. (Ed); Wachtel, Paul L. (Ed), (1992). History of psychotherapy: A century of change. , (pp. 360-390). Washington, DC, US: American Psychological Association.

Leichsenring, F., & Rabung, S. (2008). Effectiveness of Long-term Psychodynamic Psychotherapy: A meta-analysis. Journal of the Amercian Medical Association; 300(13): 1551-1565.

Longmore, R.J., & Worrell, M. (2007). Do we need to challenge thoughts in cognitive behavior therapy?Clinical Psychology Review; 27(2):173.

Man D.W., Tsang, W.W., & Hui-Chan, C.W. (2010). Do older T'ai Chi practitioners have better attention and memory function? Journal of Alternative and Complementary Medicine; 16:1259–64.

McGuire, M.T. (1965). The Process of Short-Term Insight Psychotherapy. II: Content, Expectations and Structure. Journal of Nervous & Mental Disease; 141(2): 219-230.

Ministry of Health, Sultanate of Oman (2009).Annual Health Report. Muscat.

Mitchell, S.A., & Black, M.J. (1996).Freud and Beyond: A History of Modern Psychoanalytic Thought. New York: Basic Books

Nordqvist C. (2007). Bulimia Patients Respond Better To Family-based Treatment Than Supportive Psychotherapy. Medical News Today. Retrieved from http://www.medicalnewstoday.com/articles/81481.php

Nordqvist C. (2009). Psychotherapy Useful In Treating Post-Traumatic Stress Disorder in Early Stages. Medical News Today.Retrieved from http://www.medicalnewstoday.com/releases/91194.php.

Olfson, M., Marcus, S.C., Druss, B., Elinson, L., Tanielian, T., & Pincus, H.A. (2002). National trends in the outpatient treatment of depression.Journal of the American Medical Association; 287:203–9.

Olfson, M., Marcus, S.C., Druss, B., & Pincus, H.A. (2002). National trends in the use of outpatient psychotherapy.American Journal ofPsychiatry; 159:1914–20.

Olfson, M., & Pincus, H.A. (1994). Outpatient psychotherapy in the United States I: Volume, costs, and user characteristics. American Journal of Psychiatry; 151:1281–8.

Orlinsky, D.E., & Howard, K.I. (1987). A generic model of psychotherapy.Journal of Integrative & Eclectic Psychotherapy; 6(1), 6-27.

Passerieux, C. (2013). Psychological interventions in the treatment of schizophrenia.La Revue du praticien; 63(3):356-8.

Peter Kinderman (2013). "Explainer: what is the DSM?".The Conversation Australia.Retrieved 26 August, 2013.The Conversation Media Groupfrom http://theconversation.com/explainer-what-is-the-dsm-14127

Qasem, H. (2010).Experiences in Middle Eastern populations.Selected Issues in Palliative Care among East Jerusalem Arab Resident.Asian Pacific Journal of Cancer Prevention, 11, MECC Supplement, 121-123

Qualls, S.H., & Knight BG. (2007). Psychotherapy for Depression in Older Adults:Volume 4 of Wiley Series in Clinical Geropsychology. John Wiley and Sons.

Reis, S. (2007).Psychotherapy Useful In Treating Post-Traumatic Stress Disorder In Early Stages. Medical News Today.MediLexicon, Intl., 10 Dec. 2007. Web.

Ricotti, V., & Delanty, N. (2006). Use of complementary and alternative medicine in epilepsy.Current Neurology and Neuroscience Reports; 6: 347–353.

Rosenbaum, M. (1982).Ethical problems of Group Psychotherapy. In M. Rosenbaum (Ed.), Ethics and values in psychotherapy: A guidebook (237-257). New York: Free

Roth, A., & Fonagy, P. What works for whom?A critical review of psychotherapy Research (2nded.). London: Guilford Publications, Inc.

Rüsch, N., Müller, M., Lay, B., Corrigan, P.W., Zahn, R., Schönenberger, T., Bleiker, M., & Rössler, W.(2013). Emotional reactions to involuntary psychiatric hospitalization and stigma-related stress among people with mental illness.European Archives of Psychiatry and Clinical Neurosciences. 2013 May 21. [Epub ahead of print]

Schacter, D.L., Gilbert, D.T., & Wegner, D.M. (2010). Psychology. (2nd ed., p. 620). New York: Worth Pub.

Shear, M.K., Greeno, C., Kang, J., Ludewig, D., Frank, E., Swartz, H.A., & Hanekamp, M. (2000). Diagnosis of Nonpsychotic Patients in Community Clinics.American Journal of Psychiatry; 157 (4): 581-7.

Sherer, R. (2002). Mental Health Care in the Developing World. Psychiatric Times; XIX (1).

Sivakumar, T., Agarwal, V., & Sitholey P.(2013).Comorbidity of attention-deficit/hyperactivity disorder and bipolar disorder in North Indian clinic children and adolescents.Asian Journal of psychiatry, 6(3): 235-42.

Smith, M.L, & Glass, G.V. (1977). Meta-analysis of psychotherapy outcome studies.American Psychologist; 32(9):752-60.

Somers, J.M., Goldner, E.M., Waraich, P., & Hsu, L. (2006). Prevalence and incidence studies of anxiety disorders: a systematic review of the literature. Canadian Journal of Psychiatry; 51 (2): 100–13.

Stadler, H. A. (1986). Making hard choices: Clarifying controversial ethical issues.Counseling & Human Development, 19: 1-10.

Talwar, N., Crawford, M.J., Maratos, A., Nur, U., McDermott, O., & Procter, S. (2006). Music therapy for in-patients with schizophrenia: explanatory randomised controlled trial. British Journal of Psychiatry; 189: 405-409.

Tang, A., Sullivan, A.J.O., Diamond, T., Gerard, A., & Campbell, P. (2013).Psychiatric symptoms as a clinical presentation of Cushing's syndrome.Annals of General Psychiatry; 12:23.

Tomlinson, S.M., & Cope, N.R. (1988). Characteristics of Black students seeking help at a university counseling center.Journalof College Student Development; 29:65–69.

Tseng W. (1999). Culture and Psychotherapy: Review and Practical Guidelines. Transcultural Psychiatry; 36: 131-179.

Vessey, J.T., & Howard, KI. (1993). Who seeks psychotherapy? Psychotherapy; 30:546–553.

Wade J., & Good, G.E. (2010). Moving toward mainstream: Perspectives on enhancing therapy with men. Psychotherapy; 47:306–15.

Waraich, P., Goldner, E.M., Somers, J.M., & Hsu, L. (2004). Prevalence and incidence studies of mood disorders: a systematic review of the literature. Canadian Journal of Psychiatry; 49 (2): 124–38

Weiner, I., & Richard, D. (2001).The practice of Electroconvulsive therapy: recommendations for treatment, training and privileging, Second edition, American psychiatric Association: Washignton DC,

White, P., Young, K., & McTeer, W. (1995). Sports, masculinity, and the injured body. In: Suso D, Gordon F, editors. Men's health and illness: Gender, Power and the Body. Thousand Oaks, Ca: Sage Publications Inc; pp. 158–82.

WHO International Consortium in Psychiatric Epidemiology. (2000). Cross-national comparisons of the prevalences and correlates of mental disorders, Bulletin of the World Health Organization v;78(4).

World Health Organization. (1992).The ICD-10 Classification of Mental and Behavioural Disorders: Clinical Descriptions and Diagnostic Guidelines. Geneva: WHO.

Wright, J.H., Basco, M.R., & Thase, M.E. (2006).Learning cognitive-behavior therapy.an illustrated guide. American psychiatric publishing Inc: Washington DC.

Young, L.T., Joffe, R.T., Robb, J.C., MacQueen, G.M., Marriott, M., & Patelis-Siotis, I. (2000). Double-blind comparison of addition of a second mood stabilizer versus an antidepressant to an initial mood stabilizer for treatment of patients with bipolar depression.American Journal of Psychiatry; 157:124–126.